Experiencing the New Genetics

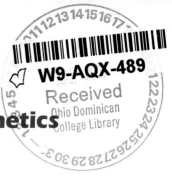

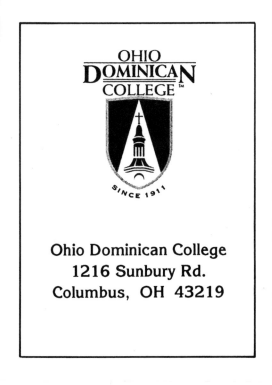

OHIO DOMINICAN COLLEGE ™

SINCE 1911

**Ohio Dominican College
1216 Sunbury Rd.
Columbus, OH 43219**

Experiencing the New Genetics

Family and Kinship
on the Medical Frontier

Kaja Finkler

PENN

University of Pennsylvania Press

Philadelphia

10 9 8 7 6 5 4 3 2 1

Published by
University of Pennsylvania Press
Philadelphia, Pennsylvania 19104-4011

Library of Congress Cataloging-in-Publication Data
Finkler, Kaja.
    Experiencing the new genetics : family and kinship on the medical frontier /
Kaja Finkler.
        p.   cm.
    Includes bibliographical references and index.
    ISBN 0-8122-3538-X — ISBN 0-8122-1720-9 (pbk.)
    1. Family.   2. Heredity, Human — Social aspects.   3. Kinship.   4. Medical
genetics — Social aspects.   5. Family — United States.   I. Title.
GN480.2 .F56 2000
306.4'61 — dc21   99-056639

In memory of all my loved ones
and the multitude of others who perished on pyres
fueled by an ideology of biological determinism

Contents

Preface

During a span of twenty-five years as a medical anthropologist, my concern has been with various issues in economically developing nations, especially problems in medical anthropology. Whereas initially my research had focused on peasant economics and politics in Mexico, where I did fieldwork for eight years, as well as other parts of Latin America,[1] for the past twenty-three years I have examined interrelated questions in medical anthropology, including the efficacy of Spiritualist healing, the cultural transformations of biomedical practice, and questions bearing on women's health.[2] In my work on Mexican Spiritualism and biomedicine, my chief interest was with how therapeutic practices, treatment outcomes, and sickness and its alleviation reveal the cultural nature of medical systems and the experience of sickness. During the course of my investigation of biomedical practice and patient response, I found that, among the poor people that I studied, the notion of genetic inheritance was one of several cultural beliefs people held about sickness etiologies.[3] Hereditarian beliefs diffused to Mexico from Europe through biomedical practice and became one of many Mexican folk etiological explanations.[4] After I returned to the United States, I became especially intrigued by the concept of heredity and its origins and I wondered how these ideas impacted on people's interaction with their families, who, after all, presumably transmit diseases to their offspring.

In my training as an anthropologist, I was required to take a comparative perspective on any phenomena I observed in another culture. Having been raised in a European culture and grown up in the United States, I was particularly sensitive to cultural differences, and in my field stays I usually compared American practices with those of other cultures. My interest was therefore piqued by my Mexican findings concerning hereditary beliefs. Inasmuch as conceptualizations of familial inheritance of disease form part of contemporary biomedicine, I turned my anthropological gaze on the source of these developments in American society, particularly on the impact of the ideology of genetic inheritance on people's experience and especially within the context of family and kinship relationships.

As a graduate student in anthropology during the late 1960s and early 1970s, I was expected to do fieldwork in a foreign land and to become immersed in a culture other than my own, an expectation that also represents a common view of the anthropological enterprise, or what anthropologists do. Reading a book by an anthropologist, an American reader socialized into the dominant culture may thus anticipate learning about some exotic society rather than about his or her own beliefs and practices, but currently anthropologists have rightly moved to analyzing their own society, cultural beliefs, and practices as well. This book thus grew out of a confluence of my past research and my present interests. But in addition to academic concerns this project also emerged out of various personal experiences. On my first visit to a physician for a minor condition, he asked me for a family medical history. I indicated that one of my aunts had died of cancer. Although she was an aunt by marriage, I did not specify and the doctor did not inquire as to the precise genealogical tie between this aunt and myself. On hearing that someone in my family had cancer, the doctor immediately insisted that I needed a complex and costly examination because I was "predisposed" to cancer, and because my condition might eventually develop into the same disease from which my aunt had died. The exchange stirred up memories of a beloved I had only thought about intermittently since her death fifteen years earlier. I realized that the physician had reawakened memories of my kinship connections to my mother's brother's wife, even though she was not even genetically related to me. Another telling and also poignant scene stood out in my mind, when I spoke with a young student about her future plans. She reported that her future might be in jeopardy because she greatly feared becoming an alcoholic. When I inquired into the basis of this fear, she responded that alcoholism was part of her genetic heritage: both her parents were alcoholics, and she was convinced that it was inevitable for her to suffer the same fate. But perhaps on a deeper level, I began to focus on the implications of beliefs in genetic inheritance and the ideology of biological determinism in which they are embedded because, taken to an extreme, it had led to the extermination of my family during World War II.

Whereas I present a *multidimensional* perspective on the repercussions of biological determinism, I nevertheless consider it a moral right to express my concern with the current proliferation of beliefs in genetic inheritance.[5] In my studies in Mexico I noted that various local beliefs and practices might have an adverse impact, but I hesitated to critique them, even when informants did so, because I was a foreigner. I felt anger and outrage when I witnessed the power men wielded over women,[6] resulting from gender ideologies and economic circumstance, or the abominable treatment to which poor men and women in general were subjected by the authorities. But since I am a part of mainstream American society and since biomedical ideologies, including beliefs in genetic inheritance, comprise, in part, my heritage, I do not feel the same constraints as I did in Mexico. Nevertheless, I have attempted to examine our beliefs in genetic inheritance from various standpoints. Ultimately, however, as in my previous work, the concepts I advance flow not solely from theoretical considerations or moral indignation but also from my association with the people I interviewed for this study. Their insights into the role that genetic inheritance plays in their lives were incisive and enriching and have led me to a multilevel analysis of the contemporary ideology of genetic inheritance.

Originally, I designed this research as a comparative study of the ways people in Mexico and the United States interpret genetic inheritance, which I would conduct by drawing on samples of people in both societies. I interviewed women residing in the southern part of the United States who either had suffered from breast cancer or originated from families with histories of cancer, and adoptees who had searched for or already located their birth parents. Unfortunately, I was unable to locate comparable populations to the ones I had studied in the United States during a field trip to Mexico in 1998. Instead, I interviewed the section heads of genetic counseling units in two of the largest hospitals in Mexico City[7] as well as the head of the breast cancer unit of the oncology hospital.[8] At all three sites I was informed that breast cancer was not usually regarded by physicians as a genetically inherited disease and that none of the physicians ever referred patients with breast cancer to genetic counselors, irrespective of whether any member of a patient's family had experienced the disease.[9] I interviewed sixteen women with breast cancer there, referred to me by a psychiatrist who heads a support group for women afflicted with this disease; *all* believed that their breast cancer was caused by a physical blow, a *golpe*, and none associated it with a family inheritance.

To compare the adoptees here with those in Mexico, I interviewed there the heads of the Association of Adoptive Parents. According to them, adoption in Mexico is an informal procedure, and most children are aware that they have been adopted; most even know their birth parents. There is no movement among adoptees to search for their birth parents, nor had the persons I interviewed ever met an adoptee who had attempted to do so. During my many years in Mexico, I had observed that children from very poor families were given as "gifts" to more fortunate members of their own families or to godparents, but the children were always aware of their birth parents. Hence, while I make reference to Mexico in the present work, given the lack of comparable populations in Mexico and the United States, my research focus has necessarily remained on U.S. society, where the contemporary ideology of genetic inheritance has largely developed.

Anthropological fieldwork in my own society felt very different from fieldwork in a foreign setting. When I carried out research in Mexico, I was totally immersed in and enveloped by the society and culture. For example, when I studied Spiritualist healing, I was required to become a participant, not only an observer, in ritual and religious healing and training to become a healer, as well as to act as an assistant to the healers. In the study of biomedical practice, I was continually involved in the activities of the outpatient clinic where I carried out the investigation of its patients and physicians.

In this study I used a multisited ethnographic approach. I was not confined by any one specific research site or encompassed by it, as I was accustomed to. The people I interviewed originated from different parts of the United States, although most resided within the university town or its environs and, for the most part, represented varying levels of the American middle class. I usually conducted the interviews in people's homes, where I was received with great warmth and hospitality, but I did not feel the same immersion here as I did in Mexico, other than being a member of the same society.

Whereas my adult cultural understandings paralleled those of the people in this study, my childhood cultural background was built on different assumptions rooted in a religious ideology. Taking into account the role genetic inheritance plays in our lives, I was led to conjure up my personal cultural background and especially to meditate on the way I was named. For instance, with few exceptions all the people in this study—profoundly religious or not—to a varying degree accept concepts of genetic inheritance concerning the length of their life span. In my cultural experience, however, it was believed that the ancestor whose name he or she bore rather than his or her genes chiefly influenced a person's life span. I was initially named after a grandmother who had died at a very young age, and therefore my father insisted that the name of a grandmother who had lived to be 95 years old be added in order that I bear the name of at least one long-lived family forerunner. Longevity thus rested with a name rather than with a gene, or with a lifestyle for that matter.

As an academician and an anthropologist, as well as an informed citizen, I learned to question my own cultural childhood beliefs, in the same way I question the dominant cultural beliefs and practices that have emerged out of the Enlightenment and out of scientific conceptualizations. The impermanent nature of scientific knowledge, including biomedical information, invites such questioning because such knowledge is transient, as ideally scientific practice ought to be, but it is also contingent on its social and cultural milieu.[10] As we will see, this knowledge exerts extraordinary influence on people's experience, not only because it is authoritative and explains suffering, but also because it plays on people's fears and vulnerabilities.

This book builds, of course, on the work of many scholars. It also moves among several disciplines. The study was guided by several hypotheses, but I employ an interpretative anthropological microscope in analyzing my findings. The data are based on illness histories and personal narratives. The phenomenological perspective I take does not lend itself to quantification or objective tabulations, and for this reason I cannot say to what degree my findings are generalizable to all Americans. However, I can say that no individual life is ever generalizable, but that one life sheds light on the universals of human existence; to wit, each human life speaks for itself and also for all humanity. I do anticipate that this work will generate hypotheses for other scholars to test on large population samples.

While all the interviews were open-ended, I began each with an explanation of the purpose of the study and with what I characterize elsewhere as a trigger question that allowed each person to respond in her own way.[11] All the interviews were tape-recorded with permission and transcribed. I extracted the major themes of each narrative from these transcriptions, and these themes are reflected in my analysis. As I discuss elsewhere, tensions usually exist in human life between individual agents and the constraints imposed on them by the societal ideologies to which they adhere.[12] In the same vein, this dialectical tension is reflected in my analysis of the interviews I conducted. For, while my culturally construed understanding regards people as agents of their existence impelled by their subjectivity, I recognize that they are nevertheless also governed by regnant ideologies, which structure their beliefs and actions and which in turn contribute to shaping their cultural ideologies and practices in an ongoing structuration process.[13] Because human beings are not passive receptacles for the cultural ideologies they learn, I take a phenomenological perspective. My point of departure is subjectively perceived and interpreted experience in tandem with the actualities and the cultural and ideological templates in which daily existence is played out. Although the subject's perspective elucidates her own life, it is necessary to interject at least one caveat: human beings themselves do not always recognize the consequences of their own ideological beliefs. Our subjectivity restrains us from seeing our existence in its totality. There are, thus, limits to which we can understand our subjectivity. Hence, when people discussed their beliefs about genetic inheritance but could not elaborate on how their subjectivity connected with their actions or on the ways in which it affected their lives and their familial relations, I brought out the anthropological microscope to assist in further interpretation.

For some people, our interaction may have led them to consider the role of genetic ideologies in ways they had not done before, perhaps because on a very elemental level we take for granted our underlying cultural comprehension and rarely examine it in the course of our daily lives. On another level, people would spontaneously refer to their family and kin relations and their basic notions about heredity when they discussed the fact that their sickness was familial; when they recounted their search for their birth parents because they desired to learn their medical history; or when they noted that they had inherited all their physical and behavioral characteristics from birth parents whom they had never met. To gain an understanding of adoptees' motives for searching for their biological parents, in addition to the interviews I participated in their monthly support group meetings during a period of six months, and I also consulted the World Wide Web, where various sites exist describing adoptees' strategies for searches.

This book is both a practical and a theoretical endeavor. It is intended to instruct about some historical and contemporary aspects of kinship and genetics, to raise questions and to analyze a prevailing biomedical ideology in American society within the context of people's experience, and to contribute to a theoretical understanding of one important facet of present day life. It will be of interest first and foremost to students and to social scientists, especially those concerned with kinship and family, medical anthropologists, scholars in social medicine, and other health professionals attentive to biomedical ideologies and their impact on human experience, as well as to cultural analysts. It is my hope, too, that the book will help the informed general reader make sense of one facet of contemporary life, especially since he or she is unceasingly bombarded by the mass media presentations that a person's health and existence are determined by genetic inheritance and family medical history.

One last point needs to be made. Some readers may find this presentation unbalanced. If so, I can say in my defense that readers may take for granted their views relating to the ideology of genetic inheritance, comprising part of our commonsense knowledge, because they form part of our dominant culture and are constantly presented in professional knowledge as well as popular accounts.[14] But the more critical view is not heard as frequently. According to some, in the 1920s and 1930s few people stood up publicly to oppose genetic and eugenic claims. At present, various serious scholars have addressed some questions raised here,[15] but ongoing critical appraisals are necessary in order for people to gain a multiperspectival perception of the subject to which I hope to contribute with this book.

Chapter 1
Introduction

In the past several decades there has been an explosion of research in genetics and genetic inheritance both in the scientific literature and in the mass media.[1] Not a day passes without some mention of genetics, genetic engineering, or genetic inheritance in the popular press, on radio and television, and in health newsletters. Indeed, the executive editor of the *New England Journal of Medicine,* Marcia Angell, could have been speaking about notions of genetics when she noted the great impact scientific research has on the public: "No sooner do we publish a study on diet or life style than news of its conclusions, though virtually none of its qualifying details, hits the airwaves. Within 24 hours, millions of people consider eating fewer egg yolks or more oat bran to fend off disease."[2] Moreover, as Turner observes, the "mass media foster attitudes of technological and scientific determinism by implying that scientific 'progress' cannot be halted"[3] and that it is a miraculous achievement. In fact, one of the most discussed scientific endeavors has been the Human Genome Project (HGP), which aims at mapping the entire human genome for the benefit of mankind. This new genetics forms part of contemporary biomedicine and forecasts great advances in alleviating disease and prolonging human life.[4]

Clearly, research in the genetic inheritance of disease and behavioral characteristics constitutes the cutting edge of modern science and biomedicine, but the scientific literature is out of reach of the layperson. The mass media present discoveries in genetics, and especially the HGP, as a dazzling new frontier, comparable to the discovery of the New World,[5] the wonders of the automobile, the mastery of electricity at the beginning of the twentieth century, and the space program of the mid-twentieth century. These reports describe the new trend toward the geneticization of existence as a fantastic advance in scientific achievement.[6] Arguably, one of the most thoughtful articles on the subject of genetically inherited diseases was written by Charles Siebert in the *New York Times Sunday*

Magazine. He writes: "Genes are suddenly thought to be responsible for everything from poverty to privilege, from misdemeanors to murder. I seem to recall watching television one night and seeing a man up on homicide charges offer as a defense the presence of a 'criminal gene,' which he claimed ran in his family." Siebert notes examples of headlines in the popular press, like the cover story in one news magazine: "Infidelity: It May Be in Your Genes."[7]

Siebert's article is one of an ongoing array of publications and broadcasts regarding the ways genetic inheritance purportedly determines all aspects of our existence and especially our afflictions. It is now thought that mental illness, stress, risktaking, shyness, social effectiveness, homosexuality, job success, exhibitionism, arson, traditionalism, and even a zest for life,[8] as well as learning problems, vulnerability to smoking, and gender differences,[9] derive from our genetic makeup, forming part of people's commonsense consciousness. While some reports do note that the "biological century will bring myriad moral and legal conundrums,"[10] most accounts fail to question the social consequences or critically examine the trend of the new genetics.[11] More common is the indiscriminate acceptance of notions about genetic determinism and the embrace of the HGP as the panacea for all ills.[12] The recent reports about cloned sheep have, undoubtedly, contributed to the propagation of "genetic essentialism," indicating that humans, too, are a product of their genes.[13]

Ideas about the genetic inheritance of disease place the family and kin group in the spotlight, requiring the scrutiny of all its members. In the August 15, 1996, *Wall Street Journal,* for example, one headline read, "One Family's Search for a Faulty Gene."[14] On the same page another headline announced, "Doctors Recommend Every Family Make Its Own Medical Tree."[15] A September 1996 *Consumer Reports* headline read, "Family History: What You Don't Know Can Kill You." The article informs the reader that deadly diseases "can be influenced or even determined by hereditary factors."[16] Family magazines recommend that individuals work out genograms and family health pedigrees as a way of predicting the future of their children. A Mother's Day card reminds the mother, "It's all in our genes."[17] Or in an article concerning colon cancer, Matthews reports that doctors tell patients that "you may think you have no risk factors, *but unless you know exactly what your great-grandmother and assorted other relatives died of, you could be carrying an abnormal regulatory gene . . .* that has been performing OK for generations until — kerplooie!" (emphasis added).[18]

As long as people are healthy and fertile, they may be aware that genes determine their health and their beings, but they may not give the matter much thought until they are touched personally, when they fall seriously ill and are asked by their physician for a family medical history. At such time the family and kin group enters the person's consciousness in a new way, and the science of the new genetics and its representation in the mass media take on fresh meanings.

At the risk of stating the obvious, the discovery of the unknown, whether in space or on the level of purported knowledge, has consequences for societal and individual levels of existence that may not always be realized at the time of the initial excitement about the new phenomenon. The opening of any new frontier, including the new cultural shift to genetic determinism, to the "biologizing of culture,"[19] has personal and political significance. The cultural currency of scientific discoveries concerning genetic inheritance currently circulating in the United States profoundly influences people's lives,[20] including their family and kinship interactions, as we will learn from the individuals we meet in this book.

My concern here is to explore the multidimensional aspects of the new genetics, which form part of contemporary biomedical practice. I address two important and interrelated questions. How do people experience the ideology of genetic inheritance, particularly within the context of their family and kin relations, and why has genetic inheritance become a major theme in contemporary life?[21]

I characterize the present day as marked by the "hegemony of the gene," which is leading to the "medicalization of kinship."[22] By this I mean that family and kin relationships are being drawn into the biomedical domain through current comprehensions that diseases are genetically transmitted from generation to generation. The medicalization of any human condition dramatically affects people's deepest level of experience, understanding, and actions, transforming the person from an active being into a passive patient. Whereas the medicalization process is not a new phenomenon in Western medical history, the medicalization of kinship is relatively recent because it is being especially promoted by the new genetics. Consider this: embedded in concepts of genetic inheritance is the notion that family and kin are the medium through which inheritance flows.

Medical conceptualizations open a window on an understanding of a society's culture and its moral beliefs, as I believe the ideology of genetic inheritance does.[23] In this book I seek to combine certain kinds of research that are usually isolated from one another. I bring together the historical development of genetic theory, which has led to contemporary hereditarian notions in biomedicine with related debates about kinship and family, because genetic transmission is embedded in these notions. Marilyn Strathern, Sarah Franklin, and Janet Dolgin have been at the forefront in addressing the impact of the new reproductive technologies on definitions of family and kinship.[24] My dual task, however, is to present empirical evidence of the consequences of the new genetics for people's *experience* and to analyze in theoretical terms the reasons genetic determinism has become so prominent.[25] By doing so, we will also deepen our understanding and gain new insights into contemporary culture and its moral notions.

Whereas outstanding books have been written theorizing about the impact of genetic inheritance ideology,[26] we lack an examination of its influence on people's experience, including their relationships with family and kin. In fact, few scholars have attended to the new genetics within the context of kinship studies.[27] As other scholars have pointed out, there has been little research with people suffering from what are believed to be genetic conditions.[28] Concepts of familial disease give new meanings to family. Pembrey observes that, with genetic diseases, "family ties can take on a new meaning in genetics and challenge our usual view of confidentiality." To whom does genetic information belong: the individual or the family? What right does one family member have to learn the genetic results of another member? What obligation do people have to tell others in the family of their own test results and inform other family members that they are at risk?[29] These are important questions that need to be addressed. Illness of any kind may cause changes in relationships within families, but in genetic conditions, because they are believed to be transmitted *through* the family, these changes may have particular potency. In Richards's words, "there is the issue of who may be held to be 'responsible' for the condition."[30] Moreover, the new genetics deserves serious treatment because, as Yoxen states, it "stands to reorder so much about our lives, our sexual relations, our basic satisfactions, our kinship, our sense of meaning to life and what we have on our conscience."[31] We need to understand how people interpret familial contributions to health and illness, an area that has received virtually no attention.[32] More specifically, we lack an understanding of how concepts of genetic inheritance influence the afflicted and other segments of the population such as adoptees, two population segments that are the special focus of this book. How do women with breast cancer relate to their families, and how does the belief that one's disease was genetically inherited influence a patient's course of treatment? If a healthy woman comes from a family in which some relatives had suffered from breast cancer, when does she become a patient? How are adoptees guided by the same ideology? Do they too become patients when they learn the medical history of their birth family?

To address these questions, I bring to bear empirical data drawn from interviews with women with breast cancer, as well as healthy women who come from families with a history of breast cancer and adoptees searching for their birth parents. These in-depth interviews illuminate the ways in which the ideology of genetic determinism is played out in people's lives, especially within the context of family and kinship relations. On first glance, one may justly ask, "What do women with breast cancer or healthy individuals originating from families with cancer and healthy adoptees seeking their birth parents have in common?" These ostensibly disparate groups of people are moved to act, albeit in very distinct domains and with different consequences, as a result of the reigning ideology of genetic inheritance, which informs their cultural comprehension. It is not uncommon to observe that cultural ideologies affect people uniformly except along class, gender, and race lines. It is frequently overlooked, however, that the same ideology will differentially guide people's behavior consonant with their *experience*, which may transcend class, gender, and race. John Dewey's definition of experience incorporates "what men do and suffer, what they strive for, love, believe and endure, and also how men act and are acted upon, the ways in which they do and suffer, desire and enjoy, see, believe, imagine — in short, processes of experiencing."[33]

Paradoxically, the same ideology may have negative outcomes for society while having varying effects on individuals. What is most intriguing is that, on a societal level, the frontier known as the "new genetics" is arguably an old frontier bordering on eugenics, one that has been reincarnated in the guise of the new and that is fetishized in contemporary society to explain disease etiologies and abnormal behaviors.[34] On the level of the individual, the identical ideology of genetic inheritance affects in a profoundly different way the afflicted and the adoptees. Concepts of genetic inheritance address problems of causality, thereby conferring a sense of coherence on those who suffer from an affliction that is fundamentally a random occurrence. Lacking an explanation of the ultimate cause, the why,[35] the afflicted individual finds genetic causality elegantly; even aesthetically satisfying and succinctly condensed; namely, that the disease was passed down by kin. Concurrently, genetic determinism affects adoptees adversely, leading to fragmentation, internal conflicts, and turmoil.

An important point I noted in the preface as well as in my previous writings,[36] deserves reemphasis here: tensions exist between regnant cultural ideologies and the individual's interpretation, acceptance, and rejection of them. This tension also exists in my analysis because it is not my intention to construe the hegemony of the gene as overdetermined by reducing human beings to cultural automatons. Nor am I unaware of the tension that exists in American society between biological reductionism exemplified in the hegemony of the gene and notions of the wholeness of personhood. Nevertheless, the interviews I conducted with women who have suffered from breast cancer and with healthy women from families with cancer and adoptees shed light on the ways in which conceptions of the genetic inheritance of disease guide people's thoughts and actions, including those regarding family and kin. On a personal level of experience, the question I posed to the participants was, "What does it mean to experience breast cancer and to know that it was inherited, or may be inherited, from a family member?" Does knowing that one suffers from an inherited disease carry the same experiential load as knowing that one suffers from a disease believed to be caused by an invasion of a pathogen, say, an impersonal virus? How does one negotiate a relationship with relatives and ancestors who presumably transmitted the affliction to the sufferer? Most important, consider that a genetic explanation of the woman's affliction touches not only her but also those whom she may regard as closest to her — her family and kin.[37]

Within the past three decades genetic inheritance has come into the foreground, supplanting more customary explanations. Science possesses prodigious authority the world over, and concepts of genetic inheritance are wrapped in its cloak. No matter how persuasive the arguments against genetic inheritance may be,[38] the fact remains that in day-to-day life people are bombarded with the view that they have inherited most diseases from their family. Indeed, while much has been written on the ramifications of the biomedical, mechanistic explanations of disease, which tend to regard it as a breakdown of the "bodily machine,"[39] there has been very little discussion of the experiential consequences of the etiological belief in genetic inheritance that bear on core relationships with family and kin.

When I embarked on the field research with breast cancer patients and healthy individuals who came from families with a history of cancer, almost all of whom were referred to me by a genetic counselor who forms part of an oncology team, I was guided by several research questions. I postulated that persons experiencing a familial disease would become conscious of their families and ancestors in a new way and would establish closer familial relationships with them, while also harboring negative feelings toward those from whom they have inherited the disease. Moreover, I expected that concepts of the genetic inheritance of disease would guide the women's therapeutic management and would preclude from their consideration alternative explanations of disease etiology. With the exception of my assumption that women suffering from breast cancer would feel anger toward their kin, all of the premises I advanced were borne out. In addition, however, the ethnographic interviews disclosed consequences flowing from the ideology of genetic diseases that I had not anticipated, including that the genetic explanation of a disease, in the words of one woman (Betty) "is easy to comprehend." While geneticists may speak of multifactorial causalities and people may, indeed, consider various explanations, in the end most of the women I interviewed emphasized genetic inheritance, a unicausal reductionist explanation that is readily comprehended. Additionally, I found that people harbor notions of predestination and a sense of fatalism normally associated with religious conceptualizations of the world,[40] while some simultaneously resort to gambling metaphors to make sense of the randomness of their affliction. The healthy women shared similar beliefs, but additionally they were also laden with ongoing anxieties that they would fall ill. These profound apprehensions convert them into asymptomatic, perpetual patients because they regard themselves as being at a continuous risk for the disease.

Genetic inheritance of any characteristic, be it eye color or a disease, is a matter of random chance. Owing to the randomness of inheritance, in the case of diseases it is often subsumed under the notion of a risk factor, although people do not always distinguish between big and little risks. If they do not, but instead see risk in absolute terms, then they have distorted the concept.[41] The concept of risk, rooted in the mathematical expression of probabilities, is a way of forecasting the future based on past occurrences.[42] Forming part of modern Western consciousness, the concept shifts human fate from the caprices of the gods to the whims of mathematical probability. Although the notion of risk is an ancient concept within the context of gambling practices, used to explain "how the card falls" or "the draw of the card," the broader concept of risk is a relatively new phenomenon in Western history going back to the Renaissance, when the idea that mathematical probabilities may rule human destiny became formalized and applied to other aspects of human practice.[43] Prior to the Renaissance, the prevailing view was that events affecting human life did not occur by chance. Such events were not subject to human control: they were predestined and governed by higher powers. They explained personal misfortunes. After the emergence of the concept of probability, the notion developed that events, particularly adverse occurrences, could be predicted, especially by identifying the risk factors. Paradoxically, the notion of risk, based as it is on mathematical probabilities, is double faced: it recognizes on the one hand that events are random, and on the other that this very randomness can be controlled to attain certainty. It permits modern humans to nurture the notion that they can control the future by controlling risks.

Reflecting the tension in present day American society between concepts of predestination and probability, among the women with breast cancer that we will meet, some indeed believe that it was the will of a higher power that had brought on their affliction. Others use the notion of risk in terms of a gambling metaphor to explain the ultimate cause of their affliction, why the disease befell them and not somebody else. But ironically, while the random nature of genetic inheritance may be regarded by some as "the luck of the draw," the notion of risk also provides meaning to the very randomness of the event by explaining "why me," a question that is often posed by people in times of great suffering. The women wth breast cancer, or healthy women who come from families with a history of cancer, experience a sense of comfort in knowing the "why" of their suffering, especially since biomedical etiological explanations eschew moral judgments.[44] Paradoxically, the concept of risk is both amoral and moral. Calculated on the basis of probabilities, it lacks a moral component, yet imposes a morality on people's behavior because they are held personally responsible for its avoidance.[45] While risk factors are presented in impersonal and amoral terms, people nevertheless interject a moral dimension when they must negotiate randomness and luck vis-à-vis their behavior. In numerous instances, people report that they have done everything correctly — they have avoided all the risk factors for disease (changed their diet, exercised regularly, ceased smoking and drinking, breast-fed their infants) — and they *should* have stayed healthy. Yet they still fell ill, a contradiction that leaves them without an explanation. The notion of risk promises that random events such as inheritance of a presumably genetic disease may be constrained. Moreover, being at risk for genetic disease places the responsibility for the affliction on oneself and one's family, giving people that semblance of control. If only the person would avoid the risk factors, all would be well and one's genetically inherited fate could be overcome. Sadly, no matter how much humans may wish to leave nothing to chance, in the domain of genetic inheritance, chance and randomness rule.

The notion of risk of getting a disease is a two-edged sword in yet another way. On the one hand, knowing that one is at risk because other members of the family have been afflicted creates for healthy women a fear of falling ill, together with the notion that knowledge of the future may enable them to master it by acting in the present and avoiding risks. Those with a family history of breast cancer must, for example, decide whether to have prophylactic surgery performed.[46] Consider, however, the painful disappointment among women such as Sandra, who acted on her understanding that she was at risk for breast cancer because she originated from a family with the disease and had her two healthy breasts removed as a prophylactic measure. Nevertheless, she developed breast cancer despite the drastic "preventive" measures she took. Conversely, within the notion of being at risk is embedded the fatalistic concept of predetermination. In this instance the notion of genetic risk dissolves for the person the boundaries between present and future, and the person may lose her footing in time, as could be seen in women who fear they will fall ill in the future and take action to prevent it. Curiously, then, the concept of risk gives some people an illusionary sense of being in control of the present and the future, a theme that is especially important in American society, by alerting them to take precautionary measures which, in the case of women who fear breast cancer, may include having a prophylactic mastectomy. Yet the notion of risk leaves others with a feeling of inevitability, because knowing that one is at risk owing to one's family medical history forecasts the future in the guise of certainty,[47] for which human beings quest, particularly in the face of affliction.[48] Still, how certain can people be of random events such as genetic inheritance?

I became interested in adoptees searching for their birth parents because of the frequent reports in the mass media and on Internet sites suggesting that they, too, are guided by genetic inheritance ideologies. The trigger question I posed to the adoptees I interviewed was "Why did you search for your birth family?" I found that along with their need to learn about their birth parents' medical histories, they had an essentialist understanding of genetic inheritance that propelled the search. Significantly, while the adoptees were all healthy at the time of the search, some, once they found their birth mothers and learned about illness in their mother's family medical history, became perpetual patients as well.

The adoptees that I interviewed considered themselves to have been molded by their genetic inheritance from persons with whom they lacked prior contact. With minor exceptions, most believed that they had inherited from their birth families medical conditions and behavioral characteristics down to the minutest details. The interviews with adoptees disclose a view of human beings as passive creatures whose interests and personalities are transmitted entirely genetically, rather than acquired by experience and by their own abilities to interpret the world around them. Their perception that one's persona is but a genetically determined passive receptacle is similar to the current sociobiological paradigm of human ontology.

To understand why genetics has become so prominent in modern life is to attend to contemporary family and kinship relations and is associated with notions of memory and continuity, for example. Belief in genetic inheritance establishes for the afflicted and adoptees alike continuity with a genealogical past, if only through the family medical history and through genetic memory conferred by the DNA. Boyarin, following Benjamin, rightly observes that "one of the ways that life is maintained is through a constant effort to retain the image of the past—to rescue the dead and oppressed ancestors by giving their lives a new meaning."[49] Generally speaking, human beings have made an effort to remember those who came before them by erecting both concrete and symbolic edifices. Connerton notes that the "ceremonies of the body, such as are exemplified in court etiquette at Versailles, remind performers of a system of honor and hereditary transmission as the organizing principle of social classification. Blood relations are signs cognitively known and recalled through the visibly elaborate display of privileges and avocations which make sense only by constant reference to that principle."[50] Family and kinship go beyond relationships of the present and of individuals; they also constitute repositories of communal and social memory.[51] While societies incorporate the past into the present by means of written texts, material objects, and ritual performances,[52] the past is also inscribed in people's memories of their ancestors, if only by perpetuating the patronymics. As among both the ancient Romans and present-day Americans, in the absence of material privileges the ancestors were and are remembered by the preservation of their names.[53] Loss of continuity of time and memory is a major theme in our culture, and contemporary families lack continuity, as other scholars have recognized.[54] Holiday rituals may serve as pneumatic devices for remembering family, but once the holiday passes, the minutiae of the present obliterate the past and modern and postmodern humans' turn to current interests and preoccupations. In fact, the present constantly beckons us to forget the past, whereas the DNA, encoded in genealogy, remembers.

Durkheim proposed that in modern society, "because the past is not transmitted with blood, it does not follow that it is reduced to nothing. It remains fixed in monuments, in traditions of all sorts, in habits inculcated by education. But tradition is a considerably less rigid bond than heredity. It predetermines thought and conduct in a much less rigorous and precise manner."[55] Contemporary American society continues to erect monuments to the past, although ceremonies of the body to commemorate it may have lost their force. But contemporary individuals' memories of the past lack temporal depth, and even names may be changed to obliterate one's ancestral past.

Durkheim, however, may not have foreseen that instead of traditions contemporary society is turning to an ideology of genetic inheritance to remember its ancestors. This ideology tends to reduce people's heredity to nucleic acid and molecules, which are devoid of honor, social classifications, moral imperatives, or even the ability to mythologize the past. Concepts of genetic inheritance tend to reinstate the unbending bonds that presumably had been lost in Durkheim's scheme of societal change. The DNA binds a person's past and future into a single family narrative. Nucleic acid and molecules serve as memory vaults, connecting people to their ancestors and reinforcing continuity with them. In the private domain, people's memories are encapsulated by family medical history and DNA molecules, which connect them to their ancestors and to their history. The DNA is not simply a symbol but a trace of molecules that stand for the past. The belief in genetic inheritance tends to reshape memory of past ancestors, gives new meanings to those who came before, and establishes a genetic connection, acting as a repository of memory for an individual's past, which may have been otherwise forgotten. While memory tends to shape our notions about past ancestors, genetic memory inexorably exposes secrets and fanciful creations of a past that never happened. People will no longer be able to re-create ancestors who never were, as may be seen in adoptees' fabrications of ancestors who arrived in America on the *Mayflower*.[56]

My concern with the ways in which concepts of genetic inheritance impact on individual experience bears on broader theoretical issues as well, especially on the tensions between positivism, with its claims of the existence of objective realities discernible through the use of the scientific method, and theories of social construction, including of disease, as advanced, for example, in the concept of medicalization. I explore this latter concept, which holds that disease lacks an objective reality.[57] For instance, according to Bowler, "without denying the important factual consequences that have flowed from the development of genetics, the history of the field will show that the new science was invented to serve human purposes—it did not grow automatically as a consequence of factual observations." Thus, "theories are invented rather than discovered." From Bowler's vantage point, genetic models are constructed to "reflect the values of the social groups whose interests are best served by the promotion of these particular models."[58]

In keeping with Bowler's perspective, in recent times, in fact, we have come to acknowledge that biomedical knowledge, like any medical system, is a cultural system,[59] that biomedicine, like science itself, is not an acultural form of intellectual endeavor but one that has emerged during a particular historical moment in the social formation of Western society.[60] Like all other knowledge systems, biomedicine is a socially and culturally constructed curing enterprise, reflecting the themes of the society and culture of which it forms a part while concurrently imposing these themes on cultural conceptualizations. Consider the most obvious example: biomedicine's model of the human body as a standardized machine and sickness as the breaking down of its component parts mirrors the predominance of technology and machines in modern society while at the same time imprinting on people's consciousness a mechanistic view of themselves.[61] The extensive body of literature shows persuasively how medical concepts are socially construed,[62] reflecting broader cultural themes, including gender differences;[63] but contemporary genetic determinism is not confined to any one-gender representation. Current hereditarian concepts are applied to all members of society, as can be seen in medical textbooks,[64] the popular literature, and the mass media,[65] and are arguably, in part at least, genderless.[66]

Fujimura is but one of various scholars who have shown that scientific knowledge, including biomedical knowledge, is socially produced. She makes a compelling case for how genetic knowledge becomes constructed when she demonstrates that, in the late 1980s, the view of cancer changed from a "set of heterogeneous diseases marked by the common property of uncontrolled cell growth to a disease of human genes."[67] This change was brought about not by new discoveries or new epistemic advances but rather by negotiated social processes.[68] Haraway, in a more critical tone, describes the social constructionist approach best when she states that "no insider's perspective is privileged, because all drawings of inside-outside boundaries in knowledge are theorized as power moves, not moves toward truth."[69]

Could it be argued that all knowledge, including ideas about genes and about disease, is socially constructed, that nature itself is a construct of culture? Can we claim that genetic knowledge, like kinship, is a social construction? After all, whichever way we construct our family and kin group, it will not necessarily impact on our mortality. The extreme cultural constructionist theoretical position claims that there is no objective reality. Yet cancer is palpable and real. People, in fact, die from it, as they do from tuberculosis and many other diseases. Breast cancer is not a social construction any more than amebiasis is, even though both diseases may have been socially produced by adverse environmental conditions. The women I interviewed who suffer from breast cancer cannot theorize away the loss of their breasts nor their pain, any more than one can theorize away diarrhea. Haraway is correct when, speaking to feminists, she observes that "feminists have to insist on a better account of the world; it is not enough to show radical historical contingency and modes of construction for everything. Here, we, as feminists, find ourselves perversely conjoined with the discourse of many practicing scientists, who, when all is said and done, mostly believe they are describing and discovering things *by means of all* their constructing and arguing" (emphasis in the original). She then adds, "relativism is the perfect mirror twin of totalization in the ideologies of objectivity . . . both make it impossible to see well."[70]

No matter how compelling the social constructionist position, and indeed it is very persuasive, scholars recognize the perils of a strictly social constructionist approach.[71] What can be said, for example, in the instance of cancer, is that whereas the disease is real, the explanations for its occurrence — its etiology — are a cultural construction.[72] In seeking explanations for their suffering, human beings the world over have constructed diverse etiological theories of disease, which can be found in the anthropological record. These include witchcraft, invasion by evil spirits, punishment by a deity, ancestral ghosts, and an inimical environment, to name the most notable.[73] Western biomedical etiological explanations usually revolve around the failure of body parts, invasion by pathogens, contagion, trauma, stress, aging, and heredity: these explanations form part of our cultural pool of understanding.[74]

To make sense of human beliefs and practices, including genetic determinism and the ideology of genetic inheritance, I draw upon a modified cultural constructivist perspective, which I believe has always been intrinsic to anthropological discourse by the very nature of its preoccupation with the concept of culture. Each society's culture is a particular construction of reality, a screen for explaining behavior and for making sense of the world in which we live, guiding people's actions, comprehension of their bodies, and interpersonal relationships; it structures people's positions in society and the realities they come to know and expect in their daily existence. In short, our culture enables us to take for granted our daily activities, our relationships, and our customary conceptions of life, including our moral footing.[75] Moreover, cultural beliefs and practices everywhere and in all periods of human history have at once elevated and deflated our existence, including our belief in genetic inheritance.

I depart from the strict constructivist view, however, because I believe that there is a reality independent of our cultural productions. Genetic transmission is not purely a cultural construction, as any sufferer of, say, Huntington's disease will attest.[76] But whether cultural ideologies are socially constructed or objectively real, it is important to assess how the individual, as agent, negotiates them, a point made earlier. Concurrently, when we examine this ideology as an etiological explanation, we must question the reasons for its ascendancy in mainstream American society at this time in its history. I propose that professional interpretations of genetic inheritance are culturally molded, reflecting important themes in our society that I will identify and that have seeped into the popular consciousness and have become part of our commonsense knowledge and cultural pool of understandings.

Genetics

As we will learn, the present perspective on the genetic inheritance of disease, embedded in genetic determinism, has exploded in Western culture since the 1960s, even though the hereditarian concept of disease appeared about a century and a half ago.[77] Several important intellectual and scientific movements contributed to its current formulation, especially the Darwinian revolution of the nineteenth century, which brought a naturalistic diachronic dimension to the idea of a biological continuity within and across species. Also, Mendelian principles, rediscovered in the early twentieth century, introduced the notion of genetic assortment of individual traits transmitted from generation to generation. The Darwin-

ian evolutionary theory of natural selection through differential reproduction gave birth to the eugenics movement, which in turn advanced a
program of selective breeding to improve human existence. Genetic determinism, as we know it today, came into full bloom in the mid-twentieth
century with the blossoming of molecular biology: it ushered in the hegemony of the gene, advancing new ways that people experience themselves in relation to their families. In addition to the hundreds of diseases
that are currently regarded by the scientific establishment as genetically
inherited, all facets of human experiences have been attributed to genetic inheritance, as I noted earlier.[78]

The pendulum swung from the 1950s and 1960s, when social and
psychological causes of disease ruled, to the 1980s, when there was a
gradually renewed interest in genetic causes of crime, alcoholism, and
mental illness and other diseases.[79] The change in medical thinking can
be traced in such basic popular texts as the *Merck Manual of Diagnosis and
Therapy*. In the thirteenth edition of the manual (1977), the table of
contents lacked entries referring to genetic diseases (although some genetic diseases were identified), whereas the same manual in 1997 devoted
all of chapter 2 to genetics and elevated it to a separate category of
"fundamentals" absent from the 1977 edition.[80]

Kinship

The study of family and kinship has been a major anthropological preoccupation since the discipline's formal inception in the nineteenth century. As a graduate student, I pored over texts depicting Australian, African, Melanesian, and South American kinship systems. While kinship
studies have waned in the light of postmodern concerns, most anthropology textbooks include at least one chapter on the different types of
kinship and family systems that exist cross-culturally. Significantly, however, with the invention of new reproductive technologies, paternity, maternity, and siblingship are taking on new meanings in contemporary
human experience, and a new language is being developed to reflect
them.[81] New genetic categories of people are being created, and thus
kinship relationships are now of greater interest to anthropologists and
to social scientists concerned with reproductive technologies.

While I identify some important issues concerning the new reproductive technologies, my focus is on the ways in which the concept of
genetic inheritance orients people toward family and kinship. Great demographic changes have taken place in the past hundred years, during
which time there emerged in Western society an aging population and a
shift in the prevalence of diseases from acute to chronic types.[82] The
etiologies of chronic diseases are poorly understood; increasingly, they

are being attributed to genetic inheritance, which leads to patients being questioned about their family medical histories. People are often encouraged to draw family trees as far back as they can remember, which, among Americans of European descent, is usually to the second ascending generation.[83] The new genetics emphasizes family and kinship relations by the very fact that an increasing number of diseases are being regarded as hereditary.

Various debates have arisen in anthropology concerning the definition and nature of family and kinship, their historical development in Western society, and their significance in contemporary life. I examine these debates because they illuminate the cultural nature of beliefs in genetic inheritance that, I will suggest in the Conclusion, are derived from mainstream Americans' comprehension of kinship. As the inheritors of Western culture, Americans take for granted that genetic ties form kinship and family. In fact, Turner asserts that out of genealogical conceptions flow people's conceptual metaphors bearing on resemblance and difference, as well as concepts of time.[84] He argues convincingly that genealogical relations impose on people notions about similarities and also separate persons from those who are not genealogically related; what is more, they also frame the focus on the genetic transmission of disease and behavior.

In response to the debates revolving around whether or not blood kinship ties are universal, I propose that kinship, however defined in different societies, can be said to demarcate, in all cultures, certain individuals by what I call their "significant same." By this I mean people who are bracketed from the rest of society by being designated as family and kin and distinguished from friends, co-religionists, support group members, or membership in other voluntary associations. The significant same groups that people create may be based on the sharing of genes or on other characteristics such as the sharing of food, breast milk, space, or affection, reflecting contemporary changes in notions of family and kinship.[85] Those who form part of the significant same group share instrumental, moral, and affective codes that embrace feelings of obligations and responsibilities, which may be limited to one or several generations of the living and the deceased.[86]

Typically, in American society, those who form part of the significant same group — family and kin — are distinguished from others because through birth they share the same genes. I hasten to add, however, that there are notable exceptions — for example, when kinship is established by legal adoption, despite its deep commitment to establishing an "as if" genealogical relation, or by assisted conception, using the new reproductive technologies that have called into question the basic assumptions about who constitutes family and kin units.

Paradoxically, the definition of family and kin, or the significant same group, is currently being broadened to include not only people recruited by birth, or connected genetically, but also those selected through personal choice. At the same time, however, the medical-genetic definition narrows the signification of family and kin to specific biological ties that are identified by the DNA. In fact, the sharing of DNA is becoming the hallmark of people's relationship with those designated as family and kin, as is seen in the adjudication associated with surrogacy disputes that bring into bold relief the genetic definition of parenthood,[87] as well as in the vignettes I will present in this book. I propose that the present day genetic determinism molds people into an idealized form of family and kinship, contrary to changing practices and despite the redefinition of family and kin in contemporary society.

The book is divided into three parts. Part I sets the stage with three chapters that introduce the reader to the theoretical issues and historical developments in the two crucial domains of life that bear on the people we meet in Part II. Chapters 2 and 3 give an overview of family and kinship beliefs and practices and the fascinating debate in the anthropological literature concerning whether kinship is socially constructed or universally experienced. Chapter 4 briefly traces the concept of genetic inheritance in Western thought and the scientific developments that have brought us to our current understanding.

Part II presents individual experiences of the ideology of genetic inheritance. We meet seven healthy women from families with a history of cancer (Chapter 5), fifteen breast cancer survivors (Chapter 6), and twelve adopted women and two of three adopted men who have searched for their birth families (Chapter 7). These individuals reveal an important facet of the role the ideology of genetic inheritance plays in contemporary life. These narratives are especially significant because each interviewee's voice is heard. We can discern from them the commonalities that reflect both the cultural nature of experience and the uniqueness of each woman's interpretation of her affliction, or reason for searching for birth parents, illuminating the complexities of her construal of lived realities. Therefore I present each participant's narrative in some detail rather than aggregate the interviews or introduce people to illustrate a theme that tends to objectify the individual and reduce the person to a premise.

Part III probes the implications of current conceptualizations of genetic inheritance. Chapter 8 discusses the role the ideology of genetic inheritance plays in contemporary life by exploring the concept of medicalization. Chapter 9 presents a multidimensional evaluation of genetic inheritance and genetic determinism as viewed by biologists and social scientists.

In Chapter 10 I address the question that, in part, propelled me to write this book—why the concept of genetic inheritance became prevalent in the latter part of the twentieth century. I advance and develop several interrelated explanations associated with aspects of contemporary life, including the American cultural construction of kinship, the current role of family and kinship in contemporary American society, remembrance of an ancestral past, and biomedical practice itself.

Part I
Setting the Stage:
Kinship and Genetics

Chapter 2
The Role of Kinship in Human Life

Contemporary scientific knowledge informs us that genetic traits are transmitted by reproduction and birth, natural processes that form the building blocks of family and kinship in American society. Whereas science and biomedicine regard genetic transmission as a universal and natural biological process that takes place in all living things, conceptualizations of family and kinship are culturally produced. In fact, as long as we remain wrapped in our cultural mantles, we may fail to see that our most profound beliefs and practices, which we take for granted as natural, including those of family and kin, are historically and culturally created. Kinship is arguably the most primordial relationship that human beings construct. People the world over infuse strong feelings into primary ties of family and kin. But even a succinct cross-cultural and historical excursion reveals the cultural basis of our kinship and family relationships. Whereas men and women copulate, reproduce, and transmit their genes to their offspring in all societies, they variously sort, perceive, and interpret their connections to them according to cultural and historical contexts. Lévi-Strauss pointed out long ago that "a kinship system does not consist of the objective ties by descent or consanguinity that obtain among individuals; it exists only in human consciousness, it is an arbitrary system of ideas, not the spontaneous development of a factual situation."[1]

Because biological processes of genetic transmission are closely intertwined with cultural conceptualizations of family and kinship, I want to raise in this chapter several issues discussed in the anthropological literature regarding the understanding of family and kinship from a cross-cultural perspective. I use references to selective cultures to discuss some debates concerning the definition of kinship. Then in the next chapter I move to a discussion of contemporary mainstream American family and kinship beliefs and practices as they have developed historically. I conclude the discussion of family and kinship by examining briefly the new reproductive technologies associated with the new genetics because they have led to a reexamination of traditional meanings of kinship and family. The issues addressed in these two chapters are important because even a condensed exploration of the multifaceted dimensions of family and kinship from a cross-cultural perspective sharpens our grasp of our own cultural conceptualizations and constructions and discloses the extent to which concepts of genetic inheritance both mold and reflect American cultural understandings of family and kinship.

Anthropological Studies of Kinship in the Past and Present

From its inception as a new discipline in the nineteenth century, anthropology advanced the notion of the cultural nature of family and kinship. The study of kinship was firmly established by Lewis Henry Morgan, who in 1846 collected ethnographic materials among the Iroquois and was astonished to find that their kinship conceptualizations differed from his own. He stated, "I found among them in daily use, a system of relationship for the designation and classification of kindred, both unique and extraordinary in its character, and wholly unlike any with which we are familiar."[2] The Iroquois possessed what Morgan termed a classificatory system of kinship that fused collateral with lineal relatives, in contrast to the descriptive system that he knew as an American. Europeans and Americans now, as in Morgan's time, distinguish between their lineal and collateral relatives, that is between their father and their father's brother, whom they call "uncle," and their mother and their mother's sister, whom they call "aunt." The Iroquois, however, did not distinguish between parents and their siblings, regarding their father's brother as their father and their mother's sister as their mother. On the basis of his Iroquois discoveries, Morgan concluded that the family was, indeed, founded on a community of blood, but that one of the earliest acts of humanity was to categorize blood kinship relations into lines of descent that were basic valued relationships. Morgan believed, as did most anthropologists who followed his interest in kinship, that a people's kinship was the folk expression of their understanding of biological relationships. For example, following Morgan, Lowie asserted that "biological relationships merely serve as a starting point for the development of sociological conceptions of kinship."[3]

Those who came after Morgan unquestioningly accepted his view that kinship ties were universally based on blood relationships; that societies whose lives were organized around kinship relationships tended to stress unilineal descent by emphasizing either the maternal side (matrilineal descent) or, in a majority of societies, the paternal side (patrilineal descent). Gross explained that under a unilineal system, "two women can be patrilineal relatives, if for example, they are daughters of brothers. Their children are not patrilineally related," because their children belong to the patrilineal group of their father.[4] These descent rules define how property, status, and social obligations are transmitted and how marriage is contracted. In Fortes's words, "descent . . . confers credentials for status and, hence, for capacities, rights, and duties, [and] . . . a specified parent is both a parent and the repository, as it were, and transmitter, of structurally significant ancestry." In discussing the Nuer, Tallensi, Tiv, Chinese, and ancient Romans, Fortes declared that "the paradigm of patrilineal descent is not just a means of picturing their social structure; it is their fundamental guide to conduct and belief in all areas of social life."[5]

Generally speaking, in most patrilineally organized societies, anyone in one's patrilineal descent group is not a potential marriage partner because individuals of the same descent group are regarded as close kin. To marry a person in one's defined kinship unit is to commit incest. In patrilineal societies, persons in one's mother's line are not formally recognized as kin and may in fact be regarded as preferable marriage partners (as in cross-cousin marriages).[6]

Anthropologists working in non-Western stateless societies, irrespective of their theoretical orientation, have asserted that the locus of people's existence in these societies is kinship and family. In kinship-oriented societies, family and kinship regulated marriage, residence, worship of ancestors, and access to land and assistance.[7] In sum, in such societies the entire reproductive, economic, religious, and ideological life revolves around the kinship unit.[8]

Kinship studies have raised numerous debates that are relevant to our contemporary understanding of the cultural nature of family and kinship relations. One such early debate revolved around theories of conception. Did people who emphasized either the mother's or the father's side as the basis of their kinship affiliation recognize the contributions of both parents to the formation of the offspring? Some scholars have argued that people in most societies recognize that both mother and father contribute to the formation of the offspring, although this recognition appears less significant than the line of descent to which the offspring belongs.[9] This debate is especially interesting in the context of the new reproductive technologies and the new genetics that I discuss at the end of the next chapter.

At this juncture, a brief excursion into the anthropological literature is illuminating. Consider the Melpa of Melanesia. They believe that the paternal substance is shared among males through the patrilineal line (agnatical); even though the mother provides the blood, the father supplies the "grease" (semen) that gives strength to the sons. Daughters inherit their strength from the mother.[10] Among the Baraya of Melanesia, the mother is not regarded as the parent whose substance forms the fetus.[11] A similar belief is held by the Zande of Central Africa, as described by Evans-Pritchard: "The spirit-soul [is] . . . What is derived from the father, in spite of what is said about the mother's cooperation in its creation, and this is what makes all children, irrespective of sex, members of their father's clan. [Thus] there is a tendency to emphasize the father's part in procreation beyond that of the mother just as the father's side of the family is stressed socially to a greater extent than the mother's side of the family."[12]

In some patrilineal societies such as China or Egypt, for example, it is not uncommon for the mother to be regarded as merely the vessel in which the father plants his seed; he alone is responsible for the new life that is born.[13] Or, in some societies the mother-child relation is regarded as nothing more than a sociological relationship of affinity and alliance rather than a blood relationship of descent. In short, the mother has no kinship ties to the offspring. Consequently, the children of the same mother but different fathers are not considered related and could even marry, whereas the children of the same father stand in an incestuous relationship to one another.[14] In contrast, in Malaysia, a Muslim patrilineal society, it is believed that both parents participate in the formation of the child. Children are created from the seed of their father and the blood of their mother. The father's seed comes from the fluid in the backbone. The seed spends forty days inside the body of the father. The first, fifteenth, and thirtieth days are when the seed falls. The seed descends to the mother and mixes with the menstrual blood, and it is the blood of menstruation that becomes the child.[15]

On the other hand, in matrilineal societies such as the Trobrianders, the father may simply "open the way" for the child to be born.[16] When Malinowski studied the Trobrianders he found that they believed that children result from the return of an ancestor through the body of a woman; the father's contribution was largely ignored. For this matrilineal society, the succession of rank, membership in all the social groups, and the inheritance of possessions descended through the maternal line. According to Malinowski, "The real kinship, the real identity of substance is considered to exist between a man and his mother's relations."[17]

Earlier anthropologists assumed that the reproductive process universally produced the family and the kin group, even when the people themselves did not stress any relationship between conception and reproduction.[18] It was usually not doubted that most societies with unilineal descent believed that the creation of the family and group resulted from the blood of the mother and the seed of the father, even though the role of one might be stressed more than the other.

Is Kinship a Universal Concept? A Debate

Until the late 1960s, anthropologists studying kinship adhered to Morgan's notion that, no matter how conception was viewed, the definition of kinship relations was universally rooted in reproduction and blood links. In a series of works, Schneider questioned whether all human societies do indeed build family and kinship ties by blood ties, and in doing so he initiated a vigorous controversy regarding the universality of kinship relations.[19] He moved the debate away from the conceptualization of kinship as a way in which people everywhere deal with the universal natural process of procreation and instead focused on how specific cultures construe relationships that in the West are referred to as kinship.[20] Schneider asserted that "whereas followers of Morgan take it for granted that sexual intercourse, conception, pregnancy, and parturition constitute the domain of 'kinship' I treat this as an open, empirical question."[21] He asked rhetorically, "does it really follow therefore that the reality of biology, the scientific demonstrability of blood-types and genetic relationship constitute a significant determinant of kinship?"[22] He answered his own question by vehemently denying that it did. Moreover, he rightly claimed that kinship could not be studied as an abstract model separated from daily existence,[23] as myriad anthropologists have attempted to study it.[24] We must not suppose that what we call kinship is universally founded on a biogenetic premise characterized by a genealogical grid.[25] Most significantly, Schneider contended that Western social scientists impose their cultural conceptualization on other cultures: "Kinship has been defined by European social scientists, and European social scientists use their own folk culture as the source of many, if not all, of their ways of formulating and understanding the world about them."[26] This is an important point, to which I will return in the Conclusion.

Schneider supported his assertions with studies he had done on the island of Yap, where he observed that birth was not a precondition for membership in the local group. In Yap, people regard themselves as kinsmen because they share a landholding unit; that is, close ties are established on the basis of shared residence rather than birth. When a person fails in his duties to the land, he loses his rights to it, and a new person may come in to establish ties to the group. Despite Schneider's vigorous rejection of the universality of kinship (meaning biological) ties through reproduction, he nevertheless seemed to vacillate on this point when he stated that "children may be given to others to raise or may be adopted, but the bond with the woman who gave them birth remains either as an important informal one, or, in fosterage, as a formal one as well." The relationship between mother and child is achieved by birth, but the child must also have a name that gives it the right to the land. Relationships can be established by people having shared a "common belly" (mother) or through a mythical ancestress and name.[27] Schneider seems to suggest that the relationship between mother and child is not denied or severed, but that kinship relations rest in the sharing of a name. There is a cultural rather than a biological connection. This is an important point that needs to be kept in mind when, in Chapter 7, I turn to the discussion of adoptees.

The importance of the name in establishing kinship ties is not unique to the Yap islanders. Veyne advances the notion that in Roman society blood ties were of little importance: "The 'voice of blood' spoke very little in Rome. What mattered more than blood was the family name." The birth of a Roman citizen was not merely a biological fact: infants came into the world and were discarded. Birth alone did not signify that a scion had come into the world. According to Veyne, the Romans thought it peculiar that Jews, Egyptians, and Germans did not expose their children to death but raised them. He concluded that "the Romans made no fetish of natural kinship."[28]

In keeping with Schneider's theorizing, Witherspoon found that among the matrilineal Navajo, kinship is not necessarily established by reproductive and blood ties. To be a mother is to have a child, but not necessarily in a biological sense, even though the mother-child bond, including the matrilineal bond, is the strongest relationship.[29] In Navajo comprehension, the woman who sustains the helpless infant is the mother. The life and substance mothers provide for their children are the primary symbols of kinship. All Navajos have two basic descent identities that derive from both their maternal and paternal origin, though their relationships to these categories differ from one person to another. In Witherspoon's words, "those of my mother's clan are my mothers." Following the form of classificatory kinship as defined by Morgan, "a Navajo may consider anyone in his mother's category to be a mother, even a man."[30] Those of his own matrilineal descent category are considered his siblings because they all descend from a common ancestor.

Yet Witherspoon also claims that the birth mother-child bond is nevertheless closer and stronger. He suggests that mothers and children, or siblings, are considered to possess an essential oneness of identity, epitomized by exogamy, hospitality, and ceremonial cooperation. To emphasize his contention that kinship is not established by reproduction and blood ties, Witherspoon stresses that the sibling order is very important in Navajo families, although it is not defined by birth. "If a child is reared by a mother who gave birth to several other children, the child by rearing only will be placed in the sibling order with no stigma attached. On the other hand, children born to the same mother but not raised by her are often left out of the sibling group unless the informant is really pushed to include all those born together even though they were not reared together. Siblings of different fathers are not distinguished in any way in the sibling order, and siblings of the same father but different mothers constitute no sibling order at all."[31] Most important for my later argument, Witherspoon makes the significant point, as others have done,[32] that "the culturally related kin universe is a moral order because it is a statement of the proper order of that universe — that is, the ideal state of affairs or the way things ought to be."[33]

In further support of Schneider's claims, Weismantel discovered that, among an Ecuadorian group she had studied, bonds between people are created gradually and mediated by food rather than blood. She found that "the physical acts of intercourse, pregnancy, and birth can establish a strong bond between two adults and a child. But other adults, by taking a child into their family and nurturing its physical needs through the same substances as those eaten by the rest of the social group, can make of the child a son or a daughter who is physically as well as jurally their own." The most critical criterion, according to Weismantel, is the sharing of food. She claims that a child becomes a member of the family by participating in daily life: by talking and by sleeping, and by being fed, clothed, and healed. Most important, "eventually [the child] will look like them, smell like them, laugh and gesture like them," and will be recognized as one of them. Procreation alone fails to make a parent among the Zumbagua of Ecuador. If a man lives with a woman throughout her pregnancy and delivery, has sex with her while she is pregnant, and feeds and cares for her and for the newborn, then he can claim to be father to the child. Moreover, labor alone does not make a woman a mother. Motherhood is associated with a woman's struggles to meet the demands of growing children, her ability to produce socialized offspring who can talk and understand what is being said. Having achieved these goals, the woman earns the title of mother. Weismantel holds that "investment of labor by an adult in the life of a child is the real criterion of parenthood."[34] She interprets Zumbagua practices as comparable to adoption practices in American society, except that these Ecuadorians make no distinctions between adoptive and blood ties.

Also in support of Schneider, Trawick, in her study of a Tamil family in South India, stresses that sentiment and love cement family and kin, especially bonds between mother and son and brothers and sisters. While she grants that mingling of bodily substances is important, she regards sentiment as crucial to kinship in Tamil thoughts and actions. She remarks, "but kinship is not only, or even primarily, a matter of relations between categories of persons. Nor is it primarily a matter of relations between physical components of persons. It is, I would argue, primarily a matter of relations between persons, whole and actual persons. In their day-to-day associations with each other, they give the system being."[35] For Trawick, kinship is a linguistic and affective system. Kin terms can be applied to people who are not genealogically related but who express a kin-based feeling toward each other. Kinship creates a longing that is often channeled by means of words or kinship terms and not by genealogical ties. Trawick has introduced a poetic dimension to our understanding of kinship relations, but her argument against its genealogical basis is less persuasive, considering that in Indian society, caste membership is defined by birth and thus by blood.[36]

It is noteworthy that many feminist scholars have embraced Schneider's rejection of biological kinship relations and, in doing so, have reinvigorated the study of kinship. Feminists insist that biology must be separated from kinship.[37] As long as a restrictive connection is made between biology and kinship and family, women's existence will be associated solely with their reproductive capacities. For feminists, kinship is not a natural fact of sex: procreation and the rearing of offspring is not a universal presocial phenomenon.[38]

Not surprisingly, Schneider has had various detractors.[39] Keesing disagrees that kinship ties are simply cultural and symbolic constructs, free of biological links: "Kinship is a network of relationships created by genealogical connections, and by social ties (e.g., those based on adoption) modeled on the 'natural' relations of genealogical parenthood."[40] Keesing grants that, theoretically, kinship need not be regarded as a natural, inalienable connection of shared substance, but empirically it is universally viewed in terms of genealogical connections.

Scheffler similarly claims that Schneider cannot make biology go away and insists that all systems use biological relations to define kinship. Relationships by birth may not be the only criterion for inclusion into a kin category, but they are one criterion, and he challenges anyone to find a report of a society where the concept of maternity is absent. Scheffler defines kinship for cross-cultural comparison as a "culturally postulated relationship by birth."[41]

In her desire to rescue the concept of kinship from Schneider's assault on it, Carsten, using data from Malaysia, shows that both blood and food form the basis of kinship. She contends that "the core substance of kinship is local perceptions of blood, and the major contribution to blood is food. Blood is always mutable and fluid — as is kinship itself." But people can also become kin not only by birth but also by living and consuming together in a house. People can become siblings when they drink the same mother's breast milk. Milk and blood are the prime sources of shared substance that constitute the kinship bond. Carsten found that ideas about relatedness are expressed in terms of procreation, feeding, and the acquisition of substance and are not predicated on any clear distinction between "facts of biology" (like birth) and "facts of sociality" (like commensality).[42] She rightly takes Schneider to task for separating biological from social experience, as if biological facts could be separated from social facts,[43] given how deeply such biological notions are embedded in a culture. Carsten suggests that kinship may not be associated solely with reproduction but that humans everywhere define some people as closer than others, based on various culturally constituted criteria.

Holy similarly asserts that in all human societies some people consider themselves "to be more closely related to each other than they are to other people, and that this mutual relatedness is the basis of numerous and varied interactions in which they are involved or provides legitimisation or rationalisation for them."[44] Holy argues that while not all peoples have concepts of descent, they all recognize, from a cultural perspective, a domain that we call kinship. He grants that in some societies people may share blood or bone or semen, but they may also have suckled the same milk or eaten the same food. For Holy, the notion of relatedness is the core of kinship that could be mediated by the sharing of blood, milk, semen, and so on. To support his definition of kinship, Holy refers to the Hua of New Guinea, where kin ties are created when people share a vital substance that could include odor, sweat, ingested saliva, food, or contact with another's excreta. Ultimately, Holy, in his search for a universal core of kinship and family, suggests that we focus on people's notions of relatedness, which may or may not be tied to reproduction and blood links.[45]

How do we resolve the controversy set off by Schneider? We can safely say that at present, most scholars would agree with Schneider, Keesing, and others,[46] that to understand the meaning and practice of kinship we must focus on how people in a given society go about identifying family and kin, without a priori definitions of what they constitute. It can also be said that people the world over delineate a circle of persons whom I call their significant same, individuals or groups who perceive themselves as similar and who consider themselves related on the basis of shared material, ideological, or affective content and moral obligations. In American society, the popular construal of the significant same was based, at least until recently, on beliefs of biogenetic connections established by procreation, as we will learn in the next chapter.

Chapter 3
Family and Kinship in American Society

Although there is a great diversity of scholarly opinion as to the nature of family and kinship, when we focus solely on American society we become more certain about their meanings and significance, which go back to at least the Middle Ages.[1] In this chapter I briefly provide a broad overview of American ideas and practices concerning family and kin from their origins to the present in order to locate our contemporary conceptualizations within a historical context. I conclude the chapter with a consideration of the new reproductive technologies and their impact on contemporary notions of family and kinship.

Contemporary American conceptualizations of kinship and family have their roots in sixth-century Europe, when bilateral kinship — meaning giving equal weight to both mother's and father's blood line — was legally established. Church law decreed that consanguinity referred to all those related by birth in the paternal and maternal lines up to the seventh degree and forbade those more closely related than that to marry. During this period, the definition of consanguinity expanded dramatically and fully included the matrilateral kin.[2] The new law prevailed over all of Europe, abolishing patrilineality and introducing a new conceptualization — that the mother also transmitted blood to the offspring.[3]

Roman beliefs emphasizing only the father's line of descent had predominated prior to this period. In contrast to Veyne, whom I discussed in Chapter 2, and according to Pomata, who admittedly is writing from a feminist perspective, patrilineality ruled a person's entire existence, although it "was fully realized not in birth but in death, when the son inherited the father's patrimony." Pomata points out that consanguinity was derived from the same father, even though, in the popular view, bilateral blood ties were also recognized. *Consanguinitas* referred to kinship between a father and his children, in part derived from the father's social power and in part from his blood: "children of the same father and different mothers share the same blood; children of the same mother 2and different fathers do not." Women played no role in determining blood transmission. Pomata states: "It is only through the male sex—as the code of Justinian tells us—that 'the rights of one and the same blood stay uncorrupted.' "[4]

Pomata's work suggests that blood ties may have played some role in defining kinship relations in Roman society, although not an exclusive one. As we saw in Chapter 2, blood kinship, generally speaking, was of diminished importance in ancient Rome. Veyne states that for the Romans the family name mattered most, and it could also be upheld by adopting slaves or free people. Adoption was prevalent in ancient Rome, and a freed slave could adopt the family name of the master who had set him free and who then became his new father. Adoption was, in fact, a major form of building family relationships and maintaining the family name. Prevailing morality taught that fathers should love their children as bearers of the family name and perpetuators of its grandeur, but, according to Veyne, the maternal and paternal "instinct" did not exist. Love between parents and children could develop in the same manner as it would between any two individuals brought together.[5]

While blood ties may not have dominated Roman conceptions of kinship, kinship established by blood was significant in biblical times, as it is today in Judaism.[6] In biblical times a child was the possession of the man who provided the "seed" for its creation. Even when boys were adopted into the lineage of a certain man, Schwartz informs us, the system still "assume[d] and [took] as its founding assumption that men are linked to men of the previous generation through their father's seed."[7] Whereas emphasis on patrilineality continues to persist into the present in American society, as exemplified by the inheritance of the father's name, contemporary society largely adheres to the bilateral kinship forms introduced during the medieval period in Europe.

Scholars, at least since the time of Maine, have differentiated "primitive" (stateless) from "complex" societies (organized as states) by the degree to which kinship has played a part in them. Maine defined a primitive society as having "[for] its units, not individuals, but groups of men united by the reality or the fiction of blood-relationship."[8] Subsequent anthropologists have followed this distinction. In comparing "primitive" with "complex" societies, Sahlins noted that in primitive societies all human endeavors are embedded in kinship ties, including economic, political and religious activities.[9] More recently, Giddens also distinguished premodern from modern society by the differential role kinship plays. In premodern societies, Giddens notes, "kinship, in sum, provides a nexus of reliable social connections which, in principle and very commonly in practice, form an organizing medium of trust relations. Kin people can usually be relied upon to meet a range of obligations more or less regardless of whether they feel personally sympathetic towards the specific individuals involved."[10] Marilyn Strathern rightly observed that no matter how complex the kinship relations of non-Western peoples may have been, Westerners usually conceived of them as primitive.[11] Arguably, the distinction between primitive and complex societies as defined by kinship organization may have possessed only heuristic value because historical data suggest that family and kinship relationships were equally significant in medieval Europe. Durkheim, in fact, observed that "the association of blood and power was of such long standing that to many it seemed like a fact of nature."[12] He also noted that in the past, depending on one's class position, one could expect to inherit from one's kin not only traits such as power, property and status but also poverty.

In the Byzantine half of the former Roman Empire, in the tenth and eleventh centuries, adoptions declined and increased emphasis was given to lineages or social groupings based purely on blood ties.[13] Similarly, historians have suggested that family and kinship relations based on blood continued to be of primary importance in western European societies at least until the end of the nineteenth century, at which time the nuclear family turned inward.[14] Until that time, the family unit of husband and wife and their unmarried children was less important than wider kinship affiliations based on biological relations. The transition was gradual, having begun in the 1500s and extending until the 1750s. During this period, there was a decline in the claims that people could make on their cousins, for example. The family began to lose responsibility for its members' crimes and actions. Kinship loyalties became subordinate to political and religious ideology after the 1640s.[15] On a local level, kin ties continued to be important well into the eighteenth century. Before the 1800s, kinship roles, such as parent, brother, or cousin, rather than individual relationships, came first in a person's life.[16]

Until the mid-eighteenth century, kinship ties were permanent. Gottlieb states: "Kinship was unique because it was a biological tie. As members of noble families were always saying, what counted was blood. Being born with a family's blood was what made one a member, and nothing could change that. Because blood flowed from the past and into the future, kinship could seem to transcend time. It had a permanence that was precious in a world of corruption and decay."[17]

Before the mid-eighteenth century, kinship meant blood relations but could also include all those living in the household, especially persons related by marriage. But the transition that took place in the eighteenth century created some confusion about the meaning of family and kin. Should it incorporate only those persons related by blood or also those related by marriage? This dilemma is reflected in the definitions offered by the French *Encyclopédie*, which initially incorporated both members of the household and individuals related by blood, then broadened the definition to include all those descended from the same stock and who therefore had the same blood. Hence, "family" referred to persons tied by blood or affinity only.[18]

By the eighteenth century, the concept of individualism had come into prominence and kinship ties began to be loosened. Significantly, prior to 1800, the emotional role assigned to the family was incidental. After 1800, new ideologies regarding family and kinship were ushered in that erased most of the older ideas and ideals. During this period, for example, nostalgia for the family and belief in family values became prevalent. The Enlightenment contributed to the notion of the home as the locus of intimacy, warmth, and comfort. The idea that people feel deeply toward the family may strike us as a cliché today, but before the eighteenth century it was not the norm. Belief in the family as an emotional unit and as a nest for the young grew stronger, coming into full force in the nineteenth century.[19]

I must stress, as historians do, that the role kinship played in western Europe varied by class at all times, as it does in present-day American society.[20] Gottlieb actually makes clear that, at least in the early modern period, large kinship groupings were a sign of aristocratic rank and wealth. She observes that "prosperous people of all ranks had more relatives than the really poor."[21] The idea of a person coming from a good family required flaunting one's ancestors and blood kin. Blood was associated with power and family honor and was supported by the legal structure. Also, the upper classes lived in large extended families, while poor people resided in small nuclear families.[22] Kinship ties were weakest among the lower classes throughout the centuries. Generally speaking, the poor counted kinsmen as those who resided within walking distance. But even among the poor, Gottlieb observes, "in general, the kin who really mattered were those with a direct link to one's parents, either generationally or laterally: the parents' parents, the parents' siblings, and the parents' children (one's own siblings and half-siblings)."[23]

Bilaterality, with an emphasis on patrilineality, was replicated in North America.[24] Legally, from the seventeenth to the nineteenth century, liberal theorists and lawyers regarded the family as a natural and therefore a "private" association, "consisting of a male, a female, and their biological children." Liberal theory also assumed that the family was created by nature through human sexual mating and reproduction.[25] Indeed, a strong orientation toward family and kinship was a defining characteristic of farm life in America, and people relied for help on kinfolk who were defined in genealogical relations among different families. In seventeenth-century America, the family was part of a wide network of community kinship relations, incorporating in-laws and other distant kin who were generally referred to as brothers, sisters, aunts, uncles, mothers, fathers, and cousins.[26] The family was a microcosm of the larger society and the backbone of the colonial period; it integrated economic, social, and political activity and placed family interests above those of the individual,[27] characteristics that are usually ascribed only to "primitive" societies.

Following the American Revolution, most states adopted specific reforms designed to reduce the power of kin groups in politics by barring nepotism. After the Revolution, in addition to nepotism laws, population growth contributed to the breakup of the family because there was insufficient land for all the children; some had to move elsewhere.[28] During the nineteenth century, family ties began to weaken in North America, as they had in Europe, and to become a matter of individual choice. The family was expected to provide comfort and safety, and the spouse romance, sexual fulfillment, companionship, and emotional satisfaction.[29]

It is instructive to note Wallace's observations from his in-depth study of life in a single town in the United States, where he found that during the nineteenth century the American doctrine of family was "sanctioned in religion, morality, and law, and almost universally accepted in the 1850s." At the time, it was axiomatic that the married pair and their children constituted the natural basis of human society.[30] The nuclear family radiated to ascending and descending generations in loose aggregations of kinship, but patterns differed along class lines. Among workers, the nuclear family was vitally necessary to the economic welfare of most adult individuals who contributed to the household. Among the managerial class, in much the same way as in England, the patronymic descent group was far more important than among the workers, and marriage alliances were an important form of consolidating a family's power. Such groups were formed of the successive generations of persons patrilineally descended from and bearing the name of an original male ancestor.[31]

Historically, then, in American society and its European predecessor, kinship established by blood links formed the foundation of family relations and also radiated outside the immediate group to larger groupings. Again, extended family ties were more important among the wealthy, who possessed property to protect and power to uphold that was legitimized by blood ties. Hence, the common distinction made by scholars between primitive and complex societies on the basis of the importance of kinship may have been exaggerated.[32] As we saw, not until the end of the eighteenth century did kinship begin to decrease in importance in western Europe. While family and kinship relations may have become attenuated in the New World colonies, scholars seem to agree that family and kinship played an important role from their beginning, at least until the nineteenth century. Significantly, the most drastic changes did not take place until relatively recently, in the 1960s, when the notion that kinship was founded solely on blood ties began especially to be questioned not only by anthropologists but also in practice.[33]

Family and Kinship in Contemporary American Society

Prior to the mid-twentieth century, kinship and family relations may not have changed as drastically as we might imagine, but changes did take place. The role of kin relations in modern times seems to have faded into the background. In contemporary society, kinship groups, unless deliberately maintained, are limited to living memory. With the possible exception of parent-child ties, people's most important relationships are apt to be outside the household with individuals not related by blood or marriage. Gottlieb even asserts that "some of us think it is faintly old-fashioned to confine oneself to the company of kinfolk."[34]

One of the marks of modern society is that kinship relations are separate from economic, political, and religious institutions, and thus play a diminished role.[35] In contemporary—especially middle-class—society, relationships are based on the economy and the production of goods rather than on kinship ties.[36] In Giddens's view, kinship relationships, on which trust had been founded, have been replaced in modern society by "friendship, [and] sexual intimacy as the means of stabilizing social ties."[37] Yet Giddens recognizes that, while rules governing kinship relations have been lost, some important ideologies about kinship based on blood relationship still survive after hundreds of years.[38]

Whereas Schneider insisted that blood relations must not be assumed to define the basic groupings that people establish the world over, he recognized that reproduction and blood ties define genealogical relations in the United States. In American cultural conceptualizations, kinship is defined as biogenetic; that is, the child is made up of both the mother's and the father's material.[39] Biogenetic substance is a symbol of oneness in American culture, and "biological unity is the symbol for all other kinds of unity including, most importantly, that of relationships of enduring diffuse solidarity," which are glued together by love.[40] Schneider claims that, while the sentiment of love is the overarching concept cementing kin relationships, there is no one single act that defines love between kin and gives meaning to biological ties other than residing in the same household. Since the nineteenth century, nurturing has become a hallmark of the modern nuclear family.[41]

Schneider, like others,[42] underscores that choice defines who precisely are considered kinfolk. In contemporary American society, where the ideology of choice rules, one is not surprised that the notion of choice is extended to biogenetic ties with regard to kinfolk and family. Strathern, writing about Britain, could be describing the United States when she observes that "kinship may also appear as a transcendent order that allows for degrees of relatedness or solidarity or liberty and for relative strength in the 'expression' of values."[43] She also points out that British individualism (and one could say the same for the United States) leads to diversity in the ways kinship is expressed in practice and what is expected from kinfolk.[44]

Alternative visions of family and kinship forms have begun to compete in America—especially since the 1960s—with the traditional ideologies of family and kin that began to develop at the start of the Industrial Revolution and became firmly entrenched in the nineteenth century.[45] These relations were characterized by biological ties cemented and affirmed by notions of affection and intimacy. Following the transformations that took place in the 1960s, alternative visions of family conflicted with the traditional ideology of family. Such families have become less dependent on biogenetic relations than traditional families, and members of such families choose those whom they would regard as relatives.[46]

The modern family of sociological theory and historical convention, consisting of an intact nuclear household unit composed of a male provider, a female housekeeper, and their children, no longer prevails in the United States. Stacey notes that "historians place the emergence of the modern American family among white middle class people in the late eighteenth century; they depict its flowering in the nineteenth century and chart its decline in the second half of the twentieth."[47] The postmodern family of the latter part of the twentieth century is characterized by uncertainty, insecurity, and doubt, and its arrangements, like postmodernism, are diverse, fluid, and unresolved, opening the way for an array of kinship relations. Stacey, in her study of the postmodern family, observes that "no longer is there a single culturally dominant family pattern to which the majority of Americans conform and most of the rest aspire."[48] In contemporary life, the routinization of divorce and remarriage generates diverse patterns of family structure and conceptualizations of its meaning. Along with other scholars, Stacey has concluded that the traditional family is no longer a viable unit because it distorts the variety of kinship possibilities that are not founded on blood ties.[49] Separation and divorce in postmodern society have generated a diversity of new kin ties associated with recombinant families that are ever changing and are subject to negotiation.[50] Today a family may consist of any grouping that is established on the basis of choice: single-parent; blended family; adoptive; gay.[51] Despite the new configurations of the postmodern family,

Gottlieb perhaps sums it up best when she states that "although it is impossible to overlook kinship as a force in people's lives, it is also impossible to pin it down."[52] The mark of a modern individual is autonomy, independence, and detachment from kinship ties, arguably excepting the nuclear family,[53] or, as Bellah et al. observe, "Kinship has narrowed and the sphere of individual decisions has grown."[54]

In contrast to scholars who have placed a nail in the modern family's coffin,[55] Finch and Mason demonstrate convincingly that, at least in England, kinship has neither disappeared nor flourished. Ideologically, kinship has admittedly lost its power, but in practice family and kinship continue to constitute significant relationships in people's lives.[56] Finch and Mason correctly argue, as others have done,[57] that kinship and family relations carry a moral load and are therefore marked off from all other types of relationships. Kin relationships cannot be viewed solely in material terms; they must be seen in moral terms. Finch and Mason state that "when we talk about seeing the moral dimensions of family responsibilities, we mean that people's identities as moral beings are bound up in these exchanges of support, and the process through which they get negotiated."[58] Nevertheless, Finch and Mason find kinship obligations fluid and not necessarily ruled by genealogical position. The only clear relationship commonly recognized is between parents and children. Unlike past centuries, when kinship relations differed across class lines, Finch and Mason, with their emphasis on the great variability of these relations, argue against the view that "working-class people in general are more inclined to value family support than are the middle classes—or indeed the other way round."[59]

Great attention has been paid to middle- and working-class families, but little has been said about elite families, among whom kinship ties are promoted and expected just as in the past. Marcus and Hall point to the conflicts that contemporary elite families may experience in the face of the dominant ideology of loose kinship and family ties. These conflicts, for which psychotherapists are sought, seem to revolve around desires for individuation versus allegiance to the family. In fact, from a psychotherapeutic perspective, strongly organized, dynastic families are often regarded as pathological. The aim of therapy is to separate the individual from family-rooted problems and to encourage breaking the dynasty's hold. Marcus and Hall note that dynastic sagas form part of popular culture, including pulp fiction, television, and films, to "complete the narrative of continuity that contemporary family life denies most people, or only provides them in a very weak form."[60] These sagas seem bent on negating people's experience of the loose ties that are found among contemporary middle-class families.

Dynastic families seem to be represented in our consciousness in yet another way. Notwithstanding the fact that a connection with people other than our kin is one of the factors that defines us as modern or postmodern beings, paradoxically, the ideology of kinship and family continues to carry a powerful symbolic load. For example, the business world, arguably the most dominant domain in modern life, has appropriated the conception of kinship: witness its incessant reference to companies as families. Investment vehicles such as mutual funds designate groups of similar funds as "families" of funds. People may still invoke kinship relations when in need, as in the Depression era song "Brother, Can You Spare a Dime?" Unions, too, refer to their organizations as "brotherhoods," and some religious and ethnic groups identify their members as "siblings." The representations of numerous institutions in familial terms may reflect the myths of dynasties or refer to a mythical coherent past that organized life around kinship and family. Family and kinship in contemporary times do not usually tend to organize a person's existence, nor is the person embedded in a kinship group that defines his or her identity. People's kin may reside far off, and physical contacts may be limited to annual holiday visits. But, to maximize the effect on its clientele, the business world has appropriated the kinship idiom, if only symbolically.

The New Reproductive Technologies

A good argument could be made that the new reproductive technologies have done more than any other factor to call into question our traditional understanding of family and kinship.[61] Scientific innovations that can potentially manipulate and influence genetic transmission and inheritance require us to rethink our definitions of family and kinship.[62] For this reason, it is important to consider them here.

From a practical perspective, the new reproductive technologies affect only the 10 percent of the population that is infertile. But viewed theoretically, they bring to the forefront questions bearing on our fundamental notions of kinship and parenthood and on the role genetic inheritance plays in people's lives. Significantly, while in economically developing nations the major concern is to contain fertility and population growth with population control programs, in economically developed nations the concern is with infertility and reproductive technologies.[63]

When the first in vitro fertilization was announced in 1978, the world was dazzled by the accomplishment. But, as is true of any innovation, after the initial breakthrough, people become accustomed to the new developments and begin to take them for granted. While in vitro fertilization technologies may have become routine by the end of the twentieth century, the latest reproductive technologies are brought into our daily consciousness by sensational legal cases that are frequently reported in the media. Such reports reveal the human problems these technologies have created which often require adjudication in the courts.

Artificial insemination by donors, which produces a clear distinction between the genetic and the social father, has been available for over a century, even though it did not become prevalent until the late 1960s.[64] But in vitro fertilization techniques and surrogate motherhood are a contemporary phenomenon.[65] Despite its high potential for failure, if both sperm and eggs are donated, in vitro fertilization has the possibility of producing a situation where neither social parent is the genetic parent.[66] Surrogate motherhood can lead to an even more complicated situation in which the social mother (that is, the commissioning mother) is one individual, the provider of the ovum is another, and the gestational mother is a third. In addition, the semen may be donated rather than coming from the social (or commissioning) father.

The separation of the gestational-genetic mother (or father) from the social mother is, of course, not a phenomenon unique to our times. The most obvious example in Western society is stepparenthood.[67] Of course, the anthropological record contains numerous examples of conception that stress the father's contribution or the contribution of ancestors, as we saw earlier in this chapter. Also, there are instances in the anthropological record where birthing and motherhood are separated. For example, the Nuer practiced "ghost" marriages, in which a woman would give birth to a child in the name of her husband's dead brother, if the brother had died before he could marry and produce a legitimate heir himself.[68] In this instance, the "blood" of the father is separated from the child, yet the dead father is regarded as instrumental in giving birth to the child. Among the Kikuyu Nandi, Dinka of East Africa, for example, a widow who had failed to produce children during her marriage could arrange to have another woman produce offspring for her deceased husband.[69] Among the Dahomey of West Africa, an infertile woman could have another woman carry a child for her, and the commissioning woman would then be called "female father."[70] Similarly, among the Nuer a barren woman could marry another woman, who then counted as the father of the children born of the wife.[71] In such instances the gestational genetic mother is separate from the social mother, who is regarded as the true mother. The instances where one gestates and gives birth to a child in the name of another woman come closest to the surrogacy arrangements currently in practice. The truly novel arrangement of the present time occurs when the provider of the egg is different from the bearer of the child.[72]

These new reproductive technologies may be more problematic for people in Western societies, where kinship is defined by biogenetic ties, than in societies such as the Dahomey, the Dinka, or the Nuer, where the mother is not the one who donates her genes but the one who pays the bride price.[73] In Western societies, the latest technologies challenge fundamental assumptions because a child's mother is no longer an obvious fact.[74] The same child may now have three different mothers: one who donates the egg, another who nurtures the fetus in her womb and gives it birth, and a third who gives primary care after birth. Owing to the fact that genetic inheritance bestows personhood on the individual in Western society, the possibilities created by the new reproductive technologies become so troublesome that sometimes they must be resolved by a legal system that is being challenged by the previously inconceivable dilemmas they produce. The courts are called upon to adjudicate about motherhood, family, and kinship, issues that have hitherto been taken for granted within the culture.

The various possibilities advanced by in vitro fertilization and surrogacy raise questions such as "Who is the mother of the newborn child?" Is it the woman who contributed the ovum and, thus, the genetic material, the woman who carried the infant in her body for nine months, or the woman who commissioned the child contractually on the basis of a monetary exchange and legal arrangement? And who will be the child's kin? A new frontier in law has been opened because previous laws regarding adoption, custody, and termination of parental rights were inapplicable for resolving disputes of surrogacy.[75] The possibility of dividing biological maternity into separate aspects that can be distributed among different women forces contemporary society and the law to rethink the meaning of motherhood, family, and kin.[76]

The legal decisions arising from disputes regarding surrogate motherhood reflect the old dichotomy between nature and culture — the one identified as woman, the other as man — that has characterized Western society since the eighteenth century.[77] Historically, a woman's relationship to her child has been viewed as natural and the man's as cultural and thus more easily established through social parenthood. Yet, with the new reproductive technologies, the notion of a separation of nature and culture is perplexing because what was once regarded as natural — that is, reproducing babies — is now the work of culture, of human-made technologies. The new reproductive technologies are not regarded as "natural" but rather as culture giving nature a helping hand. Thus, they obliterate the longstanding dichotomy between nature and culture.[78]

Dolgin presents a superb analysis of court cases that brings to light the issues involved in surrogacy arrangements and the ambivalence they have created in the courts, even though disparate court rulings reflect a shared vision of family rooted in nineteenth-century notions that limit individual choice. Dolgin followed the evolution of court decisions through the latter part of the twentieth century about who the actual mother is: she saw a gradual shift in who the "real" parents are, from an emphasis on the gestational mother and genetic father to the genetic mother and father. In the 1980s, the courts showed a preference for the gestational mother over the genetic mother because the gestational period was viewed as the foundation for an enduring or "mothering" relationship. During this period, genetic consideration played a limited role in defining the father, and, by implication, genetics played a similarly limited role in deciding who is the mother.[79]

The 1990s legal decisions suggest that the courts gradually moved from gestational, or even contractual, considerations to criteria arising from the offspring's inherited genetic makeup. Genetic considerations emerged as the chief factor linking a biological parent to a child.[80] In the 1990s there seemed to be a shedding by the courts of ambiguities concerning rightful parenthood that resulted in their favoring genetic rather than gestational parenthood. In Dolgin's words, "Thus the court unequivocally defined kinship through relationships based on a natural substance (genes). *The great importance paid the gestational role in the earlier cases is replaced in Johnson by a clear statement that families are a matter of shared substance, a matter of genes*" (emphasis added).[81] Thus, Dolgin states, genetic ties became the claim to parenthood, and gestational mothers became equivalent to a foster parent. The courts began, albeit not uniformly, to recognize genetics as a powerful factor in human relationships, and genetics now would provide the profound connection between individuals.

The court decisions favoring the genetic over the gestational mother suggest, of course, that the gestational mother carries an alien in her body for nine months, an Other, which she may easily discard. In an exchange on the World Wide Web, a question was posed to a gestational surrogate: "How can you give away your baby?" Significantly, the surrogate mother declared, "It's not my baby," because it did not carry her genetic material.[82] An MSNBC report noted that advances in medical science that enable a woman to carry a genetically unrelated child have had a profound effect on the practice of commercial surrogacy in the United States because "legal specialists and surrogacy experts agree that gestational carriers are fast replacing so-called 'traditional surrogates' to avoid the various legal problems and possible attachments of the genetic mother." This statement suggests that if the gestational mother is not genetically related, she is not the "true mother." Another surrogate mother declared, "I feel like an incubator or a house for the baby to grow." The commissioning couple indicated that they were "deeply pleased that

Summer is their genetic child. Catherine says they might have adopted but she's happier knowing her son's family medical history and sharing a genetic heritage with him."[83]

In sum, analysis of court cases resulting from new reproductive technologies suggests that the legal system initially adhered to cultural views of motherhood, family, and kinship that emphasized the traditional role of the gestational mother and the social father.[84] But, within the last years of the twentieth century, legal opinion tended to shift from recognizing the gestational connection between mother and offspring to an emphasis on genetic inheritance.

Until the 1990s, two major institutions in modern life, the legal and the medical, maintained different conceptualizations of kinship connections. The courts wrestled with notions of gestational, genetic, and social motherhood, even while they recognized genetic but also social fatherhood.[85] The legal decisions reflected the ambiguities in human relations, and they opened the way for multiple definitions of family and kinship connections, reflecting society's conflicting definition of family based on genetic and gestational social and contractual ties. Recent decisions (see *Johnson*) seem to indicate that the medical view is gradually prevailing, namely that genetic inheritance determines the person and his or her future affiliations. The biomedical perspective narrows family and kinship ties to genetically shared material alone.

Biomedicine, whose chief concern is disease and its etiology, endorses genetic relationships. The separation between gestational and genetic motherhood is moot, because it is the genetic mother and father who transmit diseases to their offspring. Thus, in the last decade of the twentieth century, the gap began narrowing between legal and medical definitions of family and kinship relationships based on the sharing of genes. Biomedicine's view of the "true" family has seemingly won out over contractual, gestational, or social considerations.

To conclude this chapter, I wish to underscore the reason why, within my broader concern of the role played by biomedicine and genetics in modern life, I have focused on the historical and contemporary developments of family and kinship and on the new reproductive technologies. Some scholars of the new reproductive technologies hail this new age of medicine and forecast the death of kinship[86] and the birth of the "orphan embryo,"[87] which has already become a reality.[88] Similarly, historians and social scientists of the family predict the demise of family and kin relations. For example, while people may reside in the same quarters in close intimate contact with their kin, they may lack any investment in the ancestry and prestige of their kin. For the majority of the population, the meaning of family and kinship is associated chiefly with affective ties.[89]

Scholars who predict the disappearance of family and kinship relations as we have known them in past centuries tend to ignore the influence of the new genetics and biomedicine on the conceptualizations of family and kin that began to prevail in the last decades of the twentieth century. Biomedical explanations reinforce our notions that family and kinship are anchored in genetic ties, flowing from past to future, possessing a permanence that transcends time. While most scholars would agree that the only clear relationship commonly recognized is between parents and children,[90] the new genetics extends kinship ties to the ascending and collateral (aunts and uncles) generations and draws the inheritance map of future offspring. The new genetics frames a vision of kinship that conflicts with contemporary notions of choosing one's family and kin independent of reproduction and blood ties. The conflict becomes evident among adoptees and in some measure among patients with familial diseases.

Family and kinship configurations respond to broader social processes. Historically, the state, the church, and the industrialization process were important institutions that molded family and kinship structures and relationships. In contemporary times, with their emphasis on genetic inheritance, biomedicine forcefully contributes to defining who is included in the "significant same" circle and to the meaning of family and kinship. For this reason it is to the conceptualization of genetic inheritance that I turn in the next chapter.

Chapter 4
Concepts of Heredity in Western Society

The historically developed traditional definition of family and kinship has culminated in the new genetics, a relatively recent phenomenon in Western scientific thought. Conceptualizations have changed over time, pointing to the historically contingent nature of what is accepted as reality and truth. Historically, it was held that the family and kin bestowed on their offspring economic and social standing, as well as such personal characteristics as physical traits, character, and health. There was a prevailing notion that character resided in the blood.[1] But while, generally speaking, people may no longer expect to inherit wealth, social characteristics, and even social position from families and kin, the hereditability of personal attributes has been amplified within the past century.

Durkheim, writing in the 1930s, asserted that heredity was a very important influence on the division of social functions. For example, in egalitarian societies prior to the development of a hierarchical division of labor, hereditary roles were of little importance, but as soon as the division of labor appeared, it became fixed into a form transmitted by heredity. However, Durkheim added, "what is certain is that faith in heredity, formerly so intense, has today been replaced by an almost opposed faith. We tend to believe the individual is in large part the son of his work, and even to scorn the bonds, which attach him to his race and make him depend upon it."[2]

With the exception of elites, contemporary American society is distinguished by the fact that some individuals may create and re-create their social and economic positions several times over in a lifetime. Each generation may begin anew, presumably improving its position and economic well-being. In fact, Gottlieb observes that "inherited wealth is regarded with some suspicion and is heavily taxed. By contrast, in the past everything tended to be inherited,"[3] linking the generations and forging ties to the past.

In Europe, until at least the nineteenth century, inheritance was a viable principle and exerted a powerful moral weight.[4] Hereditary ties linked European families,[5] whereas in the American colonies the Declaration of Independence made concepts of inheritability suspect. It was self-evident that all men were created equal, and it was no longer officially accepted that unequal status and character were inherited by birth. Following the American Revolution, laws were passed prohibiting most kinds of inherited status positions except, of course, slavery. Legal decrees and social sanctions thus diminished the importance of family and kinship ties bestowed by inheritance.

Durkheim, believing that society had progressed when it departed from hereditary notions in social and economic life, was concerned about scientific notions of heredity. He observed that, if success in science were solely a matter of heredity, there would be a great many more sons of doctors and chemists, than sons of pastors.[6] But as a Westerner Durkheim acknowledged that humans tend to recognize hereditary resemblance to parents or other relatives, regardless of how they defined their kin. Certainly, in Western society it was taken for granted that "like begets like,"[7] even though such recognition was not universal.[8] Up until the nineteenth century, the unquestioned assumption existed that individuals resembled their relatives; after that time this basic premise also became privileged as scientifically meaningful.

Historical Developments in the Scientific Study of Heredity

Historically, the scientific study of heredity was in a state of confusion before the Mendelian era.[9] Various theories existed to explain how an offspring became formed from the parent. The preformation theory came into prominence in the middle of the seventeenth century, when it was believed that the embryo grew from a perfectly formed miniature already present in the mother's ovum;[10] it was also believed that a Creator shaped each being. Similarities were indications of divine intention and of the connection of all beings, except, of course, between humans and beasts. Following the scientific revolution in the seventeenth century, a search began for laws of nature; generation became an expression of nature's regularities, which humans were expected to decode.[11] In the eighteenth century, people began to acknowledge that an offspring may look like its mother, not only like its father, contrary both to the Galenic view that semen nourished the blood and the womb and to religious beliefs of creation.[12] In fact, heredity as a causal concept was a marginalized set of facts lacking explanatory power. Even medical dictionaries lacked entries on heredity or inheritance until the last decades of the nineteenth century, when the word "heredity" first appeared in a French medical dictionary.[13]

The nineteenth century ushered in a medical revolution, along with new concepts of heredity.[14] For example, in 1823 hereditary disease became, in López-Beltrán's words, a "self-sufficient cause."[15] The word "heredity" was brought into the English medical literature between 1860 and 1870, no longer as an adjective denoting the transmission of property or physical and moral qualities, but as a noun with causal significance.[16] At this time, according to Rosenberg, "hereditarian explanations of both individual disease and antisocial behavior became with each succeeding decade increasingly pervasive and emotion-filled,"[17] and studies began to surface, advancing that insanity, mental deficiency, deafness, and blindness were hereditary and were often results of consanguineous marriages. Excessive alcohol consumption was considered an inherited disease, and it was believed that it invariably led to neurological and psychiatric problems.[18]

In the nineteenth century, Lamarckian theory of acquired characteristics became prominent, and with it economic, social, and personal aspects of heredity. The central belief of Lamarckian hereditary theory was that either acquired characteristics were inherited or people were predisposed to their inheritance. According to Rosenberg, the idea prevailed that "any unwise habitual aspect of an individual's regimen, from lack of exercise to overwork, could lead to a physical deterioration inevitably passed on to children."[19] Conception was the determining moment. If a parent was drunk at the time of conception, it was thought the child would be born retarded, alcoholic, or insane.

During the nineteenth century, it was held that cultural traits were transmitted through biological inheritance, thus combining biology with culture. Following Lamarck's theories of inheritance, changes affecting the parent's body were believed to be transmitted to the offspring. For example, new characteristics acquired by the parent in response to new habits, an altered environment, or even accidental mutilation could appear in the offspring. The belief prevailed that the sexes transmitted different characteristics, not unlike patrilineal societies elsewhere in the world, as for example among Melanesians, who believed that the mother contributed to temperament, the internal viscera, stamina, and vitality and the father to intellect and external musculature.[20] A woman's responsibility to her offspring continued throughout gestation and nursing, while the man's ended at conception. If the mother entertained bad thoughts or behaved improperly during pregnancy, it would adversely affect the newborn. For example, if she had sinful thoughts, she could give birth to a monster.[21]

Darwin's theory of evolution, proposing a link between humans and other primates, gave impetus to a theory of human degeneration, inasmuch as human beings could deteriorate to a previous animal state.[22] Thus, alcoholism and neurosis in one generation could be followed by hysteria in the next, insanity in the third, and idiocy and sterility in the fourth—which would, of course, end the cycle.[23] Heredity could cause anything, including syphilis, alcoholism, and even urbanization.[24] But as long as acquired traits were considered inherited, the notion that the environment stood in opposition to heredity was not apparent, as it is in contemporary thought, especially in popular consciousness, inasmuch as the external environment could be transmitted to offspring.[25]

Darwin's revolutionary theories of reproductive success lacked the concept of the gene, leaving the process of natural selection in the form of heritable variability without a hereditary mechanism to explain it.[26] But Darwin's theories of natural selection intensified the thinking about heredity and the process of transmission of hereditary materials. At the beginning of the twentieth century, new genetic theories were introduced, replacing the belief in acquired characteristics.

Genetics in the Late Twentieth Century

Mendel's and Weismann's theories at the beginning of the twentieth century changed the thinking about genetic transmission,[27] but it was the birth of molecular biology that profoundly revolutionized the study of heredity. Genetics flourished after World War II, especially after the discoveries made by Watson and Crick.[28] Proteins embodied in genes explained life, and genes are found on a very long molecule in the form of a double spiral, DNA, coiled up within every cell.[29] By the 1960s, it was believed that genes, defined as sequences of DNA, formed the "master molecule" determining human destiny. In Griesemer's words, "The body is slave to its master molecules."[30]

In a manner of speaking, in some measure cells replicate themselves in their own image.[31] In Granner's words, "The primary function of DNA replication is understood to be the provision of progeny with the genetic information possessed by the parent. Thus, the replication of DNA must be complete and carried out with *high fidelity to maintain genetic stability* within the organisms and the species"[32] (emphasis in the original), unless, of course, a mutation, or a mistake, occurs at random. Importantly, and this is often overlooked, even by the 1940s it was already recognized that varieties of chemicals and ultraviolet radiation can cause mutations.[33] In fact, many factors, including viruses, chemicals, ultraviolet light, and ionizing radiation, increase the rate of mutation, affecting the somatic cells that are passed on to successive generations. Granner asserts that a number of diseases, including most cancers, are due to induced mutations.[34]

Heredity is described today in terms of information, messages, and codes, a postmodern enterprise. There is the erroneous assumption that information flows only in one direction from the genes to the organism, and therefore that genes completely determine the organism's character.[35] Arguably, this assumption has led to the hegemony of the gene. The reproduction of an organism has become that of its constituent molecules. As noted by Jacob, "This is not because each chemical species has the ability to produce copies of itself, but because the structure of macro molecules is determined down to the last detail by sequences of four chemical radicals contained in the genetic heritage. What are transmitted from generation to generation are the 'instructions' specifying the molecular structure: the architectural plans of the future organism."[36] The organism becomes the realization of a program prescribed by its heredity. The rigidity of the program varies: some genetic instructions are carried out literally, while others are expressed by capacities or potentialities. However, according to Jacob, ultimately the program itself determines its degree of flexibility and the range of possible variation.[37] Thus, even variation and flexibility themselves are programmed genetically. Following this formulation, everything about an organism's existence is predetermined and genetically programmed, including its variations, although geneticists recognize that the program may be affected by unknown and external factors in the environment, chance, or human manipulation. The sequence of our DNA reveals to us who and what we are; that is, what it means to be human.[38] With DNA sequencing, some scientists have maintained that the riddle of life is close to being solved.[39]

Genetic inheritance includes, of course, the normal and the abnormal as defined by biomedicine. Over the past thirty years the number of genetic diseases thought to be inherited from family has grown astronomically.[40] While genetic diseases were, obviously, known prior to the 1980s, until then genetics was, generally speaking, a separate discipline from medicine. At that time a transition occurred, and interest turned from improving the genetic pool to employing genetic information for diagnosis, treatment, and prevention.[41] As a matter of fact, even by the late 1970s there had been exponential growth in genetic disorder designations.[42] By 1991 not only cystic fibrosis, Tay-Sachs, sickle cell, and Huntington's disease but also some 5,600–5,700 other genetic disorders had been catalogued that were known or thought on good evidence to be inherited.[43] Genes have been implicated in alcoholism,[44] schizophrenia, bipolar disorder, dyslexia, twitching of the face, neck, and shoulders, allergies, sudden infant death syndrome, insulin-dependent diabetes, arteriosclerosis, hypertension, some forms of depression, Alzheimer's disease, heart disease, Parkinson's disease, anxiety, and cancer,[45] as well as reading disabilities, attention deficit disorders, PMS, susceptibility to smoking, and even homelessness.[46]

Milunsky asserts that there exist over 250 X-chromosome-linked disorders inherited only from the mother. He states that "unlike the important and serious diseases that originate from harmful genes on a female X chromosome, no disease is yet known to result from a gene on the Y chromosome."[47] Interestingly, Milunsky's claim suggests that genetic determinism is not genderless, even though males and females both transmit the X chromosome. Not surprisingly, the nineteenth-century belief that mothers can transmit their bad behavior and bad thoughts to their progeny has become reincarnated in the contemporary hereditarian conceptualization that the mother is the one who transmits diseases to her offspring, even though the father can also transmit a "faulty" X chromosome, arguably reflecting the gendered nature of scientific research.[48]

The Human Genome Project

It is important to pause for a moment to consider the Human Genome Project (HGP) because, as a logical extension of genetic determinism, the HGP is becoming imprinted on people's kinship maps and on their consciousness. It was conceived in the late 1980s and formally instituted in October 1990, with the optimistic goal of identifying, mapping, and sequencing all 50,000–100,000 human genes to make them accessible for biological study and to unlock the secrets of all diseases, including cancer. The HGP promotes a biochemical causal model of human affliction, and it has catalogued three to four thousand single gene-linked diseases. The goal is to identify multiple gene-linked diseases, or polygenic disorders.[49] It is anticipated that by identifying all the genes involved in disease, means of correcting the faulty genes will be found. According to the web site of the National Human Genome Research Institute, "Our genes orchestrate the development of a single-celled egg into a fully formed adult. Genes influence not only what we look like but also what diseases we may eventually get." The HGP also promises to usher in an era of "molecular medicine, with precise new approaches to the diagnosis, treatment, and prevention of disease."[50] The premise of the project is that once the entire genome is mapped, cures will eventually be found for all diseases, thus having a profound impact on biomedicine. Biomedicine will move from being a reactive to a preventive practice because there will be a "cure" for each defective gene even before its effects become manifest. Great benefits to the pharmaceutical industry are fore-seen because it will be able to develop a large therapeutic repertoire to attack fundamental aspects of human disease.[51]

Theoretically, at least, the HGP foresees that biomedicine will attend to prevention rather than to treatment because genetic procedures will be able to identify individuals predisposed to particular diseases. The grand vision is to devise novel therapeutic regimens based on new classes of drugs, immunotherapy techniques, and possible replacement of "defec-tive" genes through gene therapy, as well as to promote avoidance of environmental conditions that may trigger diseases. The Genome Proj-ect's aim is therapeutic management by means of designing individu-alized therapies to replace "bad" genes with "good" ones.[52]

Molecular biology gave birth to the HGP, which forms part of the new genetics, promising people individual control over their own fate. The new genetics refers to knowledge and procedures based on DNA technol-ogy; it brings into the forefront of people's consciousness the genes car-ried by individuals and their families.[53] It anticipates that by seeking testing, people will develop control over genetically inherited diseases. By doing so they might be enabled to plan their lives to the point of opting to bear only healthy children with predetermined characteristics.

Concurrently, the new genetics is redrawing the boundaries between healthy and unhealthy people because, potentially, we are all unhealthy, or possible carriers of malfunctioning genes, as we will see in Chapter 5. The new genetics reveals asymptomatic conditions that may remain for-ever asymptomatic, as well as susceptibilities or risks for developing com-mon diseases such as breast cancer or diabetes. Most important, with the new genetics, the true patient becomes the entire family rather than the individual,[54] since to treat the individual the family's medical history and genetic map must also be known. Many regard the HGP as the panacea for all ills. But is it instead comparable to the eugenics of the nineteenth and early part of the twentieth century?

Eugenics

Galton, who introduced eugenics in 1883, coined the term from its Greek root, meaning " 'good in birth' or 'noble in heredity.' " He in-tended the term to signify "the 'science' of improving human stock by giving 'the more suitable races or strains of blood a better chance of prevailing speedily over the less suitable.' "[55] Eugenics proclaimed that moral and intellectual traits followed the same laws of inheritance as physical traits; therefore, the human body and mind could be improved by better breeding.[56] From this perspective, human heredity could be improved not via behavioral changes but by selective breeding. Eugenicists declared that they were concerned with preventing social degeneration, which they saw glaringly manifested in social and behavioral disturbances. For the eugenicists, the ills of urban industrial society, including crime, slums, and rampant disease, were all attributable to biology. Wherever family pedigrees seemed to show a high incidence of a characteristic, especially insanity, epilepsy, alcoholism, pauperism, or criminality, it was concluded that the trait must be biologically inheritable.[57]

Eugenics was not just a theoretical project; rather, it was a social program that sought to correct society's ills by advocating controlled breeding in order to eliminate the unfit and their undesirable characteristics from human society, especially "feeblemindedness, and licentiousness."[58] Eugenic theories were widely held: they were influential in the United States, Europe, and Latin America.[59] These theories had great appeal because they were cloaked in a presumably scientific mantle and because their emphasis on heredity was becoming entrenched among the middle class, especially among physicians, psychiatrists, and social workers.[60] Belief in eugenics led to programs of sterilization and affected immigration policies in the United States: "defectives" were now refused entry into the country.[61] Interestingly, undesirable immigrants, which included most of the world's people excepting northern Europeans and Anglo-Saxons, were considered to "carry a special gene for uncontrollable Wanderlust," reflecting yet another reason for these people's inferiority.[62] Eugenics emphasized the betterment of the "race" but moved its goals to medicine, culminating in German sterilization practices to eliminate "defective" races and the sick.

Hereditarian notions, including eugenics, lost their popularity in the 1940s and 1950s, owing to their association with Nazi Germany and the Holocaust. Undoubtedly, the rise of nonbiological, Freudian theories of human development in America, which attributed human failings and sicknesses to childhood events and unconscious drives, also contributed to the decline of hereditarian concepts.[63] Also, the postwar years fomented a *Zeitgeist* of the power of culture to triumph over nature. Since everything was possible, behavior became separated from genetics. In fact, the 1950s and 1960s became the Age of Psychology, which emphasized good mothering and behaviorist theories of positive reinforcement over hereditary notions of character.[64]

Eugenics, however, did not die. In fact, some scholars regard it as a direct forerunner of the current concern with heredity and the HGP.[65] While such attributions to eugenics may be excessive, it can be claimed with greater confidence that sociobiology is a reincarnation of eugenics. Sociobiology, bolstered by molecular biology, uses evolutionary theories to explicate human behavior. According to the field's founder, Edward O. Wilson, it is "the study of the biological basis of social behavior in every

kind of organism, including man."[66] Sociobiology asserts that social behavior rests on a genetic foundation, that human behavior is organized by
genetic characteristics, some of which are shared with closely related
species and others of which are unique to the human species. Wilson, like
Galton, perceives modern humanity, in Kevles's words, as "suffering from
deep inner contradictions—eager to build a better world, yet bedeviled
by the gene-based behavioral impulses of its prehistoric forebears."[67] Human genetic engineering, according to Kevles's discussion of Wilson,
"might ultimately render the human genome alterable."[68]

Sociobiology focuses on the individual organism, which seeks, through
kin selection, to transmit his or her genes at all costs, even if the individual must sacrifice himself so that his siblings, cousins, and other collateral
kin reproduce and carry his genes.[69] Central to sociobiology is the selfish
gene, which supposedly recognizes that the greater good is in and of itself
self-interest.[70] According to sociobiology, the overarching goal of any
organism is not to protect itself from death or to secure sex or power but
to spread its genes. Sociobiology focuses on the notion of genetic max-
imization strategies, mimicking the behavior of the Rational Economic
Man, who flourishes on competition and on increasing his advantage.

Sociobiologists are constantly adding new genes to their pool of genetic determinants, including most recently the "novelty-seeking gene,"
which imbues people with a desire for new sensations and a dislike of
monotony; such people lack inhibition.[71] For Hamer and Copeland the
hallmark of genetically influenced traits, including depression and other
ailments, is that they run in families.[72] Interestingly, Ridley calls attention
to Marx's well-known claim that "it is remarkable, how Darwin recognises
among beasts and plants his own English society with its division of la-
bour, competition, opening up of new markets, 'inventions' and the Mal-
thusian struggle for existence."[73] Remarkably, Ridley fails to acknowledge that sociobiological concepts imitate the market economy rather
than, as he claims, that economics and biology have both discovered
parallel workings of life. Haraway, too, discerns that "the theoretical view
of nature underlying genetic engineering and bioethics as a kind of quality control industry appears clearly in sociobiology."[74]

To conclude this succinct overview of the developments in conceptualizations associated with genetic inheritance, as we saw, the nineteenth-
century hereditarian beliefs claiming that acquired behavioral characteristics were inherited exerted a form of social control, like medical
conceptualizations in general,[75] because they suggested that if one, especially a woman, behaved improperly, her offspring would inherit the undesirable traits. Nevertheless, it is noteworthy that the hereditarian notions of the late nineteenth and early twentieth centuries differed from
our current beliefs in at least one important way. In the past, theoretically

at least, if one changed one's behavior, one's children could potentially avoid inheriting the abnormal characteristics. In contemporary conceptualization, behavioral social control has given way to a form of predestination; concurrently, one's inherited traits could be mastered by resorting to medical procedures such as gene manipulation, or in some instances be averted by diet and avoidance of other specific risk factors.[76]

In this chapter I have dealt with contemporary hereditarian concepts in genetics. Although they have a relatively short history, they are influential in explaining disease etiologies that bear on family and kinship, as can be seen in the next three chapters, on breast cancer patients and healthy adoptees.

Part II
Setting Out People's Experience

Chapter 5
People with a Genetic History I

Patients Without Symptoms

My focus in the first three chapters was on historical and contemporary issues concerning kinship and concepts of heredity. In this chapter we see the ways in which historically developed kinship relations and medically conceptualized genetic inheritance have variously reproduced themselves in seven healthy women who originate from families with breast, ovarian, or colon cancer; in the next chapter we will meet fifteen women who have experienced breast cancer. These narratives reveal the conflicts resulting from different interpretations of the disease's etiology — the ways in which the women relate to family and kin and manage their illness in light of their understanding of the genetic nature of the disease.[1]

Before I turn to the case studies, I want to briefly consider contemporary Western knowledge of cancer. After all, conceptualizations of any disease etiology are culturally and historically construed. While subjective and experiential accounts from women with breast cancer in ancient times may be lacking, it is known that breast cancer is an ancient disease recognized by the Egyptians and Greeks.[2] For example, Hippocratic medicine identified various kinds of growths and swellings that were accounted for by humoral theories.[3] The Greeks attributed cancer either to an excess of black bile mixed with phlegm (considered more benign) or to lethal yellow-and-black bile mixed with blood (believed more lethal). In Greek medicine, the ultimate cause of the humoral imbalance that led to cancer was believed to be inappropriate nutrition coupled with strong emotions. According to one of the most renowned Greek physicians, Galen (A.D. c.130–c.200), cancers arose in many parts of the body but most often in the female breast; they were treated by excision and cauterization.[4] The Galenic (Hippocratic) understanding of cancer remained prevalent until the medical revolution of the nineteenth century, when the cell theory of disease emerged to account for the genesis of tumor tissues.[5]

The late twentieth-century theory of cancer etiology is that it arises from oncogenes, normal cellular genes that go awry as the result of deregulation or mutation.[6] That is, cancer is caused by the malignant transformation of a cell through the accumulation of mutations in specific classes of genes that may be transmitted from one generation to the next. These genes provide the key to understanding the processes at the root of human cancer, including breast cancer.[7] According to current theory, about 5–10 percent of breast cancer cases are attributable to genetically inherited BRCA-1 and BRCA-2 genes. It is also widely believed that people can have a genetic predisposition to cancer.[8] Following Biesecker, Boehnke, and Calzone, "The BRCA-1 gene may be carried by one in two hundred women in America. These women face an 85 percent risk of developing breast cancer, with 50 percent of these cases occurring before the age of fifty."[9] The gene is passed down through the generations in the classic Mendelian pattern of autosomal dominant transmission, with 50 percent of the children of carriers inheriting the BRCA-1 mutation.

Theories other than the genetic origin of cancer have been advanced and do exist in the consciousness of many patients we will meet here. Alternative theories are, however, usually quickly discarded by the women in favor of the prevailing genetic theory. In actuality, geneticists speak of multifactorial components of cancer, which may include environmental, dietary, and other risk factors.[10] But, as Spanier observes, even when nongenetic factors are mentioned as possible causes, "the considerable omission of 'non-genetic influences' is quickly countered by repeating the assertion that the genetic framework offers the implied best hope against cancer."[11] Ultimately, with the numerous etiological theories of cancer currently circulating in the medical and popular literatures, implicating even mammograms, the origin of cancer, if not its pathophysiology, remains elusive, not unlike diseases previously considered hereditary, such as tuberculosis.

Of the twenty-two women who were referred to me by the genetic counselor, seven were healthy but came from families in which at least one member had developed cancer. I turn to the healthy women first because their narratives are especially instructive in the ways in which a biomedical ideology of the genetic inheritance of disease influences their perceptions of being at risk and of becoming patients and their fear of succumbing to the disease.[12] In fact, an important transformation may take place among healthy women who, as a result of this ideology, become perpetual patients without symptoms, changing their persona from healthy to sick. The ideology of genetic inheritance tends to steer people to such conclusions, especially in the instance of perceived autosomal-dominant disorders such as breast cancer, because this affliction may become visible in all generations, unlike recessive conditions such as cystic fibrosis, which may not become fully exposed in successive generations.

One additional point needs to be made before I turn to the individual women's narratives. All of the accounts I present in this and the next chapter tend to support the prevailing assertions of the genetic inheritance of breast cancer. All of the women reported having members in their family afflicted with cancer, which leads to their assumption that if it exists in the family, the disease must be inherited. But I must return to a point made earlier — that other attributions are usually excluded or only given passing reference. One could consider witchcraft (as we will see that Maya does), but such an explanation is not part of an American cultural pool of understanding, and even Maya, who comes from a society that believes witchcraft may cause disease, immediately discounts this possibility. In modern society, people holding any supernatural beliefs are usually regarded by the larger society as primitive, superstitious, and ignorant, not to speak of the disparagement of *any* ideology outside the scientific mold in mainstream American culture.[13]

Case Narratives

Dorothy

Listening to this vivacious 38-year-old high school graduate, bank employee, married, with two young children, I heard tiers of conflicting interpretations and sensed anxiety about her potential fate because of her family's medical history. Dorothy resides in a large, well-furnished home in a middle-class community situated in a rural area of the South. She conforms to the image of the ideal contemporary mother whose life revolves around her husband and children. Dorothy's maternal grandmother died of breast cancer at the age of 70; 11 years before our meeting, Dorothy's mother succumbed to the disease at the age of 48, at which time Dorothy became a born-again Christian. After her mother's death, Dorothy also became aware that cancer was a genetically inherited disease.

To make sense of why her mother and grandmother fell ill, Dorothy at first associated the prevalence of the disease in the family with the fact that the family came from an industrial community of coal mines and where one of the biggest employers was a tobacco company. Her grandfather had worked in coal mines all his life. But then she discarded the possibility in favor of a more plausible explanation given by her mother's sister, who had recently been diagnosed with colon cancer, that "childbearing gave grandmother cancer," since the woman had raised seven children, a possibility Dorothy had not discounted. She said, "I really believe in my heart that breast cancer has to do with birthing children, because I remember folk in the family talking about my mother. She was very frail after she had children, and she took medication to dry up in her breasts, leaving her with knots all over. For this reason I connected having breast cancer with having children." Dorothy believes that breast cancer is preventable if a woman does "things that one can do such as eat right or just like with mother not take the medication to dry up her milk. It dried up within her and stayed. And I just think that's a toxin." She added, "God didn't create a pill to give you to dry up your milk. You were supposed to breast-feed the children. Now I breast-fed my daughter simply for that reason, but I didn't breast-feed my son."

Even though Dorothy leaned toward the belief that breast cancer was due to a failure to breast-feed, she now believes that it is related to her family's genetic history. She inquired about genetic testing because of her little girl, who according to Dorothy has the gene from "both sides of the blood family" — from her great-grandmother, her grandmother, her great-aunt, and an aunt on Dorothy's side and from a recently diagnosed aunt on her father's side. Dorothy added, "You know it just stands to reason. It didn't skip a generation, and a lot of folk say that it'll skip a generation, which I don't know where that came from." She looked at her 11-year-old girl, who was present in the house at the time of the interview, and said wistfully, "I look at her and I think she's got a lot of physical features of her daddy's side of the family. Um, you know, but yet she's got me in her, too, which is dependent on my mother and my grandmother. And it just looks from an observation, it looks like she's got the cards stacked against her."

Dorothy misses her mother and wonders, "Sometimes I think, you know, the thought crosses your mind, why, if you knew that you had that strong genetics for cancer, why would you have children? She was 18 when she had us. I mean, these are things that just cross your mind. Well, I am glad she did, because if she didn't then I wouldn't be here. It's things like that that just cross your mind. In fact, I thought long and hard before I ever had children because of that possibility. There were two, three right straight in a row — grandmother, my grandfather, and then Mama that had died with cancer. And you have to wonder how much of a possibility do I have. And there's Mama's other sisters."

Significantly, Dorothy, who does not come from a close-knit family, having been reared in a blended family with stepsiblings to whom she feels closer than to her blood relatives, with whom she has had little contact, recently began working on her genealogy with one of her mother's sisters. Dorothy began thinking about her blood kin and had delved into the history of her family to see who was the first to have had cancer, but she could find little information.

Despite the fact that Dorothy is asymptomatic, she has had a mammogram every year, and each time she goes she is very nervous. She questioned, "Are they going to find anything?" The first time she had a mammogram, it was misread, and she received a note indicating "severe mammary dysplasia." Dorothy did not know the meaning of mammary dysplasia, and she became very anxious. She said it turned out to be of no significance, since she had the same finding for the next seven years. "But still, you're nervous and you wonder and you think about it and especially the older I get because, you know, I am turning 39 this year and I'm like, well, see what Mama was going through."

Dorothy had an ovarian tumor, which she wished to have removed and also have a hysterectomy because her mother had had one, and Dorothy was told that her mother had suffered from ovarian cancer. Despite her insistence, Dorothy's physician refused to remove the growth unless she could prove that her mother had had ovarian cancer. The doctor insisted that she get her mother's pathology report; however, the hospital where her mother had had surgery (in another state) no longer retained the records. Dorothy was very angry that her physician refused to perform the operation. She told the doctor incredulously, "You're basing whether or not you take it out on her [the mother's] pathology report as to whether she had ovarian cancer?" Dorothy was uneasy about the tumor because of her mother's medical history. "I was getting kind of paranoid about it. I mean, it worried me." If the doctor had told Dorothy that it looked like a cyst, just a plain old fibroid cyst, she would have been calmer, but he told her it was a small tumor. Dorothy thought tumor meant cancer. Dorothy reported that the doctor would perform an operation only if she could produce her mother's pathology report because, according to Dorothy, "the doctor wanted to save time and money." Dorothy felt she might have overreacted to her doctor's refusal to perform the operation, but she had done so because "it comes with age. Because the closer I get to 48, I know that I am going to be worse than I am now. I hope not." She was convinced that she too would fall ill.

I asked Dorothy why she felt that the age of 48 was so momentous. She answered, "Well, because just by association. Mother died at 48. From the time that my grandmother was my age now until I'm 48 there is that period in life that I guess subconsciously I think that's going to be my target. If I make it past 38, then 48, then maybe I am home free."

Dorothy finally decided to have children, even though she knew she could transmit cancer to them. She made this decision by rationalizing, "not so much that you're selfish but that the Lord has a plan for everybody. What's going to happen is going to happen, and I can't stop that." In the same way she cannot protect her daughter from getting hit by a car, she cannot live, in her words, "in a shell." When Dorothy finally recognized that "you cannot live your whole life trying to protect yourself from something that may or may not happen, that's when I finally let my mama go." Nevertheless, she repeated that she lives with the ever-present thought that she may get cancer.

Dorothy had considered being tested for the cancer gene, but she decided against it because "they would only tell me 90 percent or 50 percent risk," and she would only agree to have it done if she could be assured, "one hundred percent definitely." Dorothy desired certainty because its absence would diminish her life.

Looking at Dorothy's fears concerning cancer, her conflicting attempts to make sense of cancer in her family are significant. She at once accepts the medical belief that the disease is genetically transmitted while simultaneously firmly believing that her mother's disease was associated with motherhood and breast-feeding, or even with industrial pollution. But the belief in genetic inheritance seems to have won out. It has even brought her closer to her blood kin and has led her to do genealogical searches, despite the fact that she, having grown up in a blended family, felt closer to her stepsiblings than to her biogenetic relatives. Her recognition of her family medical history establishes continuity with her dead ancestors, especially her grandmother and other members of her family, but this very awareness simultaneously contributes to her fears and anxieties. Her fear that she may only reach the age of 48 diminishes her daily existence and leaves her in a state of unceasing ambiguity that she is at risk, at the same time as she embraces a sense of fatalism that sanctioned her becoming a mother.

Dorothy's situation discloses, too, how she has already become a patient by having annual mammograms and by her determination to undergo a hysterectomy and removal of her ovaries, an operation the physician refused to perform. In this instance, what is especially intriguing is that while Dorothy and her doctor both follow the same genetic model of disease, they arrived at conflicting conclusions. The physician, following Dorothy's narrative, insisted on evidence that her mother indeed had a malignant tumor, in which case he would be willing to perform the procedure, and Dorothy desired the operation precisely because her mother had one, and she feared she would be afflicted with the same disorder.

Eve

In contrast to Dorothy, Eve is a scientist with a Ph.D. in biology; but, like Dorothy, she lives with the same fears and anxieties because of her family medical history. Eve had been independently employed until she and her recently retired physician husband moved to the state, where they purchased an elegant house in an upper-class community. The couple has no children. When I visited her, boxes surrounded Eve, as she was unpacking her belongings with great energy and zest. Eve, healthy and sparking, lost her mother to breast cancer when Eve was a teenager; her mother was 34 years old when she died. Eve's mother's 84-year-old sister has cancer. Eve had two brothers, one of whom died from salivary gland cancer and the other from prostate cancer. Eve's aging father also had cancer. She attributes the cancer in her family to the fact that "my grandparents were first cousins." Both her paternal and maternal grandparents died of heart disease, and, Eve added, "that too is familial, and so it's a double whammy," particularly since the predisposition to high cholesterol is, according to Eve, genetic, as is evidenced in her family.

Eve recounted, "I am 59. My aunt and grandmother developed their cancer between 59 and 65, so now I am in that age range, and my sister, who is 54, is right behind me." Neither she nor her sister nor her cousins have developed cancer, but Eve feels that she "is sitting on a time bomb" because, she said, she is at "extremely high risk." Eve listed the highest risk factors for breast cancer as "an early onset of menses, no children, and being the offspring of a parent that developed cancer — and that's where we fit. And we are Ashkenazy Jews." She and her sister have these same risk factors, but, in addition, her sister, unlike Eve, smokes, therefore, the sister "may have a notch more than I."

Because she regards herself as at high risk and because she firmly believes that cancer is a genetically inherited disease, Eve exists with the constant fear of falling ill. Most significantly, when Eve moved to the new community, she immediately contacted and set up a cancer team, because, she said, "I am extremely anxious. I go for my mammograms twice a year and I want to have a breast surgeon that I am comfortable with, so I have a team." She was urged to have a genetic test but was reluctant to do so because she fails to see its purpose. She noted, "I do everything now to monitor myself and knowing that data, I'd only be more anxious than I already am if it came out to be that way. And if I ever needed insurance, I could be hard pressed to get it. You know, there's this big computer in the sky, and those data seem to find their way into that. I am not going to have a prophylactic mastectomy, which I have been urged to do." But, she said she agreed to provide tissue samples from her deceased mother and two other members of the family (a cousin and an aunt) for some tests.

Eve does not blame her parents or grandparents for the possibility that she may inherit the disease, because they did not know that they would transmit the gene for breast cancer, nor did her grandparents know that to marry cousins was genetically dangerous.[14] Of her blood relatives, she noted that she felt closest to her sister and her aging father, but she also became closer to her cousins because "knowing that they share the same genes provides the occasion for discussion. When I think I know something that's useful, I pass it on to the others. So basically the occasion [for seeing] my cousins is a bar mitzvah we might all go to, but we are connected through this exchange of information. Otherwise, we have very different lives. The fact that they have the same genes has created a close bond." She further commented that "we seem to have a very clear and good and accepting understanding of who the family was. Let me just say that this [disease] really has provided a lasting and a continuous bond."

The major theme in Eve's narrative was her profound fear of becoming afflicted. Despite the fact that Eve is healthy and vibrant, she acts like a patient, owing to her unwavering faith in the notion of the genetic inheritance of disease and the associated risk factors that she is convinced she possesses. Impelled by the ideology of genetic inheritance, she has acted on these fears by having frequent mammograms and, even more telling, by having arranged for a cancer team to stand ready when she falls ill. Eve recognizes a lasting bond with her blood kin because of a shared genetic inheritance, even though she emphasized that she had very little else in common with them. Furthermore, Eve's beliefs about genetic inheritance influenced in part her decision not to have children.

Kate

Whereas Eve moved to the southern town to retire, Kate, 40 years old and married, moved to the community to become a graduate student at the local university. And whereas Eve and Dorothy exist with great anxieties associated with their family genetic histories, Kate is reassured by her beliefs in genetic inheritance, which also give her a sense of mastery. Turning 40 was a watershed in Kate's life, and she marked the change when she quit a 17-year position in the computer industry to become a doctoral candidate in the health professions. At that time Kate also sought genetic counseling because her mother had a rare kind of colon cancer that is regarded as unequivocally hereditary.[15] Her father also had his colon removed, and she said, "we just have the genes for weak colons, and so that's why it's important for everybody to get checked." In fact, her five siblings have been checked as well.

Kate's 75-year-old mother had her colon removed at the age of 47. Kate said, "We have known about this since I was a kid, that this is a genetic thing and so this is something that we all have to get tested for." As it turned out, Kate was not tested, because "it's a relatively new test, so it's not 100 percent, and there were like three scenarios, and two out of the three scenarios, I'd end up having to have a colonoscopy anyway, either because the results would be unclear or because I'd be positive and I'd have to have it checked out. So basically you know I have a 2 in 3 chance anyway, and so we [she and the counselor] decided I should have a colonoscopy." Kate added, "If you have this condition and it goes untreated, you will develop colon cancer; that's like for sure. That's why they remove your colon, because if you have it, you will develop colon cancer. So if it's in your family, you need to be checked."

Kate could only conceive of colon cancer in terms of its genetic transmission. She considered diet as a possible alternative explanation of the disease etiology but discounted it. She is certain her mother's disease is of genetic origin, adding, "There are only two things that I've ever felt like genetically, I had been worried about — colon cancer and diabetes tends to run in my family. So I had a great-grandmother who had diabetes and had a leg removed."

Kate's belief in a genetic etiology gives her confidence. She said, "I think we have no history of heart disease, no history of stroke, you know, we don't smoke so there's no lung cancer, we don't have high blood pressure, we don't have anything else. Well both my father and my mother are overweight, and on my mother's side all of her siblings are overweight, so obesity tends to run in our family, but it doesn't tend to be a risk factor for anything, so I kind of feel like, well I have got these genes — that's it. Pretty much I think I am going to live a long time if I can just avoid colon cancer and diabetes. I think I've got it made. I kind of feel like it balances out." She concluded, "You know, the hand I got dealt, okay, there's a few bad cards but there are some really good cards. I have bad eyes; bad eyes run in our family but I have good skin and good hair, good teeth. I am not as tall as I'd like to be. I am short from both sides. But it all kind of balances out. In the balance, I think our genetic makeup is pretty good. I come from pretty hardy stock. I am not afraid of a heart attack, and breast cancer doesn't run in my family."

Kate feels protected from most diseases because of her genetic heritage, even when she recognizes that her family does not practice a particularly healthy lifestyle. Nobody in her family exercises — in fact, they eat a lot of fat and sugar and, she repeatedly noted, are overweight. Yet, her grandmother is 90, and Kate added, "I just think genetically I am probably in a better position than a lot of people." The certainty of her favorable genetic heritage confers on Kate a sense of being in control of her health. She claimed, "With colon cancer, if I know I catch it early enough, it can be treated and can be treated successfully, and it won't affect my life. And even diabetes, if it doesn't develop until later in life and I think even with my great-grandmother, who had a leg removed, maybe they didn't know as much about controlling diabetes; I feel like I have more control. I don't feel as much at risk. I guess I don't feel as vulnerable or as out of control as maybe some other people do."

Kate ascribes her bodily sensations to her genetic inheritance. For example, she noted that when she felt extreme fatigue she knew it was due to an "underactive thyroid" she had inherited from her mother. She also conflated the family's disease history with its personality characteristics. For example, she believes that she has inherited her stubbornness, strong will, and intelligence from both her grandmothers, who were very independent. Kate observed that personality characteristics skip a generation, so that explains why she inherited them from her grandmothers rather than her parents. She said, "I am not really all that spiritual, but there is a connection, this womanhood thing. There's some woman spirit in me," which she feels she inherited from her grandmothers. She repeatedly established the link between herself and her grandmothers, who possessed strong characters.

Kate does not feel at a disadvantage because of her genetic heritage for colon cancer and diabetes. But when I asked whether she has children (she does not), she responded, "As much as I say that, I do think that genetically in some ways I am very lucky. But in other ways I just think, 'Man, I would just not want to pass this gene down to anybody else.' It's just really hard."

In the end, because Kate's mother was the first and only member of the family to be afflicted with the disease, the geneticist speculated that the mutation might have started with her mother. In this case, Kate said, "the odds are that we each have a 50-50 chance of getting the gene, but we all could have gotten lucky and not inherited that gene." Her mother had been unlucky all her life, and her disease furnishes the evidence of her mother's lack of luck from birth on, when Kate's grandmother had great difficulties with her mother's delivery.

Kate's account reveals how she blends memory of her grandmothers with her genetic history and establishes continuity with her ancestors who are perpetuated in her genes, thus sustaining her kinship connections. She revels in her good fortune at having inherited good genes and balances them with the colon cancer. What she may fail to recognize is that although her belief in the inheritance of good genes will not draw her into the medical sphere to become a potential or perpetual patient, the fear of inheriting the disease may have inhibited her from having children. The complexities of the belief in genetic determinism can be seen in Kate's narrative and will also be seen in the next chapter, where the same suspicions that brought her to the genetic counselor gave her confidence that she is protected against all other diseases — except colon cancer and diabetes — that she considers inheritable. But, such confidence may keep her from following a healthy lifestyle, as for example watching her weight or following a healthy diet. At the same time, her consciousness of genetic inheritance does alert her to the potentiality of getting colon cancer, furnishing her a modicum of control over her behavior to protect herself from that disease's random onset, as we can see when we hear her speak of "luck" and "gambling."

Karen

Unlike Dorothy and Eve, Karen presents both in her serene demeanor and in the narrative a sense of fearlessness because she feels protected by God and her husband. A 39-year-old college graduate, married with two children, 6 and 8 years old, she initiated contact with the genetic counselor at her physician's urging because her mother and grandmother had died of breast cancer and her 77-year-old aunt has had several types of cancers as well. She observed, "My grandfather's [maternal grandfather] two sisters had breast cancer. So on both sides I get it. And then there was cancer on my father's side," although she was uncertain of what kind.

Karen became a reluctant patient. In fact, it was not clear to herself why she had decided to follow the doctor's advice and have the test done but, after thinking about it, she said, "Maybe I could take some aggressive action, more drastic action than I would. You know what I mean? A precautionary action such as what some women do—have mastectomies. I may consider that aspect. I know there's a link between ovarian cancer and breast cancer. And now I've read that. He [the doctor] told me that, too, but I knew that. And, you know, maybe have the ovaries taken out. I mean something like that. I don't have a problem with knowing."

Karen has had mammograms taken regularly since the time her mother fell ill, when Karen was 29 years old. She had gone on a routine visit to her doctor, and, she said, he "started asking me questions and he was interested in the history, the breast cancer history. He had given me various blood tests, an ovarian screening blood test, and one showed an elevated number but then there was the possibility of a false positive. And then I had an ultrasound because of my family history. So I think he was just very thorough. And it doesn't hurt to check. I think that's great because of my family history."

Karen was referred to the genetic counselor, who asked her to contact her 77-year-old aunt, whom she had not seen for many years, in order to establish a genetic profile of her relatives that could be compared with Karen's. Karen had had little contact with her family until that time—and, in fact, her aunt, whom we will meet shortly, was surprised by Karen's call. Karen felt guilty because she had not contacted her mother's sister for so long. Karen refers to her mother, father, brother, and mother and father's siblings and parents as her relatives. She does not include her cousins as her kin, even though, she said, "they [the genetic counselor] asked me questions about them. Yeah, I had a cousin that had cancer, colon cancer, and an uncle with colon cancer and my 77-year-old aunt had colon cancer." In contrast to the genetic counselor's view, Karen did not regard these people as her family. Actually, Karen has lost connections with her three brothers, who are scattered throughout the country.

Her nuclear family, her husband and children, are closest to her, and she added, "my friends, but that's not family."

Karen, unlike most of the other women, is a homemaker, and her affluent lifestyle revolves around her nuclear family and her church. As a very devout Christian, she claimed that she was totally unconcerned about her genetic heritage because "God protects me," notwithstanding the fact that she followed the doctor's urging to be genetically tested. Her physician made her aware of the genetic nature of cancer, and subsequently she had read about it in various magazines. However, she does not worry about anything she cannot alter. And besides, she added, cancer is everywhere, so she is not even convinced that her genetic heritage would cause her the problem rather than the environment. But then Karen reflected, "I do think that there is a connection and I think there is a gene, yes, in the family and I know that's not proven, so that may not be, but yeah, I feel like there are some genes in there, you know. I think that, as time goes on, medical advances will help. I guess I'm optimistic, is what I'm saying. And lots more is known now than was before." She is considering a prophylactic mastectomy, despite the fact that she feels protected by God. She said, "I feel like if I had a mastectomy, I think it would be worth it, especially if I could have reconstruction. I would want reconstruction."

She contacted only her aunt. She was not asked about her mother's brother, who suffers from colon cancer. She believes the counselor only wanted blood samples from her female relatives because of the breast cancer connection. Karen reflected that something could be done to prevent heart attacks, from which her father had died, but nothing can be done about cancer. "It's going to come, you know, no matter what. I kind of do feel that way . . . maybe in the back of your mind you're like trying to mentally prepare yourself or something."

Karen had considered the possibility that cancer could have causes other than heredity, including the environment—"something that they use on plants or that they use in preservatives, possibly. I mean, I don't know anything about that stuff. I mean, I don't read about that, but I don't—just because it's in my family, yeah, doesn't mean that you're going to absolutely get it because people get cancer that don't have it in their family. So I don't know if it's just something that happens in food, something that happens in the air that we breathe or what we eat. You know, I don't know. I don't have any real set feelings on that. I think, for me, I think it's mostly genes in my family."

She read in the newspaper, she said, that "they have, you know found a gene for breast cancer. The BRCA-1. Just newspapers, you know, magazines, articles help. Newspapers that you can get anywhere." Karen concluded by saying, "It may be that I'm an ostrich and I'm sticking my head in the sand, but I think my faith has something to do with that. I am a Southern Baptist. It's faith. It's giving your worries to God so that you don't sit there and stress about it, about your life, you know. That helps me. I feel taken care of, let's put it that way. But I always have, since I was little. That's a big part of it, I really think. And even if I were to get cancer and die, you know, then I'm going to heaven. So, I mean if you think of it that way then, I don't know, it's kind of black and white like that, I guess. I think my husband's wonderful and he takes care of me, too. Just like I'm taken care of, you know, spiritually and here on earth. I just feel that way." Karen does not question why her family has been beset by this sickness because, she said, "I feel like God has a plan and I feel that that's the way it should be. I mean, if my father had not died when I was seven I would be a different person. I just feel, it's a calmness, you know, a taken care of feeling. Faith. It really is very nice."

A close reading of Karen's narrative reveals how medical family history unites relatives who otherwise would have not come in contact with one another, emphasizing kinship ties that individuals such as Karen have sought to avoid. The only reason Karen communicated with her aunt was because the appropriate tests to assess her genetic disease inheritance required her to do so. Also, Karen became a patient with the various tests she was given, despite the fact that she was healthy and asymptomatic. Karen communicates a sense of fatalism that may be tied both to the notion of the inevitability of her genetic heritage and to her strong religious faith, which, she claims, protects her from affliction. Yet, behind that assurance of her destiny even in the next world, Karen's narrative suggests that she harbors contradictory feelings. This is seen by the fact that while she accepts her genetic inheritance as her fate, she contemplates action by possibly having a prophylactic mastectomy, which will touch her at the core of her being as a traditional mother and wife and may physically convert her to the protected child she feels she is.

Kelly

I entered a serene atmosphere when I reached the small rural community where Kelly, a 42-year-old African American woman, resides in a small, well-furnished house with her three children, who range in age from 6 to 11. Kelly, a high school graduate with some technical college education, is employed at a telephone company. She was married for two years but is currently single. Whereas Kelly is healthy, her younger sister was diagnosed with breast cancer eight years earlier at the age of 31. The sister had a mastectomy but refused chemotherapy and radiation treatment because it made her sick, so she sought alternative therapy. The sister died after having developed liver cancer. After Kelly's sister's death, her mother, who is 60 years old, was diagnosed with breast cancer. Kelly noted that her mother found a lump in her breast " 'cause she — my mother has high blood pressure and she took care of Barbara like day in and day out, you know — she really neglected herself to take care of my sister. And so, later on, after that was all over with and she felt her breast and she felt the lump and she went to the doctor and they gave her a mammogram and all that and then a biopsy and that's what it was. That was breast cancer." Her mother had a mastectomy, chemotherapy, and radiation and is doing well.

Kelly came to the attention of the genetic counselor through a breast cancer study. As a participant in the study, the researchers took her family history and blood samples. Kelly said, "I think it's something with the blood that you can check and maybe you can tell whether, you know, there's a possibility this person could have cancer. Some lady came and she interviewed me and she took my blood." Kelly wanted to know the test results. However, both her mother and her surviving sister refused to learn the outcome, and "[the genetic counselor] was afraid I might go back and say something to my mother or my sister. So I never found out." The genetic counselor never told her the results of the test because, Kelly said, "she didn't want to cause no conflict." Kelly's sister didn't want to know, "because she has been through a lot with a sick child."

I asked Kelly why she wished to know the results of her test. She replied, "It really didn't make no difference whether I signed yes or whether I signed no, so I decided to sign yes 'cause I told the counselor even if she told me, 'well, yeah, it looks like you might have cancer down the road,' I feel like this. The doctors don't know everything. And even if she told me that 'no, you're not at a high risk,' I still feel like it's a possibility that I could. So either way, you know, I just wanted to see what the outcome would be."

Kelly is close to her parents, her sister, and one aunt, and she became closer to her family after her younger sister and her mother fell ill. She said, "I felt like we were close anyway, but when they became sick we even got closer and I think we turned to God even more when they got sick. Now I go to church more than what I used to, you know, and read the Bible more than what I used to. I guess the sickness brings you closer to God, you know, because they kind of turned their life around and went to God."

Kelly, like Karen, believes it is possible for her to get cancer irrespective of her genetic history because, she said, "just looking at my family history, to me it was really ironic. I had a sister that had it. My mother had it. I had a grandfather who had prostate cancer, and I had, uh, his wife died of lung cancer, I think, or throat cancer. So, you know, it runs in the family, so I just feel like, you know, it's a possibility. Even if no one in my family had it, it's still, I feel like it's a possibility, you know. Anything. You know, with so much cancer, still it's a possibility, 'cause, to me, anybody can get it. And so it's still a possibility whether they had it or not. It's still a possibility." Kelly believes she could get cancer not as a result of the family history but because, she said, "with so much going on in the world, I figure the food, the air, the stuff they be spraying the food with . . . yes, uh huh, I feel that way. It's just so much out there in the world nowadays that causes cancer. So, to me anything causes cancer, you know—the water, everything causes cancer."

Kelly does not think about cancer, however, because, "I think if I were to just think about it, it probably would be depressing, so I don't think about it." Kelly may not subscribe to the genetic ideology; nevertheless, she has a mammogram done every year, and she began performing breast self-exams after her sister died and her mother fell ill. She said, "I do it mostly because it was in my family, but I think probably I would have done it anyway with so much of it, you know, as far as breast cancer in so many women nowadays, I feel like I would have done it anyway. I don't know if I would have gone every year or I would have started as soon as I did, you know, but I feel that it's a good thing to do as far as mammograms."

Kelly is not concerned about her children becoming ill because "anything can happen so, you know, I don't dwell on that. They could leave at a young age, a car accident or anything like that. I'm just happy they're here and healthy now. Anything can happen—a plane fall on them. Many planes come by here. A plane could fall on the house and wipe all of us out. So no, I don't dwell on that, no."

In listening to Kelly, like listening to Karen, we hear that neither of the women subscribes to the dominant biogenetic ideology: both women believe that cancer has multiple causes and might strike anyone. Kelly offered alternative explanations for the disease, and her narration of her mother's bout with cancer suggests that she attributes it to her mother's distress, hard work, and exhaustion resulting from attending to Kelly's now-deceased sister. Kelly's fatalistic perspective, like Karen's, mitigates her concern about her or her children becoming afflicted with the disease. Yet she, unlike her dead sister, became a "healthy" patient by starting to have mammograms after her sister's death because of the belief that the disease is familial. Kelly's narrative suggests, too, the ways in which genetic ideologies link families and kin in unexpected ways. The autonomous individual is no longer a master of his or her body. Whereas biomedical therapeutic management may have required taking the family into consideration, the age of genetics links family members in new ways. Diagnostic techniques and outcomes can no longer rely uniquely on the afflicted person. Test results must incorporate the family, since they are no longer the concern of the individual alone. Kelly could not get the results of her genetic inheritance, even if she so wished, because the outcome involved other family members. Significantly, both Kelly and Karen's narratives, informed by their religiosity, disclose a strong belief in predestination. It is less apparent, however, that the belief in genetic inheritance is a secular faith in predestination.

Maya

My meeting with this 50-year-old biologist, born in South Asia and married to a geneticist, with two children, in her elegant upper-middle-class home was particularly informative owing to her dual cultural background. Maya identifies herself as an American, having also internalized American values of mastering the situation. Although Maya comes from a society where large extended families are the norm, she lives in a nuclear family in America. Nevertheless, she remains in close contact with her siblings, who are dispersed in various parts of the United States. Maya sought genetic counseling when she wished to undergo hormone replacement therapy but greatly feared getting ovarian cancer. Her mother and a 45-year-old sister had died of the disease, and most recently her 22-year-old brother had succumbed to colon cancer. Maya believes that colon and ovarian cancers are closely associated, but she especially fears ovarian cancer.

Maya noted that, as a biologist, she could only think that cancer is a genetically inherited disease, unless, of course, it is, in her words, "bewitchment of our family," but she quickly discounted that possibility. She volunteered that she has been separated from her family in South Asia but that she had been brought closer to them because of the potential for sharing a common disease. In fact, Maya wished to have her sisters and her oldest daughter genetically tested, but they all refused to take the test. She believes that if one knows one is carrying the gene, the disease can be prevented by a vegetarian diet.

Maya's wish to have her relatives and her daughter genetically tested would give her a handle on the future by knowing her risk of inheriting the disease, a desire her family had not shared with her. In her case we see how genetic ideology motivated her to seek genetic testing, requiring the cooperation of her family, with whom she became closer because of the fear of the disease. The potential control she gains knowing that she may become afflicted by a genetically transmitted disease converts her and her family into patients who enter the medical domain by her wish for a genetic test.

Not surprisingly, Maya, who originates from a society where witchcraft beliefs are widely held, noted the possibility that her family may have been bewitched. As a biologist and a Westerner, however, she could not consciously sustain an unscientific view that would place her in the category of a superstitious and uneducated person, even though, I suspect, she may still maintain the belief at some level, considering that she had spontaneously given it consideration.

Alice

Alice, who is Karen's aunt, is at 77 years of age in excellent health, although she has had ovarian and colon cancer and a series of other cancers, not all of which she could even remember. Because of her current health status, I include her among the healthy women despite these various bouts with cancer. Alice's sister and mother both died of breast cancer, and her only living brother as well as her maternal and paternal aunts all suffer from colon cancer.

Alice is retired, a widow who had worked much of her life. She had graduated from a teacher's college but had worked on a tobacco farm for four years, for a telephone company, and then for the state. Alice suffered a reversal of fortune when her husband, a truck driver, made a bad investment and she was forced to sell her house and move into a trailer, where she was currently living. As I looked at Alice, I saw a feisty woman with a twinkle in her eyes, but I also saw a gracious southern lady who had seen better economic days.

Alice reported that Karen, at the request of the genetic counselor, had asked her to come in for genetic testing. Alice said that "they took a blood test of me when I was over there, but Karen had left out a lot about the aunts that died before she was born and I got the whole family written up. Aunts on my side, on mama's side and my son [at 52 years of age] died about two years ago with colon cancer." Alice related the entire family history, remembering all her relatives who had died of cancer. She concluded her account by saying that she did not believe her son had colon cancer, but rather had choked to death at the hospital.

Alice's immediate family includes her other son and his wife and two grandchildren, as well as nieces and nephews on her sister's side, whom, she said, "I very seldom see. They live spread out in different parts of the country." In fact, she has had very little contact with them except on the occasion when she gave blood for the genetic test. Alice complained that even though her niece lives close by she never comes to see her. She said, "Karen just called me because I knew a lot, but they never come to see me. But I guess she was more concerned about herself, too, to keep it checked in case she does have cancer so they find it in time. And my sister had both her breasts removed."

Alice doubts that her cancers were inherited. She is persuaded that they were caused by something she ate, and it was for Karen's sake that she agreed to have the blood test done.[16] Alice noted that she never thought cancer was familial until "lately, when everybody started talking about it. You didn't hear about it a long time ago. Nobody said it was inherited, but I think now they are trying to check further to see what's causing cancer. But since there's so many in one family died with cancer, it looks like it could be. Or maybe the water we were drinking or maybe the food we was eating, whatever."

Alice is a devoutly religious woman who believes that God wanted her to stay here and that is why she has lived so long. She is totally involved in her church and considers as her real family five widowed church members who spend their time together, one of whom accompanied her to our meeting.

Alice is a remarkable example of someone reunited with a family member only because of genetic ideologies of inheritance. Her niece's test could not have been performed without her cooperation. Yet she herself believes in the environmental rather than genetic etiology of cancer, although she realizes that hereditary explanations are a new phenomenon. She was thus prompted to contribute her blood on her niece's behalf out of kinship obligations rather than out of personal conviction.

The experiences of these seven women are especially instructive in how the ideology of genetic inheritance defines for them a relationship with family and kin. With the exception of Kelly, all the women have had little contact with their kin outside the nuclear family, following a contemporary pattern of familial relationships. Yet the belief in the genetic inheritance of disease has unwittingly brought them closer to their families, as we saw in Karen's case. Moreover, they can no longer remain autonomous individuals in their medical decisions, independent of their families: they must involve genealogically related individuals in order to establish diagnoses and predictions of their future health status, as Kelly and Alice's cases inform us. The same ideology, while not fully accepted, propels them into the medical realm, if only by undergoing frequent mammograms. Granted, the medical profession has recently urged all women over 40 to have annual mammograms,[17] but those who originate from kin groups, some of whose members have been afflicted with breast cancer, are urged to be especially vigilant and to have such exams more frequently, placing a special burden on them. Undoubtedly, the ideology of genetic inheritance alerts such women as for example Eve to take charge of their health as a form of prevention. Paradoxically, the road to prevention leads also to patienthood — and to anxiety in the present about adverse possibilities in the future. As we can see, for women like Eve, Kate, and Maya, who are not fatalistic and do not believe in predestination, the future is closely intertwined with their present lived reality. They exist in an ongoing state of anxiety generated by a fear that they will fall ill in the future. The healthy women's narratives are instructive in yet another regard. As we will learn from the vignettes of women afflicted with cancer, they, like the healthy women, reestablish closer relations with their family and kin. One could argue that the sick women move closer to their families because they are experiencing a life-threatening disease, and, undoubtedly, sickness even in estranged families might bring its members closer together. However, the healthy women's reformulation of family and kin relations suggests that the belief in a shared common genetic heritage of a disease, not only common suffering, molds family and kinship relations.

The women we meet in this chapter and the next, who have already experienced the disease, reveal the ways they interpret the ideology of genetic inheritance and how it shapes their lives on multiple levels of experience. Each woman's narrative discloses various themes which she negotiates, which guide her comprehension and lived reality, including family and kinship relations, continuity and memory, control and the absence of control, fatalism, predestination, and conflicting etiological beliefs, which give way to certainty and aesthetic satisfaction, as well as fear and anxiety. I turn to the women who have recovered from the disease.

Chapter 6
People with a Genetic History II

Recovered Patients

In this chapter I turn to the women who became afflicted with breast cancer; they have been patients already. As among the healthy women, the ideology of genetic inheritance is confirmed experientially for the patients who believed they had suffered from cancer because other members in the family had had it, a recurring theme in all the women's narratives. How else could they explain the disease? Those who entertain an alternative etiological explanation of their affliction must exist with a conflict. Almost all, therefore, adhere to the prevailing genetic inheritance ideology by employing the same evidence as their physicians to support their view, namely that other members in the family and kin have suffered from the same disease.

Although the causes of cancer are not known, to be human is to impose an order on what otherwise seem to be senseless, chance experiences. Human beings pursue explanations for their afflictions in order to ascribe a naturalness and regularity to otherwise meaningless adversity by removing a sense of randomness from their suffering. The vignettes presented in this chapter illuminate the ways in which genetic explanations guide these women's thoughts and actions to help them make intelligible the irrationality of their disease. The women's accounts disclose diverse responses to the same affliction, reflecting a central norm of American culture that lays stress on individual variation and the uniqueness of the individual. Yet, no matter how much American culture may deny having a common pool of cultural understandings, not unexpectedly, the women interviewed generally shared a similar conceptualization that breast cancer was passed down to them from relatives, reflecting prevailing biomedical notions. Interestingly, in this group class differences failed to account for the overarching attributions of breast cancer to their genetic heritage, in the same way that class differences mostly fail to distinguish family and kinship patterns and relations.[1]

Intentionally or not, the women's etiological explanations required that they recognize family and kinship when they attributed their affliction to genetic inheritance. Whereas my primary concern was to assess the ways conceptualizations of the genetic transmission of disease shape kinship and family relations, I discovered various important themes deriving from this ideology that guided both breast cancer sufferers and the healthy women discussed in the last chapter, which I had not anticipated prior to this study. Implicitly or explicitly, themes other than those associated with kinship relations emerged in the discussion, including a newly found sense of continuity with and memory of ancestors. Furthermore, as in the case of Karen in the last chapter, and Melanie, Connie, and other recovered patients in this chapter, the ideology of genetic inheritance encompasses two important if contradictory themes: predetermination and its counterpoint, mastery of one's fate, a singularly important norm of American culture. In fact, the vignettes disclose conflicting beliefs within the same individual. On the one hand, some women exhibit a sense of fatalism, of life being a crap shoot and a gamble and of not having control of one's destiny; on the other hand, the same women may indicate that knowledge of the genetic inheritance of disease gives them a sense of control because it alerts them to live a more healthful life and alerts their families to be attentive to their bodies and to signs of the disease. Note, however, that a woman can exercise control only over her own personal habits; the individual has no control over the environmental toxins that may be equally significant in the etiology of cancer, as we will learn in Chapter 9, and of which various women are aware.

It is important to stress that the ideology of genetic inheritance shapes the lives of the sick in much the same way as the healthy, with one crucial exception: the sick women no longer experience anxieties associated with the anticipation of a dreadful outcome for themselves, if not for their children. The sick women need not negotiate anymore the ambiguities of being at risk, or have the fear of the future melt into the present. Generally speaking, those whom I interviewed had come to terms with a condition that for many, such as Jana or Tina, has even become redemptive. Thus, unintended as it may be, the notion of predestination that is fostered by the ideology of genetic inheritance embraces a form of spirituality and informs the understanding of many of the women that their disease is both transformative and redemptive by leading to newly discovered transcendence, insight, and self-improvement.

I present each woman's narrative in some detail because each reveals the ways the person negotiates her experience of a disease she believes to be familial differently. Moreover, each vignette illuminates the theoretical issues concerning the ways the ideology of genetic inheritance molds people's experience, including family and kinship relations. Concurrently, we witness many different and even contradictory layers of explanations people draw upon to make sense to themselves of that which is universally and profoundly inexplicable; namely the eternal and by now mundane question, "Why must I and my family suffer?" even when the person may not voice the question openly. Actually, having been guided by their cultural comprehension, as well as by the genetic counselor, they have no need to voice the question directly, because the ideology of genetic inheritance addresses it for them. I hasten to repeat a point made in the Introduction, however, that each woman weaves together complex explanations of her disease that must not be reduced to genetic inheritance alone. Nevertheless, as the dominant ideology, beliefs in genetic inheritance orchestrate behavior and a therapeutic path. Out of the entire sample, only Leah and Tina rejected the prevailing explanations of breast cancer etiology in favor of environmental or religious attributions. Whereas the majority of the women may attribute their disease to factors other than genetics and then quickly discount them, these two women accepted alternative explanations, albeit for different reasons. I turn to these two women first because they are exceptions to the other women we will meet.

Case Narratives

Leah

Before I learned how exceptional Leah was, I was impressed by her brilliant smile. Leah is 47 years old, a college graduate, employed as a writer, and living with her male partner. Leah, one of five sisters, had been diagnosed with breast cancer three years before we met and after her younger sister had succumbed to the same disease a year earlier. Leah's 70-year-old mother became afflicted with breast cancer shortly after her sister died, as did the mother's sister. Leah recounted that because her sister had died of cancer, her radiologist was especially vigilant when she had her mammograms done and finally found a lump at a very early stage of development. Leah, like her sister, underwent a mastectomy. Yet despite the fact that several members in her family have experienced cancer, Leah believes that the cancer in her family is not hereditary because the family lacks a long history of the disease. Leah, who comes from a large family with numerous cousins and lots of aunts, reasons that if her disease were inherited genetically, there would be a higher incidence than there has been. She observed, "It's more likely to be exposure to something." Although she believes that cancer is environmentally caused, she added, "However, certainly I would advise my sisters and my nieces to be vigilant about watching for signs, but personally I don't put a lot of stock in that. What's to be done with this knowledge that it's genetic?" She answered her own question by noting that genetic knowledge only causes one to be constantly watching for signs. Consistent with her rejection of genetic ideology, Leah would never consider having a prophylactic mastectomy, nor is she interested in knowing whether she has the gene or not: "That just seems like knowledge and fear that you don't need. It's crossing bridges before you come to them." Besides, having a genetic test done would only cause trouble with her insurance company. Leah just tries to lead a normal, healthy life.

Leah was always close to her sisters, to her mother, and to her extended family, but she became even closer to them when she fell ill. She noted, "I don't know if it's so much because we gave each other the disease, but more just that we've had a common experience. You know, it's a bonding sort of thing to share this trauma." Some could argue from a popular psychological perspective that she is "in denial," refusing to acknowledge a blight on her family. However, I have no evidence that her beliefs are disingenuous. Rather, Leah belongs to a category of persons who question basic cultural assumptions, even though she would still caution her relatives to be vigilant.

Since Leah rejected genetic ideologies, or at best considered them inutile, they did not alter her relationship with her immediate or extended family. However, because of the hegemonic status of biomedical beliefs, including those concerning genetic inheritance, people like Leah who conceive of alternative explanations for their afflictions are nevertheless placed in a bind, or in what I call a "what if" state. What if the disease is genetically inherited? Then her relatives still must be alerted, even though in actuality she fails to follow the ideology.

Tina

Tina was referred to me by another patient, Lydia; they both participate in a breast cancer support group. Tina, like Leah, tends to reject the genetic model of disease. A very pleasant, active 42-year-old woman, married with no children, she is a high school graduate employed as a bookkeeper. Tina was afflicted with breast cancer at the age of 35, and, since she was the only one in her family to have the disease, she was shocked. She had a lumpectomy, but she refused any other biomedical treatment. She is feeling well, and she follows a New Age diet. She takes Chinese herbal medications for the liver, and she consults naturopaths and homeopaths. When she asked her mainstream physician what she could do to recover her health, she was told, "Get lots of sleep." She complained that "they don't really look at anything as far as diet or any of those things. But I would like to take control of things," and alternative medicine allows her to do so.

Significantly, though Tina seems to have been the only one in the family to be afflicted with cancer, her two sisters became very nervous when she fell ill. Tina recalled, "My sister told me how the doctor told her if you have a mother or a sister with breast cancer, then your chance of getting it goes way up, you know, the percentage, it's percentages." The sisters immediately had mammograms for the first time. When Tina's younger sister found a small cyst in her breast, "she flipped out over the thought that she might have breast cancer. So I think in the back of their minds, it has kind of shaken them up a little bit." But, she added, "they don't share all their fears with me, maybe to protect me or not to make me feel guilty." Tina noted that her sisters, who are younger than she, are more concerned about breast cancer than other women their age. She believes that if her disease were hereditary it would have been more frightening to her, because, she said, "if it were familial I think it would be more like that was my fate. I think if my mother had died of it, I might feel kind of more like, 'Well, here I go down the same path or something.'"

Tina is grateful now that she hasn't had any children, even though she asserts that not having children had placed her at higher risk for breast cancer. She says, philosophically, that "when you get this kind of disease you ask 'why me,' and then at some point you find, 'my life is really better because of this.'" She feels wiser and redeemed. Tina attributes her illness to having been sick as a child with infections, tonsillitis, and pneumonia and having been heavily exposed to antibiotics. Moreover, she was very thin. But when Tina went to a traditional Chinese doctor, he explained that she was born with an unhealthy liver, or that the antibiotics had injured her liver because her body was full of toxins. The doctor informed her, and Tina adopted his theory, that if one's liver is not functioning properly, it continuously recycles estrogen instead of flushing it out of the body and the body retains high levels of estrogen. Tina believes that this is the reason she became afflicted with breast cancer.

In her quest to find an answer to "why me," Tina thought out loud that since she grew up in Detroit her disease must have environmental causes, but then she discarded the possibility because her three sisters grew up in the same neighborhood and in the same house and they were well. She then mentioned books she had read suggesting that there is some deep pain she might be carrying around.[2] Tina noted, "I mean possibly emotions." But then she wondered whether it meant that "I was causing my cancer, which was a big burden to carry. They say they don't want people to feel guilty, but you do carry a certain responsibility, is what I think. It can be triggered emotionally. A lot of tension in your body, holding a lot in constricts a lot of things — the blood flow isn't there. This goes back to kind of the way the Chinese think."

When Tina fell ill, her medical history was taken and she was invited to participate in a genetic study. She was instructed to ask about the causes of death of her mother, grandparents, and aunts, from both sides of the family. These questions kept her memory of her past alive. This investigation led her to find out about her family, and she learned that a second cousin on her father's side had breast cancer. She found this odd because she had not thought that there was any cancer in her family. But then she discovered that "my grandmother died of liver cancer, but she was an older lady. My mother at 78 got a very benign form of breast cancer. They didn't even do anything to her. And then my aunt did say that she remembered her grandmother, which would be my great-grandmother, had a big lump under her arm, which, she said looking back, maybe was breast cancer." Tina referred to the media from which her aunt learned about genetic inheritance. The aunt then began thinking about "my great-grandmother. My aunt said she did remember her having a big lump in her arm." Even though Tina's family medical history suggests cancer in the family, she rejects the genetic model and customary biomedical explanations by seeking alternative healers.

Tina's experience calls attention to the ways in which notions about genetic inheritance perforce conjure up memories of family and ancestors — aunts and grandmothers — one may not have thought about until faced with a disease. In discussing her sisters' reactions, Tina's narrative indicates how, owing to hereditarian concepts, initially her sickness brought more fear than compassion to her sisters, a response that may even lead to alienation, as we will see in Lydia's case. Tina's multiple etiological attributions, which include the environment, childhood medical history, and Chinese medical theories, bring into bold relief the parsimony and elegance of the reductionist genetic interpretation that she rejects. As Betty will point out, genetic inheritance theory is easy to comprehend, whereas its repudiation requires Tina to seek a series of explanations. Before she invoked memories of other family members, Tina lacked direct experiential evidence that her disease might be hereditary, since she was the sole person she knew in her family who suffered from cancer. Then, because of her medical history and because of the suggestion of a genetic study, Tina was compelled to recall family and ancestors.

Eliza

Leah's reservations about possessing knowledge about one's genetic makeup would resonate with Eliza, even though she learned that her disease was genetic. Eliza, a 54-year-old north European academic, married, with a 10-year-old daughter, came to the United States on a sabbatical. On the occasions when we met, she conveyed an intense vulnerability and sadness in her demeanor, if not in her narrative. Eliza, whose sister and cousin had died of breast cancer and her father of a brain tumor, fell ill in Europe four years before we met. Mammograms had failed to disclose that she was harboring a cancer until she experienced seepage from her breast. She was prompted to seek an oncologist because of her family history after she had read, to her great surprise, in the newspapers that breast cancer was a hereditary disease. Interestingly, the physicians in her country had not suggested to her that breast cancer was a genetic disease.

Notwithstanding her physician, but because of the media, Eliza began to delve into her family history, about which she had previously been ignorant. Significantly, Eliza recounted that the disease had started her on a quest to determine which of her ancestors had initially suffered from cancer. She contacted various cousins whom she had not seen for years. Her search led her to an ancestor four generations back who had also been a famous poet. It was not known what he had died of, but because her cousin, also a descendant of this man, had cancer too, Eliza concluded that it must have been the famous poet who first carried the cancer gene. Eliza now took great pride in this ancestor, and she felt closer to her cousin than ever before because the two shared the same fate.

When Eliza fell ill, she did not consider her disease to be genetically inherited. In fact, she, like Connie and Melanie, whom we will meet shortly, attributed her illness to stress. She said, "I got angry when I got sick because I had a very heavy work load and I felt that it was because of it that I got sick. I felt my immune system was weakened. But then there is always discussion. Somebody says, 'your sister was sick.' Then I discovered that there was a gene that caused both ovarian and breast cancer and that this [that it is genetic] was old information." She investigated her family medical history and found that two female cousins had also been afflicted by cancer. According to Eliza, the male cousins "didn't get it because they don't carry the gene. Then I talked to my doctor and the doctor said, 'Oh no, genetic. They all say that, and what makes you think you are one of those?' And then I started talking to friends, and I learned that in 10 percent of the women it is genetic."

When Eliza arrived in the United States, her doctors examined her family medical history, ordered blood tests, and advised Eliza to have a prophylactic operation to remove her ovaries and the healthy breast because she presumably was a carrier of the breast cancer gene.[3] When Eliza received the results of the test in the United States, she said, "I felt and feel a deep sorrow. Just as if somebody is dying. A deep kind of sorrow. I have been feeling it all the time since I got the test — this empty feeling. Just like grief as when somebody dies. That's what I feel. I feel we are doomed. We are a family that was marked by this disease, and I feel sorry for my family and for the people that have this gene. That is my basic feeling."

Eliza's husband was angry, faulting her family and regretting that they had had a child together. Interestingly, unlike all the American women I interviewed, Eliza and her husband were especially concerned that no one learn about her condition, not because of insurance questions, since everybody is insured in her country, but because nobody there speaks about such misfortune, particularly when there is a child involved. It may even limit the girl's marriage prospects, an issue never raised by any American in the study.

For Eliza, the knowledge that her disease resulted from a genetic inheritance made her feel fragile but relieved because it explained to her why she got this disease, even though it was the same as, she said, "the roll of the dice." Genetic memory established for Eliza a connection with a famous poet, a connection she was proud of. Not unlike some of the other women, Eliza used the gambling metaphor, recognizing the randomness of the notion of genetic inheritance. Paradoxically, that very understanding of the randomness of the disease provided meaning because it explained to Eliza why she fell ill. Simultaneously, while for Eliza the knowledge that she carries the cancer gene doomed her during her lifetime, she nevertheless found it advantageous because it alerts her daughter to be vigilant about her health.

Jana

Eliza's sophistication and worldliness contrast with Jana's modest origins, which are commonly described as "poor southern white." The two women exude the same sorrow, however. In fact, of all the women I met during this study, Jana was perhaps the most despairing about her plight. Jana, 36 years old, was undergoing chemotherapy when we met. Her bald head accentuated a striking, high-cheekboned face, marred by dejection. Jana, the mother of three children ranging in age from 7 to 15, had returned to high school to obtain a diploma while she worked for a fast-food chain. Jana began her working life when she was 12 years old, operating a harvester cutting tobacco. When her youngest child was 3 months old she returned to work in a sewing factory, then got a job as a machine cleaner in a cotton mill, where her sister and several of her aunts were also employed. Jana worked at the cotton mill until she underwent her first surgery, a lumpectomy, when she was 30 years old. Jana regards herself as fortunate that her husband, who drives a Dumpster truck, is supportive of her, because she believes that many men often leave a sick wife since they cannot deal with the illness.

Jana related that her doctor had encouraged her to have her healthy breast removed, but she refused. For five years Jana was well. But a year before our meeting she experienced a lump in the other breast for which she was being treated at the time we met. Jana believes that she made the right decision not to have prophylactic surgery. She said, "I didn't know, first time I got it I knew what it was, I just felt a lump. The second time it felt kind of like the same thing. And then they told me. The doctor said, 'it ain't nothing but a cyst or something.' Then I got kind of worried about it—my aunts had it, breast cancer." Jana had not thought very much about why she fell ill. She said, "I don't know. Maybe it's just one of those things that people have, that you're born with." The doctor had told her it had something to do with genes, "because I had it the second time."

Jana reported that her doctor informed her that "it was a family sickness" because other members of her family had had the same disease. "You know, two [paternal] aunts had it, my cousin had it, then my 29-year-old sister, who works in the cotton mill, had it and I got it again. That's why they said I got it in my genes. That's probably the only reason I got it, because of my daddy's side—my mama's side, there's no breast cancer at all, just on my father's side." Jana said that her doctor had told her that her disease was genetic, that "it can be passed from one person to another, and then I saw some stuff on TV about it, about breast cancer and stuff. Then my sister has it too; it has to be inherited for both of us. He said it was in my genes."

While Jana accepted the doctor's attribution that her illness was due to her family heritage, she also felt strongly that her disease has to do with diet and chemicals in the food. At times she thought that one gets cancer from taking birth control pills, but she had only taken them for one year. But, repeating what the doctor had said, that it was a familial disease, she said, "I don't know what it was, then I got to thinking that my aunt got sick, so that maybe I didn't know for sure where it came from, maybe what I ate. You know, you always think because they put a lot of chemicals in the food now, more than they used to, to get the food ready faster. They raise hogs faster, plus think about it, maybe with all that happened a long time ago a lot of people were sick and didn't know what it was, so it could've been cancer." Jana also considered dejection as a cause: "maybe a period in your life when you're down and out or something, and your system gets low. [But] from what I hear on TV, and doctors say, they was pretty sure it was genetics, since I had it and this is the second time I had it and my sister had it."[4]

Jana, after having seen the genetic counselor, told her husband, "You see, they do, they're already working on it. They're working on a lot of stuff you don't know about until you get sick or something. Somebody who ain't sick don't pay attention to a lot of those things." But then, she concluded, "I don't know if they really know what gives you breast cancer or not. It could be the foods you eat, you don't ever know. It could be the food; it doesn't have to be genetic. Sometimes you just don't know, like some people who get lung cancer and don't smoke. That's why I think they don't know."

In actuality, Jana was upset when she was informed that her cancer was due to her genetic inheritance because, she said, "I don't want my children to get it. I was kind of shocked. Then I got used to it and then I thought about my girls and hoped they didn't get it, like I did. I didn't have no bad thoughts, I just thought that maybe it was just something I have to live with. There's really nothing I can do because it's in my genes, it's not like they can take them out, and you have to have them. I just hoped that my girls didn't get the gene that I got. I think about that—maybe I gave it to them [her children]. That's something I don't want to do. You know, I know if there was some kind of test that we could take, in a way I don't want my young to know if they got that gene and have to worry about if they are going to die, or get it and die or something like that. I don't want them to worry about that. I try not to think about some things. I try to have happy thoughts. I hope maybe they got their daddy's genes. You know, maybe that way they won't get it." She added, "If you know you got it or something in your body's bad, it's going to scare you more than it's going to scare your kid. You know, it would be worrying you all the time, and then if you don't know you got it—I mean that gene—it won't worry you so bad."

Jana, who regards her mother, father, three brothers, a half sister, and her children as her family, absolved her father of the responsibility of having given her the gene. She said, "But see, they say it's not in the men but in the women on my father's side." She then added, "Sometimes I wonder what side it came from, either from my grandfather's side or my grandmother's side. But it's something that you can't help, it's in your genes, it's in your body and you can't tell how far down the line it is."

Jana feels close only to her immediate family that live nearby. Her condition has served as a warning to her cousins and their children. She added, "I feel connected to the family. Then one time before, I had this feeling that my uncle and my aunt kind of didn't say anything, you know how you think sometimes that they are mad at you because their daughter died and you didn't. You know you feel that way because she died, and you feel bad because she died and you lived. People like the doctor make me feel bad because you're dead and I am still living. I'm thinking there's a reason I'm still living, I think that about my children. And I say maybe me being sick made me strengthen my faith in God, or show somebody out there that I'm sick and I can survive."

Jana, like many of the American women in the study but unlike Eliza, regards the disease as redemptive. She stated it most clearly when she said, "Sometimes I wonder why it happened to me — and you can't really explain why, either. Maybe it's something you have to face to make you have stronger faith in God. There's always a question why. You really don't know. Sometimes I think it may be something to make me stronger." Jana is a born-again Christian, and her faith sustains her. "What makes me go on is that it makes me hold on to him more. Without the Lord I wouldn't be here now; he gives me strength every day." Tears came to her eyes when she said, "I get to thinking about all that. I try not to think about that because the Lord, He put me here and he's going to take me when it's my time to go." Jana's illness brought her closer to God, but it distanced her from her friends. Her husband claims that her friends avoid her because they think that cancer is contagious.

Jana's complex narrative calls attention to her new connection with her relatives and kin because of their shared genetic heritage while concurrently creating animosities because she survived and others in the family have not. Like several of the other women, Jana is sustained by her strong religious convictions, which also assuage her guilt about remaining alive although others in her family had died. While finding redemption in her experience of cancer, the genetic knowledge provokes in her great anxiety because she fears transmitting her genes and her affliction to her children.

Concurrently, despite the doctor, the genetic counselor, and the mass media, Jana had not fully accepted that her disease was caused by genetic inheritance rather than by environmental chemicals or foods. Jana's narrative and demeanor embody the conflict she experiences between her intuitive explanations for her disease, associated with toxins in foods, and the physician's and television's messages that her breast cancer was transmitted to her by her father's family.

The fact that she had partially rejected a genetic explanation may have influenced her treatment management, as when she declined to undergo the prophylactic surgery suggested by her physician, because she reasoned that if the genes cannot be removed, nothing can be accomplished by such measures. Jana's narrative distinctly discloses the ways in which the ideology of genetic inheritance can lead to fatalism and despair, rather than mastery of one's fate, as interpreted by others we meet.

Dina

Like Jana, Dina is a profoundly religious woman. Dina, a 68-year-old gentle and gracious African American widow, resides by herself in a pleasantly furnished home and is retired from her job as a supervisor in the cotton mill where she had worked much of her life. Dina and her 39-year-old daughter were diagnosed with breast cancer at exactly the same time seven years ago, at the time of Dina's retirement. Whereas Dina, who had a mastectomy and was treated for three years with tamoxifen, has fully recovered, her daughter, who was treated with chemotherapy and radiation, died shortly after the onset of the illness.

Dina related that because the same disease afflicted her and her daughter, the doctors had told her that her family suffered from a genetic disease. Dina, however, had never contemplated this possibility. Although she thought it was unusual that both she and her daughter had fallen ill with the same disease, Dina had not thought the affliction was hereditary because others in her family had not experienced it. She said, "My aunts died old and not of breast cancer. The two who are alive are doing well. One had a stroke. So I never thought of it as being a family thing. Maybe being naïve. Not getting worried about things that you cannot do anything about." When she was told that her family suffered from this disease, Dina searched for family members who may have had breast cancer, but she could not recall anyone. At that time, she contacted her mother and learned that one of her mother's sisters had had ovarian cancer and another sister's daughter had had a lump in her breast that was successfully removed.

Dina became very close to her sisters, who live in different parts of the country, after she fell ill. She said the doctor "told me to tell them to get mammograms and their children to get mammograms because I had breast cancer and she [her daughter] had breast cancer. It could be a possibility, but anyway it was just something they need to stay on top of it." Dina repeated, "I would never have thought of this [that it is familial or hereditary], but since he told me I just thought he was concerned."

Dina agreed to be tested for the gene. She commented, "Didn't bother me. I never thought it was a big deal because I felt if I carried the gene, it was no big deal. They told me, 'you may not want to know the results,' and I thought, why shouldn't I want to know the results? It wouldn't bother me. If they had told me it was positive — I had told my sister the reason I did it, if I carried the gene and it was in the family — they could stay on top of it, mammograms, I thought it was good. I didn't see anything negative about knowing. I wanted to know." Dina's genetic test turned out negative, she said. But even had it been positive, "that wouldn't have bothered me. It would just have meant, well, I have a mammogram every year anyway. I try to eat right. It would have meant that I need to be very careful as far as eating and keep in touch with the doctor."

Dina, whose father was a pastor, said, "It was just something that had to be. Some doctors claimed it was such a coincidence"; but Dina claimed, "I always was thinking to myself this was not a coincidence. I think God was trying to tell me something, but I don't know what he is trying to tell us. We thought we could do something for the glory of God, but no, his idea was to take her." In fact, Dina had a premonition about the disease. She recounted her vision and how "my spirit had told me something was going to happen and it did. My daughter had passed away."

Dina has not questioned why she and her daughter were afflicted with the disease, because, she said, "I felt like God wanted to use me and I want to be used, for whatever. It made me stronger. I couldn't have gotten through this unless I had believed in the Lord. It is hard to lose a child."

Although she agreed to be tested, Dina does not rely on genetic interpretations of the disease. Instead, she regards her affliction as a means of communication with God, although His specific message still remained a mystery. As I listened to Dina, I felt enveloped by her sense of spirituality and by her great pain from having lost her daughter. Her suffering redeemed Dina, and she could easily, if superficially, accept the physician's view that she and her daughter had suffered from a genetic disease. To establish whether her disease was indeed genetic, she was required to reestablish contact with her kin and alert her sisters to have mammograms done and be cautious.

Connie

Connie, too, is the daughter of a pastor and is a deeply religious woman. But unlike Jana and Dina, who exude a sense of fatalism, she seeks to take charge of her affliction. Connie, a very enthusiastic and smiling 47-year-old African American woman, raised her one daughter, currently in college, by herself. Connie recently completed her Ph.D. and is employed in the state educational system. Like Dina, Connie noted that religion had helped her deal with her affliction; but, unlike Dina, Connie also became empowered by concepts of genetic inheritance.

Connie had fallen ill two years prior to our meeting, at which time she had a mastectomy and was also treated with chemotherapy. Connie regards herself as recovered, and she is feeling well. In her words, "Cancer is not a death sentence." When she initially sought treatment for "liquid coming out of my breast," the physician ignored the symptoms and refused to refer her to a specialist. She recounted her painful odyssey to obtain a referral to an oncologist from her primary physician, under her health care plan. Connie insisted on the referral because she expected to be struck by the disease in light of the fact that her mother, aunt, and cousin had died of breast cancer and her father had died of prostate cancer. Curiously, the fact that other members of her family had succumbed to the disease was a warning to her but, surprisingly, not to her primary physician. She now wishes to undergo prophylactic surgery on her second breast.

Connie believes that she has a hereditary predisposition to cancer and that her disease was caused by stress and by chemicals in her diet. Connie maintains that genetic predisposition can be "fought back by right behavior and right nutrition." One's behavior can become an antidote to the inherited predisposition. By believing that stress and an unhealthful diet influenced her inherited predisposition for cancer, Connie faulted herself for falling ill.

Before her illness, Connie had little contact with her kin, but after she became sick, she was brought closer to them, especially her only sister, who, to Connie's bewilderment, refuses to take a genetic test or resort to any preventive treatments. Other than her daughter, her family and kin were of minimal importance in Connie's life, although after she learned she had a familial disease she reestablished her genealogical connections. While Connie tended to blame herself for her illness, Connie's memory of her family history alerted her to the possibility of becoming afflicted with the disease, leading to her taking charge of her treatment by her vigorous insistence on a referral and subsequent alleviation of her symptoms.

Carol

Religious discourse dominates Carol's narrative. As a born-again Christian, Carol immediately informed me, "I did not know what the good Lord had in store for me. The good Lord is just letting me live to see my kids grown and take care of themselves. I've got two grandchildren now. So I have been real blessed." As an active participant in her church, she noted that "if it hadn't been for God's people, I don't know that I really would have survived. You go through the various states of saying 'why me,' but I had not found the answer. But there's gotta be a reason I'm going through this; maybe it's to touch somebody else's life, give them hope. And the people in the church are always there for you. They are one big family."

We met in her office cubicle at a rural day care center where this very upbeat 48-year-old night school graduate had been employed for several years as the director. Carol is married and the mother of three adult children. In her first bout with cancer, when she was 31 years old, she underwent radical and prophylactic mastectomies but subsequently developed cancer in the thoracic cavity.

When told by her doctors that her disease was hereditary, Carol was not surprised, because "my grandmother had it, my mother and mother's two sisters had it. I have a cousin that has breast cancer and her cousin's daughter that's 28 just recently found out she had breast cancer." Carol's father died of lung cancer. After listing these people, she remembered that she had a 51-year-old sister who had both breasts removed even though the cancer was localized in one breast. After identifying the people in her family who had been afflicted with cancer, she concluded, "but I've been fortunate: I've done very well. God's been good to me."

When I remarked how cheerful she seemed, she responded, "Having two parents die with it, you learn that it's almost like you can't dwell on it so much because it would drive me crazy. There is never a day I don't think about it." But, she added laughingly, "you know, you just learn to go with the flow, do what you have to do." When the doctors told her that her disease was hereditary, they stressed that her girls need "to really stay on top of it." The doctor who performed Carol's reconstructive surgery advised her that after her daughters marry and have their children they might wish to have their breasts and ovaries removed. When a second doctor suggested the same option for her daughters, she mentioned it to the 24- and 18-year-olds because "I hate to think that I could pass on to them, but it's not anything that any of us planned on. It's just one of those things that happens and if it is, it's just something that you learn to cope with and realize that you know it's not anything that anybody did because no one intentionally wants anyone to get cancer, you know. It gives me more insight that they can do things to help protect themselves better by knowing than not knowing. Making sure they get their checkups, or not to let anything go unnoticed." She, in fact, informed her daughters that in all likelihood they too would become afflicted with the disease.

Carol believes that knowing her disease is hereditary is "a cautionary measure, not that they [the doctors] can help prevent them from going through any of this." But the doctors will keep closer check on her daughters, and in this way, the girls will "just have like a head start that some people would not have, you know. And I think that's a plus. It bothers me to think that I could pass something on to my children, but like I say, it's not anything that I have done." She concluded by saying, "It's kind of scary to think you could pass something on to someone else. You have no control over that; it's just something that happens and you just deal with it. And you just hope that your children can learn from it and not feel like, you know, 'she's giving me a death threat.'"

Carol smiled when she wistfully commented, "I did everything I thought that [I should] — I didn't smoke, and I breast-fed my last two children. I did things that [made me] less likely to get cancer, breast cancer, but I just didn't luck out. I was just one of those that got it. When I was younger, you didn't think too much about it — and then when my mother got sick, and then my sisters came down with it, I thought, there's something, 'cause years ago, it used to be that it wasn't hereditary, or people speculated it wasn't hereditary. But there is more to it — it's got to be hereditary." Carol repeatedly stressed that in the past people did not believe that cancer was an inherited disease. Once her mother's sisters fell ill, she realized that the disease was hereditary, because, she said, "You can't have a family with everybody getting the same type of cancer." Thus Carol unquestionably accepts the hereditary origin of her disease, but nevertheless considers that in some areas of the country beast cancer may be more prevalent, "maybe because of the power lines."[5]

Carol grew up in a close-knit family, but she was brought even closer to her brothers and sisters after she fell ill. She and her first cousins are close, and she said, "It's just that we live so far away that we don't get to see each other like we'd like to. It affects all of us, you know. Just because a girl's got it doesn't mean that their children can't get it, even if it's males. Our kids need to know it because they're going to be having kids and things like that. So I think they're kinda waiting to see, you know, what the test results show, and then maybe they'll [her brother's children] go from there."

Carol can only recall her ancestors as far back as her grandmother, whom she cannot blame for passing on her genes to her offspring any more than she could blame herself, if she passes them on to her daughters. But she is worried about her daughters, and also her son, who could pass it on to his daughter. Carol worries that "it could pass through generations. I don't want to pass it on, but it is nothing that I did wrong."

Sharing the same genes has brought her particularly close to some of her cousins, especially Betty, whom we will meet shortly, because "we have something that our mothers had," referring to the disease and to their genetic makeup. At the time of the interview they were all waiting for the results of the genetic tests. Carol believes that genetic tests will encourage people to be more cautious, and perhaps such tests will explain why some families get the disease and others don't.

At their biennial family reunions, the first cousins all talk about whether everybody has had a checkup. Carol said, "It has made us feel that we have something in common there because we are the offspring of sisters. We still have that contact, to see what's going on in everybody's life as far as illnesses, and I think they are anxiously waiting" (for the results of her tests).

Significantly, Carol returned again and again to the subject of her grandmother and mother, to the necessity of remembering one's relatives, and to her desire for her children to know that the disease is more than likely hereditary. She added, "It's my responsibility to educate my children because it is hereditary, and to give them the best advantage of taking care of themselves and their children. Because it is something that can be handed down."

Carol's narrative indicates how the family medical history validates

empirically for her, as for others, the prevailing notion that breast cancer
is a genetically inherited affliction. She discounts an alternative explanation that focuses on the environment in favor of cautiously accepting
contemporary hereditarian explanations. In doing so, the ideology of
genetic inheritance binds her to the living members of her family and
connects her both with the past and with the future, even though she
feels most connected to the members of her church. In light of her lack
of a genealogical depth, she possesses a history, a genetic memory of her
grandmother that furnishes a sense of continuity with the past and a
legacy to her children in the future. Ironically, and poignantly, Carol,
who originates from the rural poor, is not unaware that the disease may
be her sole bequest to her children.

While Carol regards the disease afflicting her family as a matter of
predestination, paradoxically, the hereditarian ideology also empowers
her to alert her children and their physicians to attend to their health. In
this manner predestination can be controlled, even if her children become asymptomatic patients, relegated to constant medical monitoring.
Lastly, Carol's narrative reveals a modern moral contradiction generated
by the notion of risk that confronts her: although she had done everything correctly to avoid all the known risk factors, she still fell ill. Only her
church has the potential to resolve this contradiction for her, and arguably succeeds.

Betty

Betty, a 53-year-old high school graduate employed as an administrator,
mother of two adult daughters, was diagnosed with ovarian cancer and
had a complete hysterectomy. Like her cousin Carol, Betty feels morally
indignant because she had done everything right and yet she developed
cancer, but unlike Carol, Betty found God only after she fell ill. As a result
of her illness, Betty was terminated from her job and lost her medical
insurance. Her husband, a welder, who recently left her, had never carried medical insurance; consequently, Betty's immediate family became
indigent. She said, "My mother died of ovarian cancer, but I never really
put two and two together that I would have cancer. I've always been
extraordinarily healthy; I don't smoke, I don't drink, so I really never felt
that I was a candidate for cancer. My mother was a heavy smoker, so I kind
of attributed her cancer to that." Subsequently Betty was afflicted with
breast cancer, and a mastectomy was performed. Later the cancer spread
to the second breast, and she was treated with chemotherapy three times.
She commented, "They probably could have done just a lumpectomy [on
the second breast], but I preferred having everything out." Five years
have passed, and Betty said proudly, "Now I'm healthy as a horse."

Sadly, Betty is currently most concerned about having gained a great deal of weight, due to the medication she was taking to alleviate the nausea provoked by chemotherapy. She remarked, "I think the weight gain had a real impact on my husband, 'cause he was used to this skinny, very physical person and all of a sudden he got a very fat, heavy, sluggish person. And he had a real hard time with that. He thinks that I overeat." Her weight gain has been "the biggest problem emotionally for me, the fact that I could not lose my weight, more so than the physical scarring." Betty was also morally incensed that her husband had left her even though, as she said, "I was a good wife, even when I was sick, and a faithful wife, and I hold marriage in the highest degree."

Betty had not considered the causes of her illness. She said, "I think after the initial shock, I sort of accepted the fact. It happened, so it happened — let's just get on with it. I think it was probably a little frustrating at the time because I did all the right things, you know — I ate good food, I didn't eat fast food, I eat lots of fresh vegetables, I don't drink, I don't smoke, I am very athletic, I play tennis practically every day. So I did all the things I thought you were supposed to do." But "we all started thinking that it had to have been something hereditary, 'cause there were different types of cancer in the family, there were a lot of cancers. Grandmother had it, and then we don't know, of course, between our great-grandparents. We don't know what happened or how they died. They tried to put down a genealogy, but they don't remember all that much above the third generation."

Betty holds that cancer is not the end of life. "I think it was a beginning of a way of my life, and if it is genetic, and I think very probably it was, she [the grandmother] passed the gene. She passed me blond hair, she passed me blue eyes, and she passed me the gene for cancer." Betty believes she is a better person for having the disease. Neither would she have hesitated to have children, even if she had known that she was a carrier of a diseased gene, because she loved mothering. She added, "We pass on a lot of different kinds of genes among our children. You could be genetically inclined to be an addict, or be an alcoholic."

Betty, unlike Carol, had remained distant from her family during most of her adult life. She had moved away from her natal and extended families; she had been estranged from her sister for many years. But after having a genetic disease, she now attends family reunions, and she said, "It makes you curious as to if that's true, you know, 'cause we don't know how they died; but if that's true, it would make me extraordinarily curious as to how they handled that. And make me real proud of the fact the family continued." She is, however, emotionally closer to the cousins who have had cancer than to those who haven't, because, "we shared a common experience that is so life-changing. And we have shared it together."

Betty thus became closer to her cousins as a result of the disease, adding, "All of the cousins, we started spending a lot of time talking about it and realized the extensiveness of the problem in the family itself. When you really sit down and lay out the family tree, a lot of us have suffered within our own family units with our parents and several cousins. So then it kind of got a little scary. We didn't really put it all together like a puzzle until after my generation started getting sick." When Betty fell ill, she, like her cousin Carol, was told that her daughters would also be afflicted with cancer. "The odds were very great that one of my daughters would get sick, and indeed one did." Betty claimed that her daughters were like two ostriches because they would not be tested and they haven't wanted to know. Even now, after one of the daughters fell ill, the second still refuses to get tested, "the rationale being the insurance thing."

Betty has considered alternative explanations for her disease. She claimed that "during the war, there were all kinds of strange things going on. I thought about that kind of stuff. I thought maybe there was some kind of tests because our parents all lived on military bases. Maybe there was something in the air. Maybe there was some carcinogen that they were exposed to. I mean, there's a whole lot of things. But too weird for them to be exposed, my grandparents, my mother, and my father. My mother and my mother's sisters and everybody—that just seems very highly unlikely. It seems a lot more easy for me to comprehend it if it was a genetic thing. It makes it understandable. I think if it was carcinogenic, I'd probably be really mad, to know that you were exposed to something that destroyed your family like that, that you didn't have anything to do with—I mean, it's sort of different than genetics. You figure genetics are part of your family and that is part of you. Not anything you can fix or anybody else did to you. It's just part of what you're made up of. And it's a part of what your mother was made up of and your mother's mother was made up of. But something coming from the outside, that your family did not—that people were exposed to that they didn't have anything to do with, wasn't their fault, or it didn't have anything to do with the way that—it's kind of hard to explain. You know what I mean." She added that she would be very angry if she were to learn that somebody else had exposed her to hazards that had caused her disease, because "it could have been prevented. And with genetics, at this point, it can't be prevented. Now, from what I understand there are studies that they're going to be able to alter genes. And if that is true, then hopefully with my granddaughters, who I worry about now, whether or not they are genetically inclined, maybe by the time they're [born], the genes could be altered." Betty believes that with gene therapy her future grandchildren will not have to worry and suffer.

Recently, Betty began attending church. She said, "I think had I gone to church more regularly, possibly I could have — it would have been a little bit easier to keep a balance, but I didn't. But I'm starting."

Betty recognizes the injustice of her condition: she avoided all the risk factors, yet she fell ill anyway. Nevertheless, she regards the disease as redemptive. She was also drawn closer to her family and kin, from whom she was more alienated than Carol, owing to their sharing a common genetic inheritance. For Betty, as for Carol, her genetic heritage establishes continuity with her past and is a source of pride precisely because of the family's ability to survive in spite of adversity. Paradoxically, for Betty her disease inheritance is a source of strength, which she conveys in her demeanor. In fact, Betty adds a unique dimension to notions of genetic inheritance, one associated with self-esteem, a stance I had neither anticipated nor encountered in other women's narratives. Her ancestral legacy, of which she is proud, is one of survival despite the "defective family" inheritance.

Betty also calls attention to a crucial aspect of the ideology of genetic inheritance: its simplicity — its reductionism — renders it elegant. As Betty points out, the explanation is easy to comprehend. Had an outsider caused the disease, including the government, a possibility she had entertained, it would have caused her great anger. The fact that she believes her disease was genetically inherited mitigates her bewilderment about why she became afflicted, despite the fact that she had done everything correctly. She has been a good person, yet she suffers from this terrible disease that has, worst of all, resulted in her weight gain and the consequent loss of her husband. While Betty adds yet another layer to the ways in which the ideology of genetic inheritance influences people's experience, she curiously conflates the inheritance of disease with the inheritance of valued physical characteristics, failing to see that, unlike the inheritance of such characteristics, the belief in the inheritance of the disease restructures her existence by conferring on her a new status of patient.

Melanie

Unlike Eliza, Jana, and Dina, who have despondently accepted their fate, Melanie, like Connie, feels she is in charge of her condition. Genetic knowledge for purposes of prevention was an important theme in Melanie's narrative. Melanie is a 50-year-old professional working woman who raised two children to adulthood by herself but recently remarried. She had developed breast cancer six years earlier, but the cancer was caught early and, after having three surgeries, she fully recovered. After Melanie fell ill, she learned that her grandmother had suffered from breast cancer and died quite young. Melanie regretted, even resented, that her mother had not informed her of her family medical history before but added that in her house, "such things were never discussed." Melanie emphasized that had she known her grandmother had died of cancer, she could have done something to prevent it in herself. After she became sick, Melanie converted to a vegetarian diet and was treated by a naturopath.

Melanie, a highly educated and articulate woman, although convinced that she inherited the propensity for breast cancer that is part of her genetic makeup, believes that her lifestyle, especially her previous diet, had triggered the affliction. Melanie also believes that she brought the cancer upon herself by being very hard on herself emotionally and physically. In Melanie's words, "Cancer gave me a message that I was not nurturing myself."

Melanie had not had a close relationship with her family, especially her grandmother, who was a remote figure. Those with whom she has the closest relationships include her friends and her cleaning lady, who had prayed for her and to whom she felt especially connected. Friendships are of greater importance than kinship for Melanie because to share experiences rather than blood is more significant for her, as it is for many people today. But not unexpectedly, Melanie became closer to her mother and sister as a result of the disease. In fact, her sister became especially concerned about developing breast cancer because the two sisters now regarded the disease as familial, a belief that reunited them as a family.

Melanie's account clearly indicates the ways in which family links can be reestablished, which runs counter to contemporary sensibilities. She was alienated from her biological family, relying more on her domestic help than on her relatives, until she learned that breast cancer existed in her family. Her understanding of her disease in genetic terms established for her a sense of continuity with her family and grandmother, whom she could only recall as a distant figure. Yet Melanie, like some of the healthy women we have met and like Connie, embraces an alternative explanation of her disease that revolves around self-blame and punishment for not having been more nurturing to herself. This case suggests that genetic ideology may not absolve everyone from assuming personal responsibility for his or her afflictions.

Chris

Chris, a 59-year-old biologist, is married to an academic geneticist. Chris, who is of Italian descent, believes that cancer is a stigma among older generations of Italians, including her family, in much the same way as Eliza described for northern Europe. Chris experienced her first bout with breast cancer around 1982, sixteen years before the interview. Several years later she suffered another cancer episode and had her second breast removed. Most recently, part of her lung had been excised after the cancer had metastasized, but at the time of the interview she was free of any cancer and very upbeat, revealing her sense of humor.

Chris's mother had died of breast cancer at the age of 74. She said, "I cannot tell you how much cancer there is in my family. On my father's side, my great-aunt died of ovarian cancer, an aunt [father's sister] died of ovarian cancer." In fact, in her father's family there were seven sisters, four of whom had died of some kind of cancer. The daughters of these women, Chris's cousins, also had breast and lung cancer, and another had spinal cancer. Chris's mother's sister died of lung cancer, but she was a heavy smoker. In recounting the family's cancer history, Chris dolefully added, reminiscent of Eliza's and Melanie's comments that "the trouble is, they don't talk about it."

Chris had been a heavy smoker before she was afflicted with breast cancer. She continued smoking, she said, "when things got stressful. And then, when the lung cancer came along, it would be, 'Jesus, how stupid are you?' " She stopped, but she sometimes reverts to smoking. Perhaps she got lung cancer from smoking, "but then, you know, I know people who smoked heavily their entire life and haven't."

Genetic inheritance ideology leads people to question how to exist with notions of probabilities. Chris, for example, raised the question when she said, "I mean that's really an issue for me. How can people do that? Even myself. How to live when you have a probability. There is a probability that I may get ovarian cancer, which is linked [to breast cancer]. And there's colon cancer that's linked to breast cancer. I'm just sitting there saying, 'Well, those are the upcoming possibilities.' " Nevertheless, Chris refused to be tested, because "I don't trust the insurance companies." Although Chris knew about the new state law that forbade insurance companies to discriminate against people who may carry "disease" genes, she nevertheless fears that insurance companies may not wish to insure her.[6]

When the discussion turned to the etiology of her disease, Chris recounted, "In the beginning it [her disease] really wasn't something that I tried to explain to myself. I had a lump early on that was kind of associated with an injury. I remember having carried some heavy luggage and stuff like that.[7] As far as what the cause was, that never became an issue with me until I started to look how [it was] in the family and learning what was going on there. I am almost dead certain it's a gene. I work for a biotechnology center, and so I know very much how powerful these tests for genes are. And the fact that they've discovered several breast cancer genes and they can check the families for that, I am aware of that. I'd love my family to go in there and work with the medical geneticists and have their pedigree."

After the doctors took a family medical history, she told her two sisters, " 'You have the potential for breast cancer,' and what I am saying to them is, 'watch yourself. If something develops, do something early, early enough for it to be useful.' " Yet, like Connie, Melanie, and even Eliza, Chris believes that it was stress "screwing up my estrogen factor, and that is why I had the disease." But then she also believes she inherited it from her paternal side. "I mean, it's really strange that they usually say that it's your mother, your sisters, your aunts. I'm wondering if it isn't on the male side. I also wonder if it isn't the breast cancer gene but one of the others [genes]." Ultimately, Chris concluded, "I don't know where this comes from. I just think that I've got a genetically defective family."

Chris regards her sisters, cousins, aunts, and uncles as her family but had distanced herself from them when she left for college and got married. However, when one of her cousins also developed breast cancer, she and her middle sister began attending family reunions and they both reconnected with the family. In fact, Chris was very clear that the disease reunited her with her extended family. She said, "This cousin was somebody that I didn't know that well. But because of the breast cancer she had started calling me and asking me questions. I have become acquainted with my cousins really because of it. And I have been sort of drawn back in to my father's family because of it. And coming back to the family for that, I talked to all these other people. In the middle of the reunion we were comparing our medical history. It should have been a really joyful occasion. Everybody was sort of horrifying each other. My sister was standing on the edge, but I mean I really think that it brought us together that way." When I asked Chris whether she felt closer to her family because she and her family shared the same disease or because she shared the same genes with them, she replied, "I really don't know how to answer that question. It's almost as if that miserable thing that happened to you is not so bad because you've now renewed the kinship. I mean, you're a family. So that I've now redeveloped the relationships with my aunts and uncles that don't have this illness, but simply because we got together over the issue of what it is we have. Not that I wish to see them because of that, but the fact that I think that the gene sort of pervades that family makes me curious about them now. I really think it's sort of a matter of a door opened."

Chris's younger sister refuses to have a genetic test because she does not wish to believe that it is a family disease. For Chris, however, the positive aspect of her disease was, in her words, "my relationship with the extended family. I'm stuck with this. It's nice to know that I'm back in the family."

Chris is grateful that she did not inherit some other disease from her family, and she added: "My mother was a depressive. My [younger] sister's manic-depressive. Thank God I didn't get manic-depression. My husband and I laugh because we believe the reports from *Science* magazine, I guess it was, that says there's a happy note to all this: that satisfaction in life is genetically determined. Whereas my younger sister, who lives a good life, is always miserable, I, who've had all these crummy diseases, figure life is pretty decent. So I think that there's that whole other personality factor, you just don't blame people for things that happen to you. But I thank God that I didn't get the unhappiness gene and the depression and the whole mental . . ."

Whereas Chris does not regard the disease as redemptive in the way, say, Jana or Carol does, she does see a positive aspect: it brought her closer to her family. Her narrative illuminates how kinship relations become structured within the context of a person's consciousness of genetic inheritance. She clearly attributes her reconciliation with her family, including her extended family, to the conceptualization of shared genetic material. Significantly, she fails to blame her ancestors for their "faulty genes" because, after all, she could have gotten an "unhappiness gene" from them, and that would have been worse than cancer.

Moreover, for Chris, as for the other women, the notion of familial inheritance of disease fosters the possibility for other family members to benefit from her affliction by being alerted to the potential risk of falling ill — although, in Chris's case, her sister refused to act on this knowledge. Yet because Chris recognizes that she cannot cope with the fact that genetic knowledge requires her to deal with probabilities, she quests for certainty, not unlike most human beings who live with a life-threatening disease.[8] Chris, unlike many of the other women we are meeting, has not embraced a religious ideology to give her the certainty that she is protected and that she will go to heaven or that it is her fate. She is left to negotiate notions of risk and probabilities — negative odds — leaving her in an abyss ruled by random chance, while also explaining her suffering as due to her "defective family."

Victoria

Like Chris, Victoria is a secular woman who regards the affliction that befell her family as a matter of bad luck. A 51-year-old business school graduate, Victoria is married with no children and lives in a well-appointed home in an upper-class neighborhood. She has worked all her life. She had a lateral mastectomy five months before we met, whereas her two sisters had had bilateral mastectomies immediately in order to avoid a recurrence of the cancer in their healthy breasts. Therefore, she too is having a prophylactic mastectomy and reconstructive surgery as soon as feasible. At the time we met, she was being treated only with tamoxifen.[9]

Victoria believes that she and her two sisters inherited breast cancer from their father's family. The fact that all the sisters were afflicted in the left breast gave Victoria the evidence that her breast cancer was genetically inherited. Moreover, three of her father's sisters had breast cancer, and one succumbed to the disease. On her mother's side, three of her siblings were afflicted with lung cancer, but Victoria quickly added, "They were all three heavy smokers." Victoria wondered if passive smoking caused her and her sisters' disease because her father had been a very heavy smoker. But then, "that wouldn't explain his sister having breast cancer." So, she concluded, it's "just bad genes."

Victoria lamented, "We're all fairly healthy otherwise and took care of ourselves. I was diagnosed with hypertension in 1995. That shocked me because I'm not overweight. I try very hard to have a really healthy diet. I exercise. I do all the right things. I think that's genetic, I really do. My dad died of a stroke, and my mother has high blood pressure and I don't know. It's in my family—dad's side more than mother's. I just feel that that [blood pressure] is especially genetic." Genetic inheritance was the only risk factor she could find to explain her high blood pressure, unless it be stress, but she was not feeling under stress.

Victoria, who, like Chris, exists within her insular nuclear family, was brought closer to her extended family because the disease is "another common thread." In addition, Victoria said, "I think one of the reasons that I did so well through my surgery and everything was the fact that my other two sisters had been through it and I had great role models and they could answer questions for me." Victoria's first memory of breast cancer was associated with one of her paternal aunts, yet she never considered it a familial disease until her youngest sister fell ill. Her illness convinced Victoria that she, too, was suffering from a familial disease. Victoria wondered what had happened in her family that brought on her genetic heritage, even though she cannot blame anyone because no one intended any harm. Her mother, however, feels guilty because her three daughters fell ill, while she did not.

The ideology of genetic inheritance is devoid of moral judgments, which is reflected in Victoria's claim, like the other women, that her ancestors cannot be blamed for having transmitted the disease to her because they had not intended to harm her. (Nevertheless, she considers anyone who lacks such an inheritance as very lucky.) While the notion of random genetic inheritance fails to carry any moral load, Victoria, like Betty and Carol, nevertheless injects moral indignation into her experience when she expresses consternation not just because she fell ill but because she had done everything right: she followed the medical rules and still became sick. Victoria can only resort to the notion of collective family luck to assuage her indignation, but she lacks any moral buttress such as a notion of predetermination to mitigate the injustice.

Victoria lacks any religious affiliation and is completely dedicated to her job. Her coworkers are a central source of support for her. "They take care of me," she said. Significantly, Victoria depends on her coworkers rather than on family for support, reflecting one contemporary pattern of relationships in America that minimizes kinship as a primary source of social support.

Lydia

Victoria's neighbor Lydia is less serene about her condition than Victoria. Lydia is 55 years old, the mother of three adult daughters, lives with her husband, and is employed as a nurse. Lydia was the first in her family to be afflicted with breast cancer, or in her words she was "the cart before the horse," meaning that she fell ill before any member of her family in the ascending generation. When her doctors initially questioned her about her family history, she told them that there was no cancer in her family. But sadly, shortly after Lydia had a mastectomy, chemotherapy, and plastic surgery, her father's two sisters died of breast cancer. The doctors informed Lydia that she had the deadliest kind of cancer and that it had spread to the wall of her chest. But all the growths were removed, and Lydia had fully recovered at the time of the interview.

Lydia believes unequivocally that the disease "was passed along in the family." When she joined a breast cancer support group, the women immediately asked if she had a family history because most of the women in the group had a family history of breast cancer. Based on the women's questions and the fact that her two aunts had suffered from the same disease, Lydia concluded definitively that breast cancer was a familial disease. She noted, "I said, 'you know, I don't really know why I didn't put two and two together: my breast cancer must have come from my dad's side of the family.'" She knew there was cancer in the family on her father's side, but she didn't really think it was hereditary until her aunts died. Before then, "I thought my chances of having breast cancer were slim because nobody had had it as far as my grandparents go." She then recalled that her mother's mother had died of cancer, "but it was very hush-hush. I wouldn't doubt that she had breast cancer that went to the colon, but they called it colon cancer."

At first, Lydia was stunned that she had breast cancer because she nursed her children deliberately so that she would avoid getting this disease.[10] She just couldn't believe it. But then she asked herself why and replied, "I don't think there's any answers for that; just cells gone awry.

And if it is genetic, then I regret that I passed it on to my three girls. I think, you do think of that, especially the one who looks so much like me."

Before she admitted to herself that her disease was hereditary, she believed that she "was just one of those people that it hit, I just thought it was the luck of the draw that I happened to get breast cancer. You know, you try to find reasons. But it wasn't like it came to me easily that it came through the family. Now there have been people studying genetics, and we've gotten packets at the breast cancer support group. With all the publicity about cloning and the genetic study and everything, I think that's brought it to the forefront. Whereas they have been saying 'do you have a family history,' all those things you make out when you go to the doctor's office, they're kind of cluing you in that it is a familial thing, that there is a connection here." By having been asked for her family medical history, she was influenced to think in genetic terms. However, Lydia had carefully thought about other explanations. "I really believe we've got so much junk in our dairy products and stuff. I really think the environment is causing a lot of cancers. We are eating so many preservatives in our food, and the big factory farms are putting too much junk in the feed the animals [eat] and everything."

Lydia's three daughters, aged 28, 30, and 31, greatly fear breast cancer because they think it may have been transmitted to them. Lydia's family is dispersed in the Midwest, but having this familial disease has "stirred up feelings. Even though it was a bad link with the rest of the family, it was still a link. It's part of being connected, you know, you marry someone and you take them for better or worse but a family, you're into it — you have no choice — God's choice, there you are, and you take the good with the bad. There's more good than there is bad."

Lydia's family, first-generation Americans, immigrated from Eastern Europe, and they were a very close family. "Family used to be ultimately important, when I was young, the extended family, like cousins. We used to write letters back and forth"; but subsequently she lost contact with them. At her last family reunion, ten years ago, after Lydia fell ill, when she met her sisters, they feared that they, too, might become afflicted by the disease; as a result, the sisters became even more estranged than before. Lydia feels closer to her girlfriends than to her relatives. "I'm not talking about family at all, whereas in the past I probably would have. I don't know where that broke down. I always wonder, would I be thinking this way if I'd never had breast cancer?"

Lydia noted that having been raised as a Catholic, faith had always been somewhat important to her, but she became a devout Catholic after her illness. "It was such a comfort to know that God was with me." She recalled that during one surgical procedure she felt the presence of God.

Lydia recognizes the ways in which medical historytaking imprints notions about genetic inheritance that also shape people's collective consciousness and affect the descending generations. For example, Lydia's daughters are currently living with anxiety about becoming ill with cancer. From this perspective, one cannot take, as Lydia, Betty, and others suggest, the good with the bad. Good inheritance obviously is not anxiety provoking for the daughters in the same way as the possibility of inheriting their mother's sickness.

Lydia's narrative calls attention to how the idea of genetic inheritance led her to remember her family and her grandmothers, people she had not thought about in the recent past. To her dismay, Lydia's family, like Jana's friends, became estranged from her because her disease threatened them. Lydia declines to blame her family for her affliction, but her family reproaches her for the presence of the disease in their family. For Lydia, her support group, her friends, and the church have replaced kinship bonds. For her, as for Karen, "blood is water." Whereas people may desire to construct friendships in the idiom of kinship, the medical construal of genetic inheritance insists that "blood is not water."

It is also noteworthy that Lydia accepts the familial cause of her disease, but she still feels morally upset that she fell ill even after she followed all the indications to avert the risk factors, especially having breast-fed her children.

Lucie

Unlike Lydia, Lucie was prepared for her affliction because she knew from her family medical history that she would inherit the disease. Neither her smiling face nor her gait disclosed that Lucie, 44 years old, married, and the mother of a 12-year-old girl, had, only three months before, developed breast cancer and undergone a radical mastectomy. At the time we met, she was still awaiting reconstructive work on the breast. The university, where customarily all of her family had worked, including her parents, had employed Lucie, who had one year of college, for 25 years.

Of Lucie's mother's six sisters, the oldest died of breast cancer, the following one has had breast cancer for 13 years, and the third died of heart problems, although she too had breast cancer, which, like Lucie's, was confined to one area. Lucie's mother had died of breast cancer seven years earlier at the age of 65 after having participated in an experimental program at the National Institutes of Health, where she had been treated for four years before her death.[11] Lucie's two youngest maternal aunts both had lumpectomies, but no malignancies were found. Lucie concluded recounting her family's medical history by saying, "My mother's mother had cancer, but I can't remember what kind it was. I think it was colon cancer. And, yeah, hers was colon cancer, and my grandfather died of heart trouble. And my one uncle, my mother's one brother, he had heart trouble."

Lucie recounted that she "had a malignancy on the left side. Since my mother was diagnosed, we've had mammograms every year automatically. When I was 32, I started getting mammograms done. And they found a spot and they did more x-rays and in radiology they said, 'Let's wait six months and see if it grows.' Well, I was not comfortable waiting six months, with my family history, to see what was going to happen. I'm not a patient person. So, I got an appointment with one of the doctors and he said, 'Well, let's ease your mind. We'll do a needle biopsy and see what we get.' Well, they did the needle biopsy and the actual spot that was there, the lump that was there was benign, but they ended up pulling out malignant tissue and it was in early stages. So it was confined just to that breast. Then they gave me the option of having a lumpectomy and probably no radiation and chemotherapy, but I opted to go with a double mastectomy and have reconstruction because they say, in an average four to five years, it comes back on the other side, and I just wanted to be rid of it. With my family history, you know, the lumpectomy, they can think they got it, but they [can] miss, you know, a spot. So it was my option to go the route I went. And I took a drastic option. A couple of the medical people think I took a drastic option, but most of them understand and support what I did. So many people nowadays, if they even have family histories, will just automatically—my next door neighbor had it when she was very young. She had it on one side. She had to go through radiation and all that. Then her mother had it; her mother died from it. Then she had it come back on the other side. Her sister, who has only had a lump that was benign, just opted to have total mastectomy because she couldn't stand worrying about what was going to happen, you know, with the family history. I always said, when my mother was alive, we had talked about it and I always said, 'Well, I wouldn't do reconstruction. I wouldn't worry about that. That wouldn't concern me.' But then I always figured I would be in my fifties when I got hit, not in my forties, and they've come so far since my mother was diagnosed eleven years ago in how they treat and do things. So, I had no trouble making my decision. I mean, I thought of just doing a lumpectomy and just check it every six months to see if it's coming back, but it just concerned me. I wanted peace of mind, which is what I'm getting from the mastectomy. I'm much more comfortable knowing that it's gone and there's, you know, my chances of it coming back are maybe one percent; whereas, with a lumpectomy, [there's] a higher percent [chance] of it coming back."

As if to reassure herself, Lucie repeatedly referred to the fact that it was her option to have the mastectomies done, that the plastic surgeon was all for it, and that it was a good decision, even though she was concerned about how she looked until the reconstruction was completed. She added, "But, you know, they said it had to be a decision I had to make. They couldn't, you know, they could only give recommendations. They recommended the lumpectomy and waiting six months to see if anything came back or that kind of stuff, but I wasn't comfortable with that. And then the doctor said, well he could understand with my family history being as high as it was, some people are diagnosed and it's the first time it hits them. They've never thought of having cancer. I mean, I'm thinking about with my mother. She always thought, she said, 'I never thought I'd have cancer. I always thought I'd have heart trouble.' And I think a lot of people haven't had an opportunity to think about cancer, and, all of a sudden, they're diagnosed, 'you've got cancer.' Whereas I've had enough time over the last eleven years to think about it and know that I just don't want to worry about it. It means going a drastic route and taking three or four months of my life and having to adjust to surgery and changes and all that. I'd rather do that and then be comfortable the rest of my life than wondering every six months, 'Is it going to come back? What's going to happen?' "

Lucie's decision, supported by her husband, was based on her family history. She believes she inherited her cancer from her mother's side. "All that history was on my mother's side, even though the father's side I don't think actually kicks in that much.[12] As far as I can gather, the father's side isn't as important as the mother's side but my father's mother had breast cancer. She actually died from heart failure, but she was diagnosed with breast cancer at age 84. She died at 89, but she went through radiation. This was back in the early '70s. She was a nurse in the war, and she was treated at a VA hospital. She ended up living five more years, and the breast cancer is not what got her; it was heart failure that got her. She just agreed to be a guinea pig for them to learn from it, which is what my mother was, in a way." She continued, "If I had done the genetic study that they were asking me if I wanted to be in. I know they had an article not long ago about most people who think it's genetic, it really isn't genetic. Well, about a month or so ago they were talking about it—just because you have one or two people in your family doesn't mean it's genetic—but I can't help but believe that if I was in the genetic study, it would come back that it was [genetic]. My sister is going to do the study, hopefully. And my sister is very interested in the testing, but she's concerned because she had so much trouble insurance-wise when she had her lumpectomy, which was eight years ago. She and my brother-in-law are in private business, and they have their own insurance policy. Well, insurance would not cover her. The insurance red tape. So, the concern is, and I'm sure they're used to this in the studies they do over there [in the School of Medicine of the university], what happens if insurance finds out? You know, a lot of insurance companies will not insure a person if they're tested. And so if you go through this gene study and you end up with the gene that says you're gonna get breast cancer, you're probably going to get breast cancer, then what's going to happen with your insurance?"

In thinking about the etiology of her disease, Lucie said, "I think it could be genetic for some people and then I think for some people it's just, maybe it could even be the food you eat." She believes that in her case it is genetic. She remarked, "You know, that business they say about the food you eat. I don't know that that's true per se, but it could be. I don't think there's one thing you can say that causes any type of cancer. I mean, I don't believe that lung cancer is going to only come from cigarette smoking — there are people that smoke cigarettes for years and years and never have lung cancer, and then there are ones that smoked and did have lung cancer. So I just think in each person it's going to be a different reason why it happens to you. I don't look at things like it's cut-and-dried — I believe I have it because it's genetic. But I don't think that could be the truth for everyone."

Lucie felt that, in addition to her genetic inheritance, she had all the risk factors that could have contributed to the onset of the cancer, including having had her daughter at age 30 and not breast-feeding. Moreover, it could also have been diet. She noted "the terrible things we grew up eating. I mean, I would say that, I would classify my whole family as a country family, which means you grew up on country cooking, you know the fats, cooking with all the fats and the grease and all the things that are supposed to be bad for you now. That's what they grew up on. And that's what we grew up on because that's the way my mother was taught to cook and that's the way she cooked. And I'm sure that probably ties into it also. I don't doubt that. I think the studies that they found where you eat the healthy foods and eat the good stuff for you and you'll live longer, I think that's probably true. Because some of mother's family who was full of the fats and the bad things for you, they had the heart trouble and they had the cancer trouble. So, all of them along the way have had something happen." Even so, Lucie believes she fell ill "because of the family history. I felt like my time would come. Mine wasn't just because my mother had it. I think, and I could be wrong about this because I'll never know the facts, I think if it was just my mother alone diagnosed, it would be different than the fact that I had all the aunts that were diagnosed. And her sister that had the kind I had, had it on one side and then, about five years later, it came back on the other. And I just think it was more than just my mother. It was having aunts; it was having my father's mother, which I didn't know at the time. I didn't know that until after I was diagnosed.

One of the geneticists said that really the father's side doesn't weigh that much, it doesn't really kick into the figuring. Now I don't know if that's true or not, but knowing that that grandmother had it, all the aunts that had lumpectomies, so far benign, but, you know, this sort of was a pattern there. I think really if you want to survey the females of my generation, the cousins that are with me, I think you would probably find most of them think they will probably get it. I mean it's just, with our family history, we would get it."

Significantly, Lucie, having had endometriosis, had had a hysterectomy. She said, "They took everything out and they thought they got it [endometriosis] all and it came back. They put me back on hormones, which just got it all stirred up again. There were apparently cells left, so it grew again. I was put back on hormones because I'd had the hysterectomy, and the hot flashes and all were real bad. I kept saying to my doctor, 'my back is hurting like it hurt when I had endometriosis.' And he said, 'there's no way it's come back. It's too early. It couldn't have come back.' He kept saying that, and finally they did an ultrasound and it had come back. But by then it was so far, it had just spread everywhere. When I had my surgery a few years ago, they had to remove parts of my colon. It had just gone in there and just wrapped itself all around everything. He was able to just remove enough and get everything sewn back so it worked, so I was very lucky."

Lucie was put on estrogen therapy for two years. The doctor put her back on it six months after that surgery because "my hot flashes, I mean I have really bad hot flashes. I have them now. Because, see, I was concerned about breast cancer. And he said, 'We're going to follow you. You're going to have mammograms all the time. I think you really need to put this back on [estrogen therapy].' He said, 'I don't think the endometriosis is going to come back again.' And so then, see, then they found the breast cancer, so now I'm off of it [estrogen] again." At the time of the interview, she was not taking any medication.

Lucie sees her cousins often, adding, "We can't help but think about it [the disease] when you look at our history. Now, my friend in the office who, I mean she's the first one in her family to have it. Well, if I was in that case I'd have to wonder, 'why me?' I mean, 'what made me have it? There's no history, so why is it here?' You know, that kind of thing. She had no history at all. Whereas I've got history, so that's what makes me think I would get it. I expected it. And I think my sister expects it. It's just the family thing. I mean, it's one of those things you get from your family. I don't feel bitter towards anybody in the family for it. I mean, it's just part of life. It's just the way the cards were dealt, I guess."

Lucie is closest to her husband and daughter and sister. But she said, "Our family communicates a lot. We have a family reunion once a year.

And, like my aunt in Florida had been sick for a while before that, so we had been calling down there. Different people take turns calling around and talking. I've got cousins in Virginia that I e-mail with. One of the cousins' sons, the one that had the type like I did, he has kids my kid's age and we get together and the kids do things together. They've grown up together. We've tried to keep them a lot because I grew up with my cousins that were here."

Lucie's account instructs us in how her genetic inheritance reinforces her connections to her family, especially her deceased maternal aunts, as well as to her paternal side of the family, whom she had not even remembered before. The genetic memory replicates itself in Lucie's constant reference to her association between her breast cancer and her family. There is a sense of inevitability in Lucie's account that reflects her intense awareness of her family medical history. She, like the healthy women we met earlier, had been a patient even before the cancer made its appearance, although she can also recite other risk factors. But it was her belief in the heritability of the disease that determined the type of treatment course she chose: radical prophylactic mastectomy of her healthy breast. While Lucie is not unaware of other etiological explanations, her belief in genetic inheritance leads her to discount the possibility that her disease was due to other factors. In fact, she need not search for other reasons, not even conceivably that the disease is associated with her estrogen treatments or the very fatty diet on which she and her family was nurtured. The ideology of genetic inheritance comforts her because it explains why she was afflicted. Lucie was comforted—unlike her coworker who similarly fell ill but who could not explain "why me" because she lacked a family history. In light of how the cards are dealt, it explains the randomness of her affliction.

Katherine

Katherine, like Lucie, had anticipated her affliction for the same reason but at a later age. At 62 years of age, statuesque and authoritative, Katherine is a widow, a mother of a married daughter, and an academic in the health professions. When we met, she was wearing a turban to cover her bald head, but it also revealed her very striking, symmetrical features.

Nine months before our meeting, Katherine had gone for a regular mammogram; a lump in her breast was discovered. She described her condition as "ductile cell carcinoma, infiltrating type, and I have a sister that has the very same cancer." Her sister, who is now 60 years old, found she had cancer when she was 44 years old, but unlike Katherine's, her sister's metastasized several times.

Katherine insisted on various treatment regimens. She had a lumpectomy with removal of all the surrounding tissues, chemotherapy, radiation, and tamoxifen treatment. Evaluating these treatment outcomes, Katherine claimed, "So as far as I know, I'm cured. I don't want it to recur. Now, our father, he had two sisters with breast cancer. And they had mastectomies and they did okay. They lived to be a good age. His father died of colon cancer, and his mother died of old age. He was from a family of ten. Two were killed in World War I and the other eight, every one of them had cancer. Yes. My father died of colon cancer, like his father. His mother died of colon, stomach, and pancreatic cancer, but I am pretty sure it was colon. His younger brother died of renal cell kidney [dysfunction]. And two sisters had breast cancer. And one sister had leukemia. Now the sister who had the breast cancer also had renal cell cancer. But that was encapsulated and it hadn't metastasized, so they took care of that by surgery. So quite a few in this family have had cancer. Different types."

Katherine's mother had died of pancreatic cancer and her maternal grandfather of throat cancer, but her maternal grandmother died of old age. One of her grandmother's sisters died of leukemia. When Katherine finished recounting her family's medical history, she said, "Aside from that, there was no cancer in my family. That's as far back as I can trace it in terms of the cancer, but my father's family had more of it than my mother's family. I have a brother that had colon polyps which were precancerous, and they were removed and he's done okay. And my sister, who had the breast and the kidney also, had polyps removed. And no problem there."

Katherine, who arrived in the United States from northern Europe with her family in 1947 when she was 12 years old, recalled, "There's eleven of us, and nobody else in the family so far has had cancer. It was sort of no surprise to me that I got cancer because of our family history. Well, one in nine women will get breast cancer; with the family weakness for cancer and the history, it doesn't surprise me. And I'm surprised that not more of my siblings have been affected by it, given our history." In fact, Katherine noted that she had anticipated it, because "I do believe that, that it's, that we're genetically programmed to have certain illnesses, and cancer was the thing in my father's family. And since both parents died of cancer, why is it a surprise? It just isn't a surprise. I mean, I basically am a very healthy person, I think. I walk three or four miles a day and I eat right and I have a positive mental health attitude — I look at the bright side of things. That's not to say that I haven't experienced stress. I have. Plenty."

Katherine, like Melanie and Eliza, considers stress as a possible cause of the disease. "I think the weakness is there, and I think stress plays a much bigger part than people give it credit. And I think that they're finding this out from people who have cancer that they have stresses in their lives." She identified several stressors that she had experienced, including difficulties in selling a house, problems with family members, and, most important, her daughter's epilepsy. Katherine projects herself as a "take-charge person" and said, "I felt exhausted for the first time in my life and so I think that that may have triggered that, indeed there was a [cancer] cell there, perhaps—we all have them, I think—and your immunity [is compromised]." But ultimately, Katherine believes she has inherited the disease from the family. Her condition is not, she observed, "like schizophrenia, not like bipolar disorder, but there is a genetic weakness, and, given enough stress and environmental conditions, yeah. I believe that [it is genetic]. I had already thought this is something that we're going to have to watch in our generation. Both parents dying of cancer. Grandparents dying of cancer. Aunts and uncles dying of cancer. Because of the family history, I think I'd be a fool not to wonder, 'might this happen to me?' when, you see, both parents died of cancer." Considering all this, she concluded, "You do everything that you can. You eat right, you exercise, and you take reasonably good care of yourself. You don't smoke, you don't drink, you don't do the kind of high-risk behaviors that make for a problem." Knowing that they had a family history, Katherine and her siblings were alerted to do "everything right. They all have an exercise program. None of them are overweight. None of them smoke. None of them drink, and they have a positive outlook on life."

The disease Katherine believes she inherited forms part of her overall inheritance. Like Betty, Katherine regards inheritance as "balanced. I got from them, I think, intelligence. I got from them good looks. I got from them, motivation, stick-to-itiveness, high energy. And those are the good things. And, yeah, I can't [say] we're perfect specimens. We have genetic endowments that are superior, so I guess that's just the way things go. Now, if there was any kind of, if I had contributed to my daughter's epilepsy in any way, that would have really stressed me out no end. But not really. There's no history in the family, and so cancer is just something that you do your best [with]." Katherine reported that she had received the results of the BRCA-1 warning gene, "and it was negative. And I think they're working on the BRCA-2 gene."

After I explained my study to Katherine's daughter, who was present for a few minutes before Katherine arrived in the house, the woman immediately responded by saying that genetic inherited diseases "make you reflective about your heritage." When I repeated what her daughter had said to Katherine, she rejoined, "Well, I'm not of childbearing age. I imagine if I were a young woman of, say, about 30 who was diagnosed with cancer, in looking at family, I would have been maybe upset and angry that I got this because I was handed this genetic endowment that was a curse more than anything else, being young. But I've lived my life and I've had a good life, a difficult life, but I see this as just one more thing that I need to get through. But as I see it, it's not the end of my life. I have a sense that I'm going to be around for a long while. And it's just another invitation to grow emotionally and spiritually is really how I look at it."

Katherine emphasized that, while she was not surprised to get the disease, she also thought, "but I got it early, and let's do what needs to get done in order to get well," adding, "I don't see myself as having gotten ill. I really don't. I had these cancer cells growing, and I grabbed ahold of it and had them excised. The cure was what made me ill. Yeah, I was cut, mutilated, poisoned, and burned for the cure. But the cancer itself, no. And I don't think of myself as still having cancer. I also know that there's no guarantee that I won't get it back, but I have done everything within my power to make sure that it doesn't come back. But I still have a chance that [I'd get it again], unless they took out every node in my body and [those nodes are] negative."

Having the disease gave Katherine new insights. "My first reaction to it was, when I got the diagnosis, was kind of disbelief. God, what does that feel like, to say I have cancer? Well now I know what that feels like. And I was kind of numb. Then the next thing I felt, the next day, was some anger. That my life, that my life is the way it is, that I have to go through this alone [she has been a widow for 14 years], and that my daughter was out of the country [at a university] and I was a little bit sorry for myself. Why did this have to happen to me? Isn't it enough that my husband died, that I have a child that isn't well, that dah dah dah dah dah. So isn't it enough that these things have come my way? I had two marriages. My first marriage ended in divorce, and then I met this other man, who was a very good, stable, kind, loving person who not only loved me but loved my daughter unbelievably. So he died of lung cancer, and, yeah, I felt sorry for myself, but I was also aware of the fact that I needed to watch my own health because stress causes problems with immunity. I know that. And I felt that very much I needed to take good care of myself after he died. I went through tremendous grief. I really truly did. I think I grieved all the ungrieved losses of my life during that period of time. I left my country when I was 12 years of age, and that's a horrible time to have a child move anyway. I not only lost my home, I lost my friends, and I lost my culture. And we came to America and it was a strange and frightening place for me to be and I didn't acclimate to it really. I got to feeling real depressed at 13, 14, and 15. So I grieved my parents' deaths and, of course, then grieved my husband's death as well. But then I talked it through with friends, did some weeping, and by Sunday morning I woke up with, I'm going to get through this. I'm going to do whatever I need to do in order to conquer this. And so I talked to people at work who work in oncology and I said, 'All right. I'm going for this interview with this team. What do I need to ask?' And one of the people, who is a breast cancer survivor, said, 'I'll come with you, Katherine.' And I said, 'No, you won't. I want to present myself.' And so they wrote out the questions, made sure I understood them, 'cause my background is psych, it's not med-surg anymore, and we thought through what my options were and then when I met with the team, I knew what points to ask about my illness, my cancer. And I got all of those questions answered, and then I talked about what the options were and, after, they told me what the options were and told me that I should take a couple of days and think about it. And I did and then I went to the doctor and said what I want: "I want the surgery, the chemo, and the radiation. And I was okay from that point on, when I knew it was going to be done."

As in Lucie's case, the fact that Katherine knew it was a familial disease influenced her therapeutic choices. She noted, "Given my sister's experience, she just had surgery, breast reconstruction, and chemo. She didn't have radiation. And I knew that the type of chemo that I chose, it's pretty tough. It's one of the toughest in terms of side effects, because it knocked out — my white count went all the way down to 300, and my neutrophils, the fighters, went down to 100, and they're normally 5–7,000.[13] And I was very vulnerable. But I also knew that there are medical ways to cope, and when the first treatment made me so sick, I said, 'You've got to find me another management here, another way to manage the nausea and the side effects.' And they did. And I got up every day, put my makeup on, and I went to work. I didn't last long, but I did it."

Katherine insisted on the most drastic type of chemotherapy because she knew breast cancer was a genetic disease. She requested to participate in a study because, she said, "I wanted to participate in any kind of medical research because I have a daughter, because I have nieces, and also because I knew that I'd get closely monitored if I were in a medical study. So I am in a medical study." Katherine inquired about a mastectomy because of "family history. And I asked about having a mastectomy as opposed to a lumpectomy, and what the surgery oncologist told me was that the rate of death for women who get a recurrence of their cancer was the same for mastectomy as it was for lumpectomy.[14] And so I said, I asked then, 'Okay, what's the comparison with recurrence, if the deaths from it is the same?' They said they thought that it was pretty much the same also."

Katherine, who had moved away from her natal family to live in various parts of the country, depends more on her friends than on her family. But she was brought closer to her sisters because "I think that having a second sister with this, in their minds, increased their vulnerability and so they rallied round. 'Let's help you in every way we can.' And so they talked to me, and they called me very frequently, and one said she'd come down, and I said, 'You don't need to. One of my friends from a different state is going to come down to stay with me.' "

Katherine, like Lucie and the others, is very much aware of her family history because of having become afflicted with a disease she believes was transmitted to her by her family, but she does not hold them responsible for her disease. Katherine, too, interjects a moral dimension into her narrative when she voices in despair her frustration with the fact that after having done everything right, she fell ill — even though she was certain that she would inevitably fall ill. For Katherine, as for Lucie, it was not "if I get sick," but "when I get sick," as a consequence of her firm belief in genetic inheritance. Katherine was the only one to note that she would have been angry with her family had the disease affected her at an earlier age when she was still in the reproductive phase of her life. Intriguingly, however, she expressed no concern about her daughter. Consistent with her emphasis on genetic inheritance, Katherine equates inheritance of the disease with the intelligence and good looks her family bestowed on her. She forgets, as Betty and others do, that the personal and physical attributes she inherited and of which she is so proud did not turn her into a suffering patient even before she became symptomatic, as the notion of inheriting the disease has done.

Suffering, in Katherine's Christian tradition, nevertheless redeems her, as it does many of the women we have met. It is also important to keep in mind that genetic inheritance ideology led her to instruct her family to live a healthy life in order to mitigate the effects of genetic inheritance. By doing so, Katherine also became closer to the family with whom she previously had minimal contact. Moreover, for Katherine, as for so many of the women, the concept of having inherited her disease brings into her consciousness the ancestors who bequeathed her her genetic inheritance.

Sandra

I conclude this chapter with Sandra, whom I met in her luxurious home, which she had constructed shortly after she fell ill, when she turned to housing development to "challenge my cancer." As soon as I arrived in her house, Sandra, a 54-year-old, married, vivacious woman, announced, "I have an interesting cancer [case] because I had had prophylactic mastectomies. So I am a person with no breasts who got breast cancer." Sandra, referring to her mother, who had died of heart disease at the age of 42, said, "She might have developed breast cancer [if she had lived]. My grandmother died of breast cancer when she was 70, which metastasized to her liver. Her sister died in her 50s of liver cancer, which we now believe was a metastasis of a breast cancer because she never went to the doctor until she was at death's door. She would never have done breast exams or anything, so she died of that. My father just died of Parkinson's last year. I have very, very few people left, but I've always been afraid of breast cancer."

Sandra's mother, like Sandra, was an only child. "I come from a very small family, and I found out about my familial history when my grand-mother's niece came to my father's funeral. I hadn't seen her for years. Turns out that she had had breast cancer. Her older sister had died of breast cancer. She has another sister who has breast cancer." Sandra's grandmother's nieces and great-nieces all had breast cancer. After learn-ing about all the family members who had cancer, Sandra concluded, "There is a strong family history, which was a big surprise to me. I didn't know all of them had had breast cancer," because she hadn't had any contact with them. When Sandra learned about her family history last year, she assumed that "there has got to be some genetic link. And I'm almost positive my great-aunt died of this. It was a revelation that this disease had shown up so much in my family." She regrets more, she said, her "fat legs that came from my grandmother than my breast cancer. It's one of the things you get. You get fat thighs, you get pretty eyes, you get breast cancer."

The people closest to Sandra include her husband, her two children, and her grandchildren. She had always lived apart from her family, but now she found them through the disease. In fact, she began feeling closer to her family when she had learned about her family medical history. "I thought about the cousins more, my mother's cousins more, because I hadn't seen them for 25 years. And I did, I thought, 'that's amazing.' And I really would like to see them, but not because of the breast cancer. Just because I hadn't seen them for a long, long time and then I remembered when I was a little kid playing with her daughter, it just sort of . . . You see, I have almost no family left. I have one aunt." Sandra's father's family was very small, too; so, she said, "It was kind of nice to find out that I have got some more family out there if I just looked around." Sandra came to this realization because she shared a common hereditary disease. She de-clared, "It made me want to contact this cousin who came and find out whether her sister died of liver metastasis."

Sandra feels fortunate because she has an adopted daughter. "So she's not going to get this breast cancer." She is relieved that her grand-children are not genetically related to her. "Now, that doesn't mean they won't get breast cancer, but you know my daughter is adopted and these are her children, her two little girls. And so, they are not going to inherit it from me, at least." Sandra is pleased that the genetic factor was halted with her. She gave birth to a son, and she knows that men can also get breast cancer, but they will not require prophylactic mastectomies. Like

Leah, she refuses to be tested because "there's nothing we could do with the information that would be of any benefit to him."

Sandra never asked herself, "why me," because she, like Lucie and Katherine, had anticipated the affliction. In fact, Sandra observed, "they used to say that it was an injury that brought it about, but of course we know it doesn't. So I grew up with this almost dread of breast cancer. When I kept having these lumps, I decided to have a prophylactic mastectomy. They scooped the breast out and did silicone implants. I remember the surgeon saying, 'Well, you won't get breast cancer now.' " Reminiscent of Lucie's treatment regimen, when Sandra began having hot flashes, the doctor suggested estrogen therapy. He was not concerned about cancer because, he assured her, " 'You don't have any breasts.' I also do not have a uterus because I had fibroids and had a hysterectomy when I was 40, so this seemed like a no-brainer." She took estrogen replacement therapy for two years, and then, "I got this little pea below my chest wall." Initially, Sandra ignored it, believing she was totally protected from breast cancer. But it turned out to be breast cancer. She recalled, "It was sitting up on the chest wall. Now they had to take the back muscle because that's where it was sitting."

Sandra easily got through the surgery, but when she went to the beach and had to wear a bathing suit, she discovered that the prostheses "go boing, they don't hang right. So then you have to get like the old falsies because they are hard. So then when you lie on the beach, one [breast] lies down and one sticks up. I don't want to deal with that, so I had a tran flap reconstruction."[15] She felt very well. "They described it as a 'favorable cancer.' And if that's not an oxymoron, I don't know what is." Had she known that there was still vulnerable tissue left, she would have refused to take estrogen replacement therapy. The doctors didn't seem to know that, either, because "they assumed if you had no breasts you couldn't get breast cancer."

Despite her family medical history, Sandra is convinced that the estrogen she was prescribed caused her breast cancer. Her view is that she had inherited the propensity for cancer, which was brought out by the estrogen. Otherwise, she was always healthy. She ate well and was very active. She added, "But when you go to any gynecologist, particularly male gynecologists, they will pooh-pooh this idea that it [estrogen] could cause breast cancer, because otherwise my body was healthy."

Sandra's account reveals that owing to her family medical history, she rediscovered and became closer to her biological family. She established a new connection with her kinship group, and she also remembered relatives from the past.

Ironically, Sandra, like Betty and Katherine, gives equal weight to her family's entire legacy, her fat legs and her cancer, as if the two legacies were of the same magnitude. It merits repeating that inheritance of fat legs does not necessarily bring kin closer together or convert the person into a patient.

Sandra indicated to me that her daughter is now searching for her birth parents. Interestingly, Sandra is also interested in knowing about her daughter's birth parents in order to learn "what they look like." When Sandra observed that her daughter did not look like her, she quickly reminded herself that her biological son did not resemble her either, but this acknowledgment did not impede her from considering that her daughter needs to find her birth mother in order to discover who she looked like. Sandra's comments about her adopted daughter's search are particularly relevant to the subject of my next chapter, which focuses on adoptees who had searched or were searching for their birth parents. As we will learn, these searches emerge out of an ideology of genetic inheritance. However, for adoptees the very same tenets produce different, arguably less positive, consequences than for the women with a family history of a disease.

Before I turn to the adoptees, it is important to reemphasize the multifarious themes, set on a template of similar understandings, that we encounter in these narratives. All the women in this chapter seek to make sense of their affliction, but they give individual interpretations of its meaning. With the exception of Tina, Leah, and Dina, who reject the belief in genetic inheritance outright, the women negotiate with themselves various interpretations, although a few, like Jana, Chris, and Lydia, for example, are also conflicted by alternative explanations centered around environment, stress, and diet. The women accept, with varying intensity, that they had inherited the disease from somebody in the family, to which, with the exception of Lydia, they became closer because of shared inheritance. As we saw, Lydia's suffering became a danger signal to her sisters. The women were also led to remember relatives whom they may not even have known or thought about. For Chris, Melanie, Katherine, Victoria, and Lucie, for instance, the ideology leads them to view their sickness as a random event, a matter of luck, whereas Jana, Betty, Dina, and Tina regard it as their fate and a form of redemption. The same ideology encourages Katherine, Liza, Connie, Melanie, and Carol to take charge and alert other members of the family including the descending generation to take preventive measures. Interestingly, when we move to the adoptees we will find greater uniformity in their comprehension of genetic inheritance ideology.

Chapter 7
People Without a Medical History

Adoptees

In the last chapter we saw how women with a family medical history of cancer were variously guided by the ideology of genetic inheritance of disease. The majority of patients we met accepted notions about genetic inheritance while also entertaining alternative explanations of the disease. Of course, some of the women may have relegated alternative interpretations to occasional musings; only a few rejected, if incompletely, the belief that their affliction was produced by genetic inheritance. When patients act, informed by the ideology of genetic inheritance of disease, they perceive their actions as beneficial to themselves and their families. Or, as we saw in Sandra's case, she was relieved to know that her adopted daughter is genetically unrelated to her, which protects Sandra's daughter and grandchildren from affliction. Thus, a nongenetic family connection was regarded by Sandra as a supreme advantage. Unlike cancer patients, adoptees who search for their birth mothers are also informed by the ideology of genetic inheritance; ironically, however, their actions may result in conflict and distress,[1] and their lack of genetic connection to their families may be a source of great sorrow. Moreover, the people we met in the last two chapters became especially conscious of their family and kinship ties as a result of their family medical histories. However, adoptees in this study experienced an ongoing consciousness of family and kinship owing to their *lack* of a medical history and their contingent relationship with their adoptive family associated with the ideology of genetic inheritance.

Adoption is, of course, not a recent phenomenon in Western history. In fact, in Rome it was a privileged form of establishing kin ties, as we saw in Chapter 2. As a matter of fact, Veyne observed that "the frequency of adoption is yet another proof that nature played little part in the Roman conception of the family."[2] In ancient Rome, adoption took place at any age in order to preserve the family name, which was central to the society.

The Roman notions concerning kinship stand in marked contrast to contemporary understandings of the meaning of adoption.

Because American culture has always emphasized blood ties, adoption has never been the favored mode of establishing kin ties. Adoption began to acquire its contemporary meaning about 150 years ago; according to Minow and Shanley, "The growing acceptance of formal legal adoption from the mid-nineteenth century on reflected the notion that binding relationships between parent and child could be created by volition and consent, as well as by biology, *although adoption did try to mirror the 'natural family' through efforts to match race and religion as well as to seal from view the adoptee's family of origin*" (emphasis added).[3] Although views of adoption were changing, the significance of biology in the definition of family precluded the legal recognition of adoptive families until the twentieth century. Dolgin states, "By the late nineteenth century, statutory law provided for adoptive families in the United States and Great Britain, and only in the twentieth century were such families afforded real protection by the law. To some extent, the legal recognition of adoptive families represented an early acknowledgment that the love and intimacy that are supposed to characterize the parent-child relationship need not be anchored in biology. For decades, however, the law continued to insist that adoption be structured 'in imitation of biology.' "[4]

In this chapter I present vignettes of people who have searched, or are searching, for their birth mothers[5] and who either were members of a support group or had friends who had similarly searched.[6] Their searches bring into bold relief the ways in which kinship and genetic inheritance ideologies in American society drive the adoptee's endeavor. The adoptees we will meet struggle with fragmentation in the lived world, characteristic of postmodern times, resulting in conflict between their belief in genetic inheritance as the true definition of kinship and the love and intimacy that defines an adoptive family. This conflict is revealed in published reports about adoption. In fact, there is a substantial body of literature, not uncommonly written by adoptees or adoptive parents, that explores why people search.[7] With some variation, the discussions found in the literature preview some of the central issues discussed by the adoptees I interviewed.[8]

Robert Andersen, an adoptee and a psychiatrist, identifies two types of reasons adoptees search: intellectual and emotional. The intellectualized reasons for searching are to complete their genealogical charts and medical histories, whereas the emotional reasons are the desire to see, touch, and speak to their blood mothers, fathers, sisters, and brothers and to know their parents' occupations. Were they teachers, secretaries, nurses, astronauts, neurosurgeons, helicopter pilots, or prostitutes? He muses:

Does it matter if one's birth mother was a harlot instead of a nurse? I think so. Would you rather have a racehorse out of Winning Colors . . . or the mare down the road? What do people mean by the phrases: Blood is thicker than water; chip off the old block; like father, like son; it's in the blood? What is meant by the proverb, 'The daughter of a crab does not give birth to a bird'? Why do so many singers have children who can sing, athletes have children who are athletic, professors have children who are bright, and alcoholics have children who drink too much? . . .

Our genes largely determine our biology, psychology and characters. Although environment plays a role in human development, it merely interacts with biology; it does not eradicate it (emphasis added).[9]

Andersen, whose book was recommended to me by many adoptees, speculates that his mother may have been a prostitute, which he believes may be an advantage, because "possibly I come from a line of survivors. Maybe my genes help me to be pragmatic, businesslike, or unconventional." He unequivocally stresses that blood is the adoptee's heritage, and those who never know their heritage are the poorer for it: "A lack of generational continuity adds a degree of vulnerability to all the adoptees' interpersonal relationships. In fact, some experts believe this discontinuity constitutes the core of adoptees' psychological problems," because adoptees are viewed as having come from nowhere, without roots or family tradition.[10]

Writing with some skepticism about the adoptees' search phenomenon, Elizabeth Bartholet, an adoptive mother, claims that adoption is a stigma because of the principle that blood ties are essential to parenting. She recognizes that in American society "biological origins are central to our destiny" and that "it is only genetically linked parents who are truly entitled to possess their children and to whom children truly belong." Along with Andersen, Bartholet similarly observes that the assumption of the search movement is that "adoptees must forever suffer the loss of their birth parents and the related loss of genetic continuity with the past," and that they are prone to " 'genealogical bewilderment' as they struggle to live a life cut off from their genetic origins."[11] In short, according to this literature, adoptees are in pursuit of their genetic sameness, which is taken to be equivalent to their true family, their significant same.

Bartholet, like Andersen, asserts that adoptees suffer because they are cut off from their biological links and because generational continuity is destroyed. She observes that "sperm donors, their offspring, and birth mothers in surrogacy arrangements increasingly voice complaints of the pain they suffer from being cut off from genetic forebears or descendants,"[12] although she rightly claims that parenting cannot be equated with procreation. She wisely observes that a sense of immortality does not come with passing on one's genes but with the parental relationship with a child and how it shapes that being. She concludes, "All adoptions require parents to transcend the conditioning that defines parenthood in terms of procreation and genetic connection."[13]

Before I move to the adoptees' narratives, I must emphasize that the majority of adoptees do not search for their birth parents. According to Lynn Giddens, former Coordinator of the Center for Adoption Education of North Carolina, 1.9 out of 4 adoptees search for their birth parents; that is to say, 47 percent of those who were adopted search. The 53 percent of adoptees who do not search purportedly have various reasons, including denial of their real feelings, loyalty to their adoptive parents, lack of interest, or lack of mental energy. In Lynn's words,

You have to have some form of stability to be able to even undergo the process. Dysfunctional people would certainly find it difficult to start and finish, because it is an emotional and time-consuming process. It seems to be people that are comfortable — most of the people who I see search are comfortable with themselves, and they want their answers to finish formulating their image of themselves and their past and their background. People who are very unhappy with themselves normally don't search, from what I see. The argument is that such people are too busy trying to survive the consequences of that. People search at considerable emotional and financial cost. The emotional search is draining and also there is an ambivalence of not wishing to hurt the adoptive family's feelings.[14]

Along with Andersen it could be argued that the search for a birth parent fulfills an existential need for human beings to know "where they came from," meaning who brought them into this world. If Andersen's argument is correct, it would refute Schneider's assertions that the significance human beings give to blood relationships is simply a social construction. Would an individual coming from a society where blood relationships are not given cultural currency wish to meet, nevertheless, the woman from whose belly he or she had emerged? Would a Navajo, a person from Yap, or a Roman, for that matter, even be curious about the woman who brought him or her into the world? Or would persons from these societies find such concern with physical origins incomprehensible? These questions cannot simply be theorized; they require empirical data from societies such as the Navajo or Yap to enable us to tease out whether an individual's desire to know the person who gave him or her birth is a universal existential human preoccupation or whether this quest is molded, like kinship relations, by cultural conceptualizations. In the absence of empirical data, I hypothesize that while the notion that blood is thicker than water is not universally accepted, the interest in knowing from whose loins one came forth may be universal, Schneider's compelling arguments notwithstanding.[15]

Our current state of knowledge allows us to advance the notion that adoptees in America may have been curious about their birth parents from the inception of the practice of closed adoptions because of the way the culture emphasizes blood kinship. Significantly, however, the search movement came into bloom beginning in the 1960s,[16] not coincidentally around the same time when conceptions of family began to change, when our collective consciousness concerning genetic inheritance came into the forefront, and when notions about diseases as genetically programmed began once more to take root in biomedicine. It will be recalled from the discussion in Chapter 4 that eugenics and concepts of genetic determinism applied to human behavior and human sickness had lost their luster following World War II, not to become prominent again until the 1960s.

Certainly, adoptees' desire to obtain a biomedical and genetic history is one significant reason for them to embark on the difficult project of searching for their birth parents, supporting the notion of the medicalization of kinship, which I will develop in the next chapter. But I hasten to add that the desire to obtain a medical history is not the only reason for searching for various individuals. As we will see, although adoptees share several reasons for searching, some have additional, idiosyncratic motives. To listen to the extraordinary efforts each adoptee expended to find his or her birth mother is to be deeply moved by the odyssey. Searching requires resourcefulness, stamina, and an ability to cope with potential rejection.

Unlike the women we met in the last two chapters, the adoptees in this study almost all shared the same notions of the predominance of biology. They believed that genetic transmission influenced their health status and shaped them as individuals even down to their quirks of personality. Their complete acceptance of the ideology of genetic inheritance motivated them to seek their birth parents to discover their *real* being and to learn about their medical histories. The fifteen people I introduce in this chapter all shared similar longings to know their genetic parents and to learn about their biological parents' medical histories. All were invariably questioned by physicians about their family medical histories, and biomedical ideologies frame their lives, as do conceptualizations of genetic inheritance.[17] Yet, as we read their narratives, we also learn specific concerns of each of these conflicted women and men.

The people in the group, overwhelmingly women,[18] ranged in age from 20 to the late 50s. They were all seemingly in overall good health, but their relationships to their adoptive parents varied. With one exception, all the individuals were adopted when they were two to three months old; and, with one exception, they all knew, from an early age, that they had been adopted. Most were born to poor women, but, not surprisingly, all were adopted by middle- or upper-middle-class families. If we accept the fact, as I do, that class differences tend to promote cultural differences, then, from a developmental perspective, one would not expect these individuals to share interests or experiences with their birth parents, if only because the birthing mothers and their biological adopted offspring experienced dissimilar opportunities and life chances. Yet, as we will see, most of those who found their birth mothers are certain that they and their birth mothers possess the same interests, habits, beliefs, and practices, underscoring the adoptees' conceptualizations of themselves as genetically and biologically molded beings. They all conceive of themselves as passive receptacles that lack any agency: biology has sealed their beings. While the accounts reveal how the ideology of genetic inheritance of disease and of personality characteristics has influenced the adoptees' day-to-day experiences, it is important to listen to their separate narratives in order to grasp each nuanced voice, which also disclose individual motives for searching. I turn first to those who have found their birth mothers. Their accounts reveal the ambiguities and dissonance between the realities of their lives and the ideologies by which they are guided.

Case Narratives: People Who Found Their Birth Parents

Kristen

I begin with Kristen, who recently became the new leader of the support group. Articulate, determined, and extremely knowledgeable about adoption laws, Kristen is 31 years old and married with three young children. She has two years of college and lives in a well-appointed middle-class subdivision. She began her search, lasting seven years and ten months, for her birth mother when she was 21 years old. Kristen at last found her birth mother about eight weeks prior to our meeting. She initiated her search shortly after her first child was born, primarily to obtain a medical history but also to know from whom she had inherited her personality and why she was given away.

Kristen claimed she was obsessed with procuring her medical history, especially since she was suffering from Raynaud's disease, which she described as a circulatory disorder characterized by muscle aches and weight gain or loss. In Kristen's case, she had gained twenty pounds in the past year. In her understanding, Reynaud's disease is the precursor of lupus in at least 35 percent of the sufferers.[19] Kristen commented, reflecting the sentiments of almost every adoptee I met, that "when you go to the doctor you do not have a medical history and you are not a person."

Kristen recounted that because she lacked a medical history it took two years for Blue Cross/Blue Shield to approve her need for a hysterectomy. She was being treated for endometriosis and her doctor wished to perform a hysterectomy, but Blue Cross would not authorize the procedure. Kristen maintained that if she had had a medical history she would have received the procedure immediately rather then having to undergo tests for two years.[20] Furthermore, Kristen observed that it was very important to have a family medical history because she would know what she was passing on to her children. She said, "You don't know what I could have given them that would hurt them."

Kristen contacted the agency that had handled her adoption to advise them of her Raynaud's condition and to request her medical history. When the agency found her file, she was informed, in Kristen's words, " 'Well, do you know that your maternal grandmother died of lupus?' And I was like, 'What? Whoa, wait a minute, you're sitting on this information, you never told me.' I got very upset." When she received the information about her family, Kristen called her doctor and told her that she was adopted and that her maternal grandmother had suffered from lupus. Kristen said the doctor "got real quiet, and said, 'You need to find your family. You need to be getting physical documents about your family history.' " The doctor also told her that there is a strong maternal genetic link with Raynaud's disease and lupus. Kristen noted, "All on the same branch of diseases. After I found out, I was like a demon. I was not only dealing with my children's health, my curiosity, but I was dealing with my health."

Upon learning that her grandmother had suffered from lupus, Kristen requested a lupus test. It was false positive, meaning, Kristen explained, that "I have lupus, but you know they're like you show no signs. I very well could have lupus next year. But to determine that I definitely did not need to start medication, my general practitioner sent me to several specialists to rule out that it is a [genuine] false positive. So I don't have to be on medicines." But Kristen is currently on a one-year recall visit schedule for blood tests for lupus because of the information she had gathered about her genetic background.

When she found her birth mother, Kristen learned that her maternal grandfather had died from a heart attack when he was 34 years old. She said, "When I found my birth mother, she's opened her entire life to me, her medical records, my grandmother's medical records, my great-grandmother who's 93 and still alive had gotten her doctor to get up stuff for me. And my great-aunt Lois has done the same. And the whole family is riddled with arthritis, my grandmother died of lupus, my mother has connective tissue muscle disorder, and so I was able to call my doctor back and say, 'This is what I've got in my background.' And the doctor started laughing, saying, 'God, no wonder you're gonna test positive for lupus, you're always gonna test positive for lupus.' " The doctor, a rheumatologist, told Kristen that with her background and genetic makeup, " 'You're asking for a lot of problems,' " — that she will become afflicted with arthritis later on, and that the "Raynaud's disease will get worse — and I was started on medication for that. I was also told, 'You will have to watch yourself, because of the genetic background there.' " Kristen is convinced she has inherited all these disorders from her birth mother.

Kristen lamented that she wished she had learned sooner that she came from a family with lupus because it would have explained her circulatory problems, her cold fingers and toes, especially in wintertime. Had she known that this condition was part of her family heritage, she would have been assured sooner that she "was not crazy," she said. In fact, Kristen reported that the doctors had not taken her symptoms seriously until she was able to show that others in her family had suffered from the disorder. The medical history not only recounted for Kristen her family history but, significantly, affirmed her sanity.

When Kristen found her birth mother, she also discovered that she had a half sister with cerebral palsy, and she wished she had known that before she had children. She commented, "It would have at least been tested when I was pregnant. It wouldn't have changed anything, but I would have been prepared emotionally."

Kristen discussed her strong resemblance to her birth mother: she looked just like her. Even more astonishing to Kristen, her birth mother, like her, possesses, in Kristen's description, "weird mannerisms." Kristen gave the example that her "foot was always shaking, legs crossed. Where did I get these expressions from? Her facial expressions were the same. We are so much alike, it's very scary. Looking at her is like seeing myself in twenty years. I am referring to character, our personalities are exactly alike, but I hope not physically. She has taken a lot of medicine for a medical condition." Kristen noted all that she had inherited from her birth mother, "because how hard I struggled to be what my adopted parents wanted me to be, the perfect little lady. I would try, I couldn't do it. I mean, it was not just too hard. It wasn't me." Kristen thinks and feels like her birth mother, giving the example that "my adopted mother doesn't hug. She's not very affectionate. When I met my birth mother she was the same way as me — very touchy, very huggy, very open with her emotions, her feelings, and on the other hand, my parents have never figured out why I'm so touchy." Also, Kristen added, "I was not raised to be opinionated, mouthy, such a strong person, but that is who I am and that's who I'm most comfortable being. And to find out that my birth mother [Kristen refers to her by her first name] is the same way, it really makes me think that we're more genetic on who we are, than how we're raised."

In order to find herself, Kristen needed to find her birth mother. She continued, "I am nothing like my adopted family. My beliefs, I'm very liberal. My parents are dyed-in-the-wool conservatives. It's either black or white. Our political beliefs are not the same; our religious beliefs are, but in the way we deal with things on a day-to-day basis we aren't alike. You put me and my adopted family at a family reunion, and I stick out like a sore thumb. I look different. I act different. I am a very strong-willed, very independent woman, and none of my aunts or female cousins are strong. I fight for my political beliefs, I fight for my rights, and I'm not going to give it to you; and if you don't like it, oh, well, don't ask my opinion again. My family's not like that at all. Either side." After having met her birth mother, Kristen knew that all that came from her biological mother. In fact, Kristen finds it extremely curious that after having been separated for 31 years from her birth mother, they are so much alike.

To obtain medical records, Kristen searched for her birth father as well, especially because she has reason to believe that "there was high blood pressure and diabetes in his family, and I want to have the medical history." Members of her father's family had died of heart disease; and Kristen added, "If his mother was crazy, then I may need a psychiatrist."

Subsequently, Kristen found three men who could have been her father, and she had asked them for a DNA test. The test showed that none of the men was her father. Kristen was distressed by these findings because the man who presumably was her father denied it and refused to share his medical information, whereas one of the men whose DNA had not matched hers insisted he was her father and wrote her into his will. Kristen was less enthusiastic about a potential inheritance and more distressed that she lacked her father's medical history.

Significantly, while Kristen believes that she was shaped by her birth mother, the people she regards as closest to her include her adoptive mother and her husband and children.

We can glean important themes from Kristen's narrative regarding the role genetic inheritance plays in a person's recognition of kinship. Kristen's commitment to a biomedical ideology that focuses on genetic inheritance informs her intense desire for knowledge of her medical history and her understanding that her entire being is actualized by her genetic makeup. From a biomedical perspective and the perspective of the adoptee, the medical history confers a personhood not only of one's existence in the present but also of one's past. The people who share her genetic heritage are those who have bestowed her with her being rather than the people who have raised and educated her. Consider also that Kristen confounds various facets of her person with genetics, including physical resemblance and political activism.

Like many of the other adoptees we meet here, Kristen's emphasis on medical history anchors her person in her patienthood. Her biomedical understanding of genetic inheritance requires her even to be on an annual recall schedule and to take certain medications. For Kristen, as for the other adoptees, kinship means biological connection, validated by a medical history that firmly establishes her continuity with past and present, with her birth mother's mother and her birth mother, whom she had finally met after 31 years. The medical history, by recapitulating genetic inheritance, turns into a kinship history and an ideological map of the past. Importantly too, having her biological family's medical history affirmed for Kristen her sanity. Only when she could demonstrate a genetic history did her doctor take her symptoms seriously and acknowledge that her ills were not "in her head."[21] In this instance, a genetic medical history is equated with mental stability.

We cannot second-guess any human being's motives, and we must accept what we are told unless we have evidence to the contrary. But if adoptees feel conflicted about searching for their birth parents, the need for medical records justifies the search for them. Kristen actually acted on the medical information she received; her desire to obtain her medical record emerged not out of a rationalization but from her conviction about the genetic inheritance of disease and about her personality characteristics. In fact, Kristen, like a few of the patients we met before, also conflates the abnormal and the normal with her belief that she inherited from her birth mother not only her medical conditions but also her entire personality and being. Furthermore, Kristen's narrative reflects the notion that we encountered in the breast cancer patients, that by knowing her medical history she could be prepared in advance, a form of controlling the future, if not her children's inheritance, at least her emotional state.

Sadly, Kristen's account reveals, too, that owing to the ideology of genetic inheritance, not uncommonly adoptees experience fragmentation, which militates against their finding a sense of coherence in their lives. For example, on the one hand, Kristen's definition of family is consonant with the prevailing biogenetic definition of kinship in America; but on the other, she feels closest to her adoptive mother, with whom she claims she has nothing in common.

Loreta

Loreta, whom Kristen succeeded as the head of the adoption support group, is exceptionally knowledgeable about adoption matters, having founded this group many years ago. Loreta, 45 years old, was working on a Ph.D. dissertation in human relations and studied "post-traumatic stress disorder symptoms under closed adoption records" for her master's thesis. She associates the stress of relinquishing a child with a post-traumatic stress disorder because, she said, "I believe that what I'm seeing from the birth mothers is, relinquishing your own flesh and blood gets back to genetics, because the act itself is unnatural. The act of giving away your own."

Loreta began thinking about her birth parents when she was 12 years old, but she did not initiate her search for her birth mother until she was 28, after she gave birth to her son and four years after her adoptive mother died. When she found her birth mother, shortly after she started the search, she learned that her birth mother was 17 years old when she gave birth to Loreta; she was of lower-class origins, whereas the father was 43 years old and from an upper-class family. Her birth father had died when Loreta was a year old. Loreta noted the class difference between her birth parents; because of this difference, she feels she has little in common with her birth mother's family and a lot in common with her father's children, to whom she feels close. Significantly, Loreta linked class status with genetic inheritance when she noted, "I am more genetically connected and enjoy my birth father's side more than I do my birth mother's side. I don't know if it's because of their educational attainment or what, but we have more interesting conversations, more stimulating conversations, share general philosophies on the world. They're similar. My birth mother's side and I don't. I think personalities are the same because we share similar personality traits. We look alike. I look just like my birth father. We have similar demeanors. They're reserved people, basically. I'm intemperate, which comes from my birth mother, if I'm pushed. But basically that side of the family [my father's side] is very quiet, very reserved."

Loreta launched the search because of "an innate desire to know who you're connected to. I think it goes back to genetic imprinting. My theory is that it goes back to the days of when families represented the unit for the tribes. And that there's some imprinted memory theory. It's imprinted that we instinctively know our own." Loreta supported her theory with twin studies that, according to her, have shown that twins "used the same toothpaste and their first daughters were given the same name. So, I think that basically it boils down to with your own you instinctively feel a kinship connection that passes through." She added, *"It's a memory code in the genes."*

Loreta pointed out the dilemmas adoptees face because their daily existence is contrary to the ideology by which they live. She observed, "I think that society gives double-edged messages, one being 'blood is thicker than water.' You've heard that all your life. I have, too. So they have to make allowances, though, when you're talking about adoption, because all of a sudden they go, 'oh, sorry.' Because if society really believes that, we're cooked. Well, basically I think adoptees know that's the prevailing opinion. You instinctively want to be, see your own. You instinctively feel like you belong somewhere, but where? is the question for adoptees. And people who share the same blood and genes are like you. My personal opinion is apparently society doesn't think highly of not being connected genetically. Because I think that would explain why adoptees overcompensate for the loyalty issues they extend to the adoptive parents. Overcompensate. Yeah, and they are trying to prove that in their case it's not right, true, that they do mean just as much to their adoptive parents, that the bond there is just as strong."

Loreta noted that she shares with her birth mother "the same genetics; we share the same medical history; we share the same ancestry; we share certain commonalities of taste, personality traits. We like the same color; we like to move our hands when we talk sometimes; have high-pitched voices when we get excited. We usually are shy people, introverted people, and rise to the occasion only when necessary."

Besides her "innate" desire to know, Loreta was very concerned to secure her medical history, although I hasten to add that Loreta, unlike Kristen, regards the medical history as a derivative reason for searching. Even so, Loreta stressed, "because of the medical history I got up on my high horse and decided to find. I mean I was always curious, but when I started experiencing medical difficulty is when I decided it was constitutionally in my favor to go for it. I mean, there was no, there wasn't anything to constrain me from believing I had the right to do it, which is what the need for medical information gives adoptees — permission. If you just sit down and say, 'Yeah, well I just really wanted to know. I was just curious' — that doesn't sound like a good permission point in society's eyes. So we train ourselves to find whatever will convince the other party that we don't need permission to do this."

Then, concurrently, Loreta claimed that she had a child only because she searched. "I wouldn't have had him if I hadn't searched, because I had seven miscarriages. He was my eighth." Her birth mother's medical history aided her in the decision because "after we were having miscarriages one by one, they said there was something genetically involved. So when I found her, there were some things in the medical history — asthma, rheumatoid arthritis — that targeted blood tests that had never been done, and they were able to figure out that I had inherited the arthritic gene, rheumatoid, and it was causing the immune system to shut down during pregnancy. Once they did the blood test and it came up positive, they were able to give me medication from the time of conception on so that I carried eight months. They recognized that there was something in your immune system that was inherited and that they could do something for it. As a result, I was able to get pregnant."

Loreta's birth mother informed her that her birth father had died of prostate cancer when he was 44, that she herself had had uterine cancer at 30, and that her sister (Loreta's aunt) had had breast cancer at 58. Because of these disclosures, Loreta has semiannual mammograms and an annual Pap smear to allay her concerns about uterine cancer. She added, "Those are important things to know. I mean, I was conceived with someone who actually shouldn't be doing anything [referring to her birth father's prostate cancer]. In fact, it's a miracle I'm here, because normally prostate cancer, when it reaches terminal stage, infertility sets in. But only males inherit it. It carries for them genetic implications but not for me." Loreta has become a patient as a result of these discoveries.

In addition to having inherited her health status, Loreta believes that she has a unique connection to her birth mother. She noted, "I like her, in fact I love her. We don't, we probably would never be associated socially, which was my preference, not hers. She would have taken me home and kept me in a cradle from now on if I'd given her that right. But we share a bond in the sense that she's there if I need her. I'm here if she needs me. Well her lifestyle is different from mine, so that we didn't really have a lot of avenues cross over. My adoptive mother was more educated and stressed education more than my birth mother's side. My birth father's side are on the same educational level as I am, but not my birth mother's. And, so, just knowing she's there and who she is, it's just a good feeling."

Loreta cited other motives for searching that revolved around her biological makeup. She said, "I get the fact of knowing that I've got Cherokee in me and that my child probably qualifies for the Indian Welfare Grant for college; if so, I desire to investigate it more, because my mother's half-Cherokee. You could look at her and tell, too. So there's implications like that that are very important and just simply knowing who's who," referring to her discovery that she unknowingly dated and almost had sexual relations with her first cousin's son. This suggested to Loreta that "you'd find possibly blood has mingled with blood many a time. I think it's a chemical reaction. You like your own, usually. Sometimes you don't. There's a chemical reaction at times to be with your own. Believe me, if I'd married my cousin and found it out ten years after the fact, I would not be very happy. Because I would think genetically that it would probably take three to four generations for birth defects to show up, sort of like in the Lumbee Indians. They've intermarried so much that the birth defects now are actually showing up pretty regularly, so I don't think that. I just think that it's not something I'd want to do, to marry a cousin."

Loreta combines her genetic history with her ancestors' biographical past and her current personality characteristics when she says, "I think one of the things that's important is there's a lot of talk about history, there's a lot of talk about genetics, uh, genealogical searches . . . we feel connected by our past, or who came over on the *Mayflower.* My son's already asked me which one of my relatives came over. Now we can say adoptive relatives and name them, or we can say blood relatives and see if there's a few names. If it's adopted, you don't feel as spiritually connected to these people as you do if it's a blood relative." There is "a spiritual connection. I've done research on my grandparents and my great-grandparents, and I'm more inclined to do research on them because I know that's where I evolved. I'm not as inclined to do it on my adoptive family because there is really not going to be [the same] . . . when I did the genealogical search on my husband, some of the family traits that were spotted in 1600–1700 is what I spot in him today. In my husband. And in my son." She said her husband's side of the family is very high-strung, and so is her son. "For example, my husband, his father's side in Alabama were very hard, strong, hardheaded people. They don't like a lot of interference from people. They've just got that personality. And so when there was a write-up about World War II and there was a segment recorded by one of the townsmen that his family did not like the community bothering them and that they wouldn't have even gone to war had they not been bothered by the Yankees so much knocking on their door and that they went to war because they made them mad, not because they had any real belief in the war. And traits like that, I think personality traits, I see it in my husband and I see it in my son. In fact, we were talking to a child psychologist because . . . I have some concerns being an only child that he doesn't have a lot of interaction with children, so I wanted to get some tips on should we force him to go to Cub Scouts and this and that. So we've met with her a couple of times, and this morning we were talking about genetics, and my husband made the statement that my child has a cantankerous part about him, which, he wasn't raised that way, but he's got it. And the child psychologist asked [whether] anyone in your family has that, and he said, 'Yes. My father was just like it.' He says, 'It's scary.' And it is, because my son has never been raised, but he gets very grouchy, very judgmental, very cantankerous, irritable. Just personality-wise. A genetic copy of his father, yeah. His grandfather was just like that."

Similarly, Loreta sees in her birth mother "some of her traits that I've worked on most of my life, such as my temper, my irrationality when I get angry. My rage. My low self-esteem. She's got low self-esteem, but then that could just be a birth parent–adoptee issue," because Loreta's adoptive mother was "totally different. Fortunately, she was an educator, so she had patience to work with me, to try to get me to train myself, as she put it, to learn self-control, which I've worked on since I was a child."

Loreta distinguishes between what she calls "associational" and blood relationships. She has an associational relationship with her adopted siblings, with whom she shares memories, unlike with her birth siblings. Loreta claims that an associational relationship "is what love basically is for adoption."

When I asked Loreta whom she regarded as her family, she responded by generalizing: "I think the sad part for adoptees, we don't end up sometimes feeling we actually have family except . . . I mean, I had a family, which would have been my adoptive family, but they're all dead. And my adoptive brother committed suicide. So they're all dead, so I don't have a family, so my family now remains my son and my husband. I've seen some adoptees who jump in with mom, dad, brothers, sisters as if they had never been gone a day in their life. The clock stopped the day they were placed and picked back up when they found. They consider the person mom, dad, brother, sister. I, on the other hand, don't. I don't have that connection. I feel, I sense that she is related to me genetically, but not on a, I would not, I don't have a close associational relationship because of choice. But then my husband says the reason that is because she reminds me too much of myself and I'm not happy with some of the things I see."

In speaking about her birth siblings, Loreta commented, "My mother has three children younger than me. My birth father's side, all my siblings have been to graduate school. On my birth mother's side, they're all happy with high school diplomas. So there was a lot of jealousy on my birth mother's children because when they met me they thought I was, considered myself a little, I don't know. Snooty, is that a term? I believe one of them did say 'snooty.' Oh, she thinks she's better than us. No, it didn't really cross my mind, but I could tell that was a genuine fear of hers." Loreta recounted that her birth mother would have been happy to have her move in with her. But Loreta said, "The unfortunate part was, when I met her, it answered my questions. I liked her, but it's not probably someone I'd want to move in with unless I was homeless. And so, of course, because I did like her, because I was genetically connected to her, I was able to compromise with her and give her this once or twice a year. I talk to her occasionally. Maybe three or four times a year. But if I give her too much, she'll expect more. One of those Catch-22s; you don't want to give too much 'cause then you end up, they think you're going to come for Thanksgiving and Christmas."

Loreta's analytical posture toward adoptees' situations and reasons for their searches reveals her profound allegiance to genetic determinism, in the spirit of sociobiology. Loreta does not doubt for a moment that I.Q., shyness, and conscience are inherited characteristics. She noted, "I have seen some adoptees who have absolutely no conscience, and it shocks me. And their adoptive families, on the other hand, can be just as moral and as conscientious and driven by it and I'll sit there with this big question mark in my mind. Then we'll end up helping them with a search and, once they do the search process, we find a birth parent like that."

Loreta recognizes that because of society's constructed beliefs, adoptees are placed in grave contradictions between societal ideologies of genetic inheritance and life experience as adoptees. Out of the constructed ideology flows an important theme in Loreta's life: her need to know her medical history, a knowledge that connects her to a past, arguably a mythical past that creates a spiritual connection and changes her ethnic status to her advantage — to Native American. Loreta, in fact, has elevated genetic links to a spiritual connection, unifying biology with spirituality, with biology becoming an expression of spirituality. The same ideology also influences important life decisions, such as whether or not to have children or to become a patient.

It is generally recognized that adoption calls forth class issues, since most adoptees, including Loreta, are offspring of poor mothers adopted by middle- or upper-class families. But Loreta restates the class differences in genetic terms when she claims that her closer connection to her paternal siblings is an expression of her genes, consonant with her view that a blood kinship is an expression of a spiritual connection. Loreta credits her feelings of closeness to her genetic link with her educated father's children rather than with her impoverished birth mother's family, ignoring that such feelings are associated with shared education and class position. Significantly, she attributes all her negative characteristics to inheritance from her mother, further reflecting her class bias.

Pamela

Unlike Kristen and Loreta, Pamela is less certain what she inherited genetically from her birth mother. Pamela exudes intelligence and modesty in her demeanor. Now, age 39, she lives with a female partner and has worked for the past 15 years as a supervisor while also pursuing an advanced degree. Pamela recounted that until she was 18 she never considered searching, although she had been curious about whom she resembled ever since she was 12 years old. She was unaware that people search until she read a newspaper article about a person who helps people to find their birth parents. After arduously searching for 15 years, Pamela found her birth family in a nearby town. Pamela reported, "No member of our society should have to go through what we go through just to find out where we came from. The digging for it and the looking and all that. And when you run against a brick wall and you run into someone you thought was a good lead, and it's nothing. You cannot imagine how you plummet. It just drags you to the bottom." There is less urgency for her to find her father.

Pamela underwent the grueling quest for two reasons: to discover whom she resembled and to uncover her medical history. There is no resemblance between Pamela and her adoptive parents, and, she added, "There is a great loneliness when you live among people who look different from you." She explained that it was important to know one's likeness, otherwise, "you feel you sort of dropped on the planet somewhere. You don't have an origin. And then I wanted to know why I was given away. I wanted to know what the circumstances were."

Included in her need to know her birth mother, Pamela stressed, was the importance of knowing her medical history: "And then as you get older you begin to wonder about health questions and heredity and things like that. But it's a given that you want to know who you look like. And I was also curious as to who do my interests come from. The things I like to do. I like to read, I like to study, I like the piano. I like foreign languages. Those kind of things. Where did all that come from? So that became a growing issue. I was curious about that because my dad and I are extremely close. We're very much alike in our temperament—I mean, almost identical. We love to read. We love to learn. We love to do those kind of things. But I always had a very strong interest in foreign languages. And he never had that same interest. So I always wondered, well, where does that come from? I love meeting different kinds of people who come from different places, and I want to know what their experience is like. I was curious about that too. In high school I was very athletic. Basketball team. Track team. I was in the band. Had musical interests, and I wanted to know where those came from," because her adoptive parents were neither athletic nor musical.

Pamela found her birth family, even though none of them knew she existed. She discovered that her mother had been killed in a car accident, but she became very close to her birth mother's sister. Once she had found her birth family, she discovered that she had inherited many of her personality characteristics from them. At the same time, after meeting her birth family she considered that perhaps her different talents were not inherited from them—that perhaps she had acquired the talents from her adoptive parents. She added that her birth family "hadn't had the same educational opportunities that I've had. One of the questions my aunt asked me when she met me was, 'Did you finish high school?' And I was really taken aback by that. I was just sort of stunned. Like, 'Are you kidding?' But that was a big deal to her. Their life circumstances were very different than mine."

Pamela, more than the others in the study, vacillated between what she believed she had inherited from her birth and adoptive families. Her gray hair and ambidexterity must have been inherited from her birth parents. But then she thought about her aunt, and she reflected, "She shares with me, she has a real decency about her. About how she treats people and the things that were important to her. Family history is really important to her, and it's extremely important to me. I mean, I've got two families now and both of which are my families. But I think the sentimentality. She's a very romantic kind of person, and I'm definitely that. She is very shy, and so am I." Pamela concluded that she and her aunt have the same personalities, especially because both are introverted, but the two women have different outlooks on life. Pamela assessed, "I am more optimistic than she," immediately adding, "they're very poor. Very poor. They have not had any educational opportunities. There isn't much work where they are. But my grand-uncle is artistic and good with his hands, and so am I."

When she met her birth mother's sister, she asked first about the women's health history. Pamela reported, "I wanted to know, what was the family's history of breast cancer? I was very concerned about that. And I was also concerned, is there any diabetes in the family? Is there any heart disease? Those were the three biggies. Those were the risk factors for what were really important to me. The other things I really didn't think very much about. I didn't think about things like Parkinson or Huntington's, any of these catastrophic kind of things." Pamela was preoccupied about these diseases because the doctor asked her family history of cancer, diabetes, and heart disease, and she had to respond by saying, " 'I don't know' every single time. And I do a lot of reading, and it's pretty obvious that it's genetics. More and more, I think we are going to determine that [it's genetics] that's real, there's a greater role in your health history than we're aware of. So I wanted to know. I have half the picture. I only have my birth mother's family because we don't know who the father was. But we're working on that." She continued, "My mother was 13 when I was born. And I was very aware that at thirteen, whatever genetic or hereditary or what kind of health problems could be in the family wouldn't have surfaced at that age for her. So that concerned me. Every time you go to the doctor, the first question they ask is, 'What is your health history?' I would answer, 'No, I don't know.' And you just get frustrated by it because you get asked that every single time, everywhere you go. And so all those things after a while begin to build up. I discussed it with my parents and let them know that I was searching. My mother was supportive of it. My father was not."

Pamela wishes to learn about her father to discover his genetic history, "because once again now the doctor, this morning, 'What is your family history?' " Pamela responded, " 'Well, I can give you half of it.' You know, she looked at me pretty funny, and she goes, 'What do you mean you can give me half of it? You always say you don't know.'" Pamela, happily, is now able to say that she knows at least half of her medical history. Because Pamela's natural family is very large, she was confused about which member suffered from what disease. She said, "I mean, I literally have to write out a family tree and who is this 'cause the family is so large and who's married to whom and there was some history of skin cancer. Obviously, that concerned me. I've always been real careful with the sun, but I'm much more careful about the sun now."

Even though Pamela was close to her adoptive family and proud of it, she said, "I never really could claim it was mine. This isn't mine. Where's mine? What does mine look like? Well, one of the things I found out is that my blood history goes back pretty far too. And then I came back to my adoptive family and told them, 'Hey, I've got this too.'"

Pamela divulged the contradiction she was experiencing when she was told that a person automatically feels an affinity for blood kin. But Pamela disagreed with this view. She observed that she could have gone to school with "some blood cousins, and I had no idea who they were." But she immediately followed up this statement by saying, "The first time I met my aunt, I felt emotion. Connecting in a way I'd dreamed of doing for a long time. But there wasn't love there. There was no shared history." Importantly, Pamela became closer to her adoptive family once she found her biological relatives. She commented, "For me, I am free to love them in a way that I was never free before." Owing to her shared experience with her adoptive family, Pamela felt more comfortable with her adoptive family than with those she called her "genetic relatives." Significantly, Pamela observed that she lacked a proper vocabulary to describe her newfound relatives.

Pamela is still in pursuit of a sister who was also given away for adoption. She wishes to find her because she has always wanted to have a sister and because there is the possibility that one of them may need an organ transplant someday.

Pamela vacillates between her belief in genetic history and continuity and her recognition that she shares most of her interests with her adoptive family. On the one hand, she insists that she must have, in her words, "originated from somewhere genetically," and yet, unlike most of the other adoptees I interviewed, she also recognizes that due to drastic class differences between herself and her biological relatives, shared experience overrides any kind of blood kinship.

Pamela, like most others in the study, calls attention to the role medical family histories play in framing the ideology of genetic inheritance, an ideology that propels people like Pamela to take agonizing measures to find their biological relatives. She in fact noted that she had learned that all the diseases of concern to her were genetic because she was incessantly asked about her medical history by doctors and because she read about it in magazines. Pamela added that if she had ever considered having a child, and she hasn't, she would have "every check [medical] that there was to make sure the child was going to be OK." Her newly acquired knowledge of her medical history also guides her actions, including staying out of the sun because she had learned that members of her birth family suffered from skin cancer.

Pamela's account also discloses that she, like most of the other adoptees, seems to believe that her persona was passively purchased. Her personhood must originate somewhere; it was either formed by the adoptive parents or inherited from the biological parents. There seems to be little realization of the person as actor, as an individual who may have developed interests and a persona through her own ability to interpret her experience. Following the sociobiological paradigm of human existence, genetic ideology tends to foster the view that one's being is but a passive container.

Risa

Risa, a seemingly bubbly 46-year-old college graduate and mother of a 22-year-old son, was twice married but currently lives by herself. Risa is on the staff of the local university. Risa, whose birth mother was 15 years old when she gave birth to Risa and whose birth father is deceased, began her search when she was 19 years old; she finally found her birth mother a year before our meeting. Risa searched for her birth mother because she was lonely and because she desired to have a medical history.

Risa was very rebellious and, like Kristen, very different from her adoptive parents, even though both women claim to love their adoptive parents. When she found her birth mother she asked her, " 'Does this mean I can't believe I am an alien anymore?' I lived in a fantasy world. I did not deal with the real world until I found my birth mother." Risa was a clairvoyant, a fact she could never disclose to her adoptive parents, and she wished to know how she acquired this attribute. She longed to find her parents to discover the truth. Risa said, "If I found out that other parts of my family were like this, it would mean that I was not as weird as I thought I was."

Risa's adoptive parents wished her to become, she said, "a sorority girl, a nice, sweet middle-class girl who was supposed to get married, have kids, be happy, and have a little picket fence, garage, cars, and take the kids to PTA." Instead, to her regret, Risa turned into a hippie in the '60s, and, in place of having a Ph.D. beside her name, she has "divorcée." Risa, who grew up in a town of 300 people, became a political activist in the

'60s, and she asked, "Why did I come up that way?" She wanted to know why she became an extreme radical.

After meeting her birth mother, Risa considered that perhaps the seeds for this radicalism were planted by her adoptive mother and father after all, despite the fact that her adoptive father, a Methodist preacher, preached that people must listen to the government. Risa, however, turned to biological explanations when she said, "When I met my birth mother I found that my birth mother is very hard-headed and she is very strong-willed. They were from Germany on my mother's side, and Germans are very strong people. I think genetically they're survivalists. I do think genetically I got that survival attitude from my birth genetics." Like Risa, her birth mother never behaved as was expected of her. Her birth mother went off with a well-known folk singer. Risa did "that kind of thing," and she believes that her birth mother's behavior was transmitted to her genetically.

Risa was told that her maternal grandmother was a bona fide psychic. When she discovered that her mother's brother's daughter was a psychic, Risa felt an immediate connection with her birth family. She said, "I don't have to feel like I'm—what do you call it—some kind of weird being, because I have a cousin that's like me. And even down to the multileveled experiences of psychic message [that] go through." Risa mentioned that her birth brother was a psychic as well, but she could attribute his behavior to his being from California; the cousin, however, had grown up in a rural area in the East close to where Risa grew up. "Of course," Risa added, "my grandmother was like that too," confirming for her the genetic origin of her psychic abilities.

Risa wished to learn her roots. She discovered "that I had brothers and sisters really not adopted. A reality of knowing that there was a birth father and mother." Risa noted that she feels close to the people with whom she shares genetic ties, even though she has not been around the family. She explained, "It's got to be a psychological remembrance that is involved with New Age kind of metaphysics, including remembrances of past lives." The birth family left her a legacy that exists in their blood and that was transmitted to her through the genes, as a form of energy transmission. She felt the connection, "even going into the graveyard. And being with and seeing the grandparents. And seeing my great-great-great-granddaddy that was."

Most important, Risa's state of health precipitated her search. Risa becomes depressed, and her doctor had told her that her heart skips a beat and that that was probably genetic. He was concerned that she find her family. Both she and her son are being treated for high blood pressure, and she has been experiencing bad health for awhile, including stomach and colon dysfunction.[22] She learned that her birth father had died of a heart attack. Risa believes that she inherited high blood pressure, and "cancer is all over my birth mother's family. And she even had difficulty discussing it."

Risa lamented that had she known her family medical history before, she could have shielded her son from experiencing difficult times. Now, both she and her son require "high blood pressure medication the rest of our lives." Risa reiterated a familiar refrain: if only she had known there had been so much cancer in her family, she could have started taking preventive measures much earlier. As it is, she has already had two biopsies. But then Risa added that not only her birth family but also her adoptive mother's brothers and sisters suffered from cancer as well.

Risa, like Pamela, became closer to her adoptive family once she found her biological one, who welcomed her into the family with painted signs on the occasion of a family reunion. Yet, for Risa, as for most of the other people in the study, her adoptive mother, her deceased adoptive father, and her son are the people closest to her.

The ideology of genetic inheritance creates dilemmas for adoptees, including Risa. Risa could not reconcile her theories of the inheritance of disease with her experience with disease in her adopted family. Nor could she decide which characteristics she had inherited from her birth family and which from her adoptive family: what was the source of her rebelliousness, activism, and strong will? Certainly for Risa biological history confers a continuity with the past that she had not experienced before, attested to by her experience on visiting the graveyard. Like Loreta, Risa attributes spirituality to the biological connection, with biology having become a form of religiosity. Moreover, knowing her family medical history permits Risa, like the others, a modicum of control over her health by practicing some preventive measures, a power that genetic inheritance ideology bestows.

Risa's narrative illuminates an additional dimension to the belief in the inheritance of personality characteristics. It substantiated that she was a normal human being by confirming that the clairvoyant powers she possesses are not a sign of derangement. Again, as in Kristen's case, genetic inheritance ideology has rescued Risa from regarding herself as mentally ill. The powers she inherited from a grandmother established yet another connection with her genealogical past and with a living cousin who shares the same characteristics. Interestingly, too, Risa informs us how scientific beliefs about genetic inheritance have become incorporated into New Age metaphysics, suggesting that genes transmit a specific energy from generation to generation. This has undoubtedly endowed New Age theories with great legitimacy.

Roberta

Roberta, like Risa, searched for a past and longed to assure her birth mother that she ought not regret having given her away, because she was healthy and happy. Roberta, 32 years old with a B.A. in physical education and nursing, lives with her sister, who had also been adopted. Roberta began questioning where she came from and why she was given away when she was 16 years old. She found her birth mother about two months before our meeting.

Roberta was made conscious of inherited characteristics when her adoptive mother called attention to Roberta's musical talents. Roberta's mother told her, "Well, they said your natural mom had music talent, and you must have got it from her 'cause you didn't get it from me." After her adoptive mother told her this, Roberta felt relieved that, as she put it, "I had a history. I was born, I wasn't just popped out of a Social Services filing cabinet drawer. I came from somewhere and she recognized that, so it was like no big deal that I was adopted. Now I have a history, and I know it. Well, I can tell you who, um, I can tell you that my dad, my adoptive dad, was from German descent and I can tell you how his great-great-grandfather got here. And I can tell you what my mom's grandfather did as a career, and on the nurture side that has something to do with me. *But on the nature side, that's not my history.* That's not where I come from. Now I don't have stonecutters in my history like my adoptive mom has in hers. So it was neat to find out some of that. And I think some of it is just not knowing."

When I asked Roberta how she acquired her newfound history, she responded, "I guess genetically. Because I did come from somewhere else, because I was not just hanging out in the filing cabinet drawer until my adoptive parents adopted me. I did come from somewhere, and I think that's important. I don't know as much about heredity as I wish I did. I hated science in school, so I really didn't pay a whole lot of close attention [except to] things like the dyslexia and being gay. My half birth sister is also gay, so that was a real tickle because it has a higher incidence in like identical twins or paternal twins over siblings, and then higher incidence between siblings than the general population. You know, one study showed that it [gayness] is hereditary or genetic or at least familial. So it was really neat to find out, and that was one of the things my adoptive mom got tickled about when I told her. Cause, of course, every parent who finds out their kid is gay goes through this 'where did I go wrong? I raised you in church. What did I do?' And when she found out that my birth sister [actually half sister] was also gay, she was, like, 'You did come that way.' You know, it was almost like a relief for her that, even after all these years, there was something back there that still said, 'You didn't raise this kid right.' And then to find that out kind of let her off the hook, like I did come that way."

Roberta indicated that "a big driving force [to find her birth mother] was heredity as far as medical care. I wanted to know. It's awful to go into a doctor's office, a new doctor, the first thing you're given is one of those sheets that you fill out. You know, 'Have you or your parents or family ever had diabetes, hypertension?' and I would always have to write, 'Don't know.' That was one area I didn't have a history, 'cause all Social Services said was 'everybody's healthy.' Yeah, right. I don't know any family where everyone is healthy. And so I have never even allowed myself to consider having kids because I was not going to bring kids in without knowing what they were set up for. And a lot of people say, 'Well, they can test now,' or 'There's treatments now. You can't let that stop you.' It's like I'm watching my [adoptive] mom be eaten up by diabetes. I don't want that passed down from me. Schizophrenia is hereditary. I don't want — I don't know that it's not in my family and skipped me and, if I have a kid, there are just some things I didn't want to take a risk on. So it's been really neat the last six weeks, two months, considering having a kid, 'cause at least on my [birth] mom's side there is some diabetes, but it's several steps back. Her dad, his dad, and his dad. And there was some cervical cancer, but that's no big deal either. It's like, 'Whew, maybe I will have one.' " But neither Roberta nor her newly discovered siblings or their offspring suffer from diabetes. Roberta continued, "They're not educated enough to be able to tell me what type diabetes. Was there diabetes from a young age, or were they 60 and weighed 300 pounds? And if they had lost the weight, they wouldn't be diabetic. And my birth sister had cervical cancer. So it's pretty clear otherwise. Watching my mom with diabetes, it was like I said, 'The one thing I don't want to find is diabetes,' and the first thing out of my birth mom's mouth was, 'Well, there's diabetes.' And it was like, oh no! Not that one! I'm pretty safe from schizophrenia now. I'm past 30."[23] Before learning about her medical history Roberta had not considered having children, but now that she has her family's medical history, she is contemplating having a child by artificial insemination.

Roberta hesitatingly believed that she resembled her birth mother. She added, "I think that was probably me recognizing some of my features in her face. So I think, even though I did not recognize it enough to go, 'Yes, she looks like me. Oh, I see it.' I think at some level, I was recognizing features and that was giving me the familiarity that I was feeling. Because they're all totally different than I am. They're at a different place in life, and socioeconomics, I guess, had a lot to do with it. None of them have graduated [from high school]. Well, I've got two siblings, a brother and a sister, both half, they're twins. Neither of them finished high school, much less went to college. Neither of them has a profession; they have jobs. Just as they see things differently than I do. Right down to what I noticed—everyone, including my half sister's son, has what I call four front teeth. You know, two front teeth were prominent and the two next to them were inching behind them, which is the way mine were before nine years of braces. And so I'm the only one that had braces. I mean, just totally different experiences. I grew up with, at least my childhood from 12 and down, the storybook house, everything but the white picket fence, the PTA, mom and the dad who taught me how to cut grass."

Roberta reflected how she felt after she met her birth mother. "You look for somebody for years and years and years. I think there's an excitement and there's nervousness but not really a connection. It was kind of neat finding out the similarities that we had. We're both very crafty, handcrafts, needlepoint. That kind of thing. We're both musical. She plays several instruments, and so do I. I think she plays piano, organ, and something else. And I play clarinet, sax, bass guitar. I saw a lot of our same personality traits. I need to dominate the conversation. I have a need to be right. I call it self-preservation; in her I called it selfishness. That's where I felt the connections. I could tell she was nervous and apprehensive, and she was behaving as I would have behaved if we were in reverse roles. Very reserved, very tight. Her whole body was tight, almost to the point of uppity. And those who know and love me say I can be so uppity I'm intimidating. So there was a lot of personality."

Roberta maintains that the characteristics she described are transmitted by heredity. An example is "the way she seemed to handle problems. You know, she shuts up about them. She keeps it in herself. She swallows it. And that is my base personality. But yet I open my mouth and I hear my mother's words coming out, so it's really—nature versus nurture has always been a fascination for me, and I definitely think it's both. I think she gave me a core personality, and mom swears I came stubborn. But I think my adoptive mom molded it. My half brother has what I believe to be dyslexia. Yeah, that's her son. And I have dyslexia. But he didn't get any help with his and dropped out like in the eighth grade. And I asked my birth sister, 'Did either one of you have any learning problems?' because I was curious to know. Because it does seem to be at least familial, and it tends to run in males; dyslexia is much more prevalent in males than it is in females. So I was really interested to know if he had it. And she said, 'No. Mama just always said he had the stupids,' which is not what my mom said about me. She said, 'You're too bright not to be getting it together.' And had me tested and got me in specially. So, I came with a thing, which in this case is dyslexia, but my adoptive mom is the one who molded me, if that makes any sense. You know, I came with a stubborn personality, but mom is the one who taught me how to turn it into perseverance."

Roberta maintains she inherited her personality from her biological mother because, "well, I guess your mom carries you for nine months. I feel more connected with her. I mean, it takes, what, 20 minutes maybe to be a dad? So I haven't really thought much of the genetics of him which — and she showed me a picture of him, the only one she had was a yearbook picture, and he looked so dorky. Like, no, I don't see any of me in him. And maybe I'll have something to connect to if and when I ever meet with him. But there has been far less fascination with finding him than my birth mother, and I think it is the nine months as being connected. Because he like found out she was pregnant, 'Nope, I'm not getting married' [to illustrate, Roberta snapped her fingers], joined the Marines, and was out of there. So she's the one that couldn't jump on a bus and leave town, so I think there's more of a connection there. So, I don't know. There may be a lot to tie me to him heredity-wise."

Roberta found her father's address and telephone number, but she hesitated to call him. She explained, "I've . . . with the information that I was given, I kind of expected to find out that my father was dead because he, it was told to me that he was in the Marines and this was 1965, so Vietnam was going on. He was not a high school graduate, so I figured he must be a grunt, you know. And most grunts were dying during that time. And so I kind of didn't focus on him at all; I just took it for granted he was dead. What I found out is that he's not dead, but I haven't called him yet. And I've had the address now for probably two months, six weeks, two months, somewhere around there. It hasn't been real important."

Roberta was delighted to find a sister she had always desired, even though she lacked the same sense of kinship toward her as to her adopted sister, or even to her birth mother. Roberta reflected on the meaning of family by saying, "No, you could say it's of connection, but not of close-ness. I was raised that you know your parent is the one that goes to the first grade recitals and your parent's the one that takes you to the emer-gency room at 3 A.M. when you've got a raging fever. That's your parent. They're the ones that clean up the car after you've gotten carsick. That's parental things. And that's taken over my adult life, too. I have people that I consider family and those are my partner and then I have two very close kids, uh, friends who have three kids and those kids call me 'aunt.' And I consider them my nieces and nephews and I would do anything for them, as I would for their moms. They are family. If I were hurt in an accident, I would want them to be allowed to visit me. I would con-sider them more of a family than like even my adopted mom's sister or my father's sisters. Family is who loves you and takes time with you and that kind of thing." But Roberta quickly added, "I think there is a con-nection with the blood and the heredity, but like I said, it only takes 20 minutes to be a dad and ultimately it only takes nine months to be a mom technically or legally, or however you want to call it, but what it takes to be a parent is eighteen long, tedious years of devotion and whatever. And, yeah, to me family is who loves you and supports you and who's there for you and who you're there for. I mean, I've got cousins that could care less if I'm alive or dead. Adoptive cousins, my mom and dad's nieces and nephews."

Roberta proudly showed me pictures of her birth family; she pointed out her gay sister and the sister's partner and said, "What's funny is we have the same taste in women."

Roberta's narrative discloses the collective cultural consciousness that talents and personality traits are inherited, a notion instilled in her by her adoptive parents. Roberta, however, is not fully guided by a genetic paradigm, accentuating for her a sense of fragmentation. For her, family signifies, as Schneider long ago observed, love and nurture. Significantly, Roberta is fully conscious of the disparate class position between herself and her birth family, which explains many differences between them, including whether one has the "stupids," or unobtrusive dyslexia. For Roberta, history means both a genetic and an experiential history, and she recognizes that she is not a passive vehicle through which genes do their work. Roberta is thus unique among those I interviewed because she is able to separate genetics from her lived experience, unlike most of the other individuals, who tend to conflate medical conditions with behavioral and personality traits by attributing all to genetic inheritance and who mistake class differences for genetic differences.

Whereas Roberta is aware of the limits of genetic inheritance, the medical history plays a role for her that is similar to the one accepted by the other adoptees we meet here. It advances a genetic conceptualization of disease and influences courses of action—in Roberta's case, whether to conceive a child. Unlike Pamela, who feels comfortable with being a lesbian, Roberta and her adoptive mother are both relieved of a sense of culpability for her lesbianism by attributing it to genetic inheritance. It legitimates Roberta's sexual status and removes the responsibility from her adoptive mother for Roberta's sexuality. According to Roberta's view, homosexuality thus is not a choice but a genetic state, as Hamer and Copeland argue, but that recently was refuted.[24]

Monica

Monica, a 40-year-old married mother of three children ages 11, 9, and 7, is a high school graduate. Monica assists others in finding their birth parents. She found out who her birth mother was three months before our interview and 13 years after she initiated her search, although her mother had already died. Monica retains contact with her mother's sister and with five siblings. Monica, the middle child, sickly from birth on, was the only one of six children who had been given up for adoption. She was 7 years old at the time, and the family could simply not afford to pay her medical bills. Her foster parents, elderly farmers who had already raised a family, adopted Monica.

Monica indicated that at one time people didn't speak openly about wishing to search for birth parents. She said, "In the '60s and '70s they didn't talk about and you didn't hear of searching like you do now." Monica became aware of searching possibilities in the early '80s: "Like, 1980–81, somewhere in through there, I started hearing about people searching. Before then you kind of asked around and people didn't know what to do, didn't know how to go about it. And then, you started hearing it on television, and people then started finding out what to do."

Monica was concerned not to hurt her adoptive parents by searching for her birth mother; but she wished to obtain her medical records, because "I've had a lot of medical problems and my little boy has asthma and I have asthma and I've had two lumps removed from my breast, so I was concerned if there was cancer in the family and different things. So I did find out there is cancer in the family, that my grandfather had cancer and my aunts had cancer." Monica's mother died of a heart attack, and she believes she may have inherited the disease, because "I asked them if they had any heart problems and there is high blood pressure. And I told them that my heart flutters and one of my sisters said hers did, and so did one of my brothers." In fact, three of the siblings said that "their heart flutters, so it could be, but it's something now that I'm aware of and I can watch for and start taking better care of myself." Having the medical history helped Monica to watch for heart disease and cancer. She observed, "I can keep up with my mammograms regular, instead of just, okay, I'm going to let it slide. I know I'm going to have to keep on it. I know I'm going to have to take care of myself with the heart and exercise. And it's something I can tell the doctor and we can watch for." Monica was especially worried about getting breast cancer because the doctor told her she might inherit it and therefore she needed to watch herself.

Monica searched also because, in her words, "It's like a hunger and you just want, you want your family. It's like, how can I describe it? It's like taking a puppy away from the litter, from its mother, and how they cry. You know how they are when you take a puppy away? A child is like that, too. And even though we're grown up, you still have that little girl inside. And I can remember laying in bed and crying when I was little, wanting my mother." The adoptive mother didn't fill that void [even though] she took care of me, you just have this need for your birth mother."

In Monica's case, her search was more poignant because her adoptive parents were constantly reminding her that she had been adopted. Monica said, "And see, they never did let me forget that I was adopted. I was always reminded, 'we've done this for you. We've done that for you. If it wasn't for us you'd be in an orphanage.' You know, this type of thing."

Monica felt an immediate closeness to her siblings, as if she had never been separated from them. She felt they have a lot in common in appearance: "Our hands are alike, our feet, our eyes, our ears, we have the same nose, the same lips. The things like how she [her sister] decorates her house is how I decorate mine, the colors. We have the same interests." Monica found a lot in common with one of the brothers, as, for example, "this streak of humor in us and I mean we just, we just click together. And it was so funny 'cause as soon as he picked me up at the airport we started. And you could say that we have the streaks of temper." "In fact," Monica added, "I got to meet a great-aunt. She's living and she asked me, she says, 'I want to ask you, do you have a temper?' And I said, 'Well, they tell me I do.' And she said, 'Well you got it honest,' she said. 'Your mother had one and your grandmother did, too.' And my grandfather, he's living. I got to meet him. He's 99. It's turned out to be a really good reunion because I never heard of anyone accepting that quickly. I mean, it was just instant. Like, when I called, Michael [a brother] is the one I located first and I called him and we just started talking." Monica was amazed to what degree she and her siblings were alike in all respects. She noted, "I mean, it's like I rub my chin when I'm thinking and Monica Ann does, too. The way I laugh." Monica, however, recognizes that when she met them they were all looking for things they shared. Monica was less interested in finding her father.

Monica's narrative makes it clear that she believes having her birth mother's medical information allows her to take precautions against cancer and heart disease. In Monica's case, the very medical symptomatologies link her, as they do others, to kin. The family's medical history mediates the connections with the birth family. When Monica learned that her mother had died of a heart attack, she immediately linked her mother's disease to her experience of heart murmurs; other siblings, too, established a connection with Monica by claiming to have the same symptoms.

Monica, compared to the other people we met, is less in turmoil over the conflict between blood and adoptive ties, because her adoptive parents constantly reminded her that she had been adopted and that she had been a stranger in her adopted family, giving impetus to her search for her "real" parents. In Monica's case there was less effort by her adoptive parents to establish "as if" biological ties, eliminating for her the conflict regarding who was her true family. She, unlike the others, was adopted at a late age, which may have influenced her relationship to the adoptive parents as well.

Monica, too, conflates family medical histories with physical and behavioral characteristics. She makes no distinction between the similarities between her and her siblings' physical appearance and the fact that they also decorate the house in the same way. Her genealogical memory thus incorporates her bad temper, her physiognomy, and her detailed behavioral characteristics.

Liz

Liz, a 27-year-old married, employed college graduate, is a biracial child. She is the only one of three children in her birth family to have been given up for adoption. According to Liz, her adoptive father, a college professor, could not confront his alcoholism problems. In discussing the problem with her adoptive brother, she asked him, "Do you think about alcoholism? Do you understand that it's genetic?" Liz, having never felt connected to her adoptive parents, from whom she is estranged, began her search for her birth parents mentally when she was in grade school and, she said, "I started physically looking for them when I was, I think, 19."

Liz searched because she was unhappy at home. "I felt like I wanted to see what these people looked like. I wanted to know if my personality could be different, more like them, because I was curious about who am I like if I'm not like these people." Race was a cardinal issue for Liz, who claimed she has been considered black, and that she looked darker in the past. She declared, "Biracial people can change like this because my mom and dad look so different from each other. My father is black like brandy and my mother is white, so over time I've looked like anybody, you can kind of look more like your father and start to look like your mother. My skin color at different times looks different. I don't know why, but it's changed colors as well. But the thing was, I was a black child. I was never, ever called mixed race, ever. Like even when I went to psychologists or something, they'd be, like, 'it's a black female.' Or going to the doctor's record: 'This is a black female.' I lived a life of a minority child in a white town — um, big Afro hair. I can still get that back if I want, but it's not easy to comb through. I looked really different. Everybody there was Norwegian and light, very white-skinned and light hair, straight hair, and I mean, I definitely looked different. People would touch my hair — Oh, it's so neat,' because it was a big, tight curl. Very tight. And so I always felt different, which was not fun, because when you're a kid you want to look like everybody else. You want to fit in. So, at home like I would be called names or something. I would be called the 'n' word, words that are used, derogatory, toward black people. And they even would call me African or Cambodian or Ethiopian. They would say, 'because you're so skinny' — I was a skinny kid, but, because of the way I looked, too. And then like sometimes they [children in school] would see like an encyclopedia would have an African woman in it, just really dark, thing in her nose, half-naked, and then they'd go, they'd all laugh and point at the book and then I would come over and they'd go, that's me when I get older."

Besides her different appearance, Liz claims that she is also different from her adoptive parents in most other respects. She said, "You know, I'm much more emotional or, I guess more feminine and more nurturing than my mom and caring, kind of a people-pleaser person. And my mom is not like that. She's very aggressive and more harsh. We didn't have much in common. She didn't like the same things I liked. We didn't enjoy anything the same, so it was like we just really had nothing to bond with each other. It was really strange. So, I was ready to go out and see if anybody else was like me, physically, emotionally, in every way. So that's why I looked."

Liz had found her birth parents seven years earlier. It was more important to her to find her mother first. She knew her mother was white. Liz said, "In my mind, she always just kind of looked like me, and she looks like me in some ways, but then I'm like a blacker version 'cause she's pretty white, she has whiter skin and everything. But we have different features. She's shorter than me, too. I'm leaner and taller, like my dad. I have cheekbones, too." Liz and her birth mother became best friends. She found her father and his family shortly after she met with her mother.

Liz discovered a great deal in common with her birth mother. The two women have the same habits—for example, "We both bite our nails, we like horses, we both love riding horses, and we both like nature. We both are very emotional, and many times we're emotional where we begin tearing and cry, and we're both creative, and we're both very feminine in some ways. I'm not much of a boyish type, you know. I like to do the girlie thing. And we both like doing those kinds of things. She's very nurturing and into pleasing people, helping others. She does those kinds of jobs, which I like to do, and I mean there's just so much, I can't tell you. There's so many things we have in common." Liz believes she inherited all the characteristics she had listed from her birth mother, in addition to "temperaments and some of our skills, like we're both not super verbal people, like this verbal I.Q. and all these other things. I'm not one with a super-huge vocabulary and all. You know, academically I've done okay because my learning is more visual. I see things in a different way than my family did. They spoke a lot of big words and they do a lot of book-smart stuff, but I wouldn't say common sense. And my birth mother has a lot of common sense."

Because Liz was so different from her adoptive family, she stood apart. She said, "I mean, I don't know where all these differences were, and then, when I saw her [birth mother] and how she was, her intelligence is like mine. And my birth father, too. I can see a little bit of me in both of them, but I could not see it in my adoptive parents. No. And we interact the same way with people. It's really weird. And other characteristics, like how things are inherited like depression. Those are inherited things, and what is depression? It's a lot of characteristics, it's a lot of emotions, and I don't know how you can put into words where it comes from completely, but they're finding that those kinds of things are very much inherited. So in her [birth mother's] family, depression has been there in different generations. Not alcoholism. Like, alcoholism is in the family that I'm not related to. So they pass on alcoholism, where my birth mother's family is more the emotional, like anxiety, depression, those kinds of things you can work through, you can learn how to deal with them. But, yes, I have been much more emotional than my family, much more able to get depressed. And it was because of my childhood, too, what I went through, but I handled things differently than the rest of them. And I'm much more laid back compared to my family, I mean as far as the way I do things. It's much more just less jumpy or something. I just don't know how to explain all of it, how I'm so different from them and then how I'm so much the same as my birth parents, other than to say that there's got to be some genetics."

Liz found a great deal in common with her birth father also. She indicated, "We're both very good at sales and we like to sell stuff. My [adoptive] parents hate retail, they hate shopping and they hate selling and they hate buying and we never could do anything like that together and they don't like those kind of fields at all and I was like the only one that's ever done anything like that. It's just weird. I don't know why, but I'm very different than my parents and the things I do have always been different. There's something in my personality that doing this is an okay thing to do. My parents would be like, 'Oh, you're sleazy. You're selling things. You're not being honest with people.' " Liz and her birth father also share the same sense of humor. She noted, "We'll joke the same way. My parents would do a lot of the academic jokes and I didn't understand what they were joking about. A lot of them were about famous people or some kind of historical thing and I was, like, 'I don't get it.' With my birth father, we would just joke about something in our conversation and we'd say it sarcastically. Like we have the same sarcastic humor. And we would just laugh before — we wouldn't even have to explain the joke. We'd just laugh about the same thing. If we said it in a certain tone of voice, he would know I was joking; my parents would not know I was joking. So that's kind of interesting, 'cause he hasn't even known me that long and we'll just know, like."

Liz feels a kinship relationship to her birth mother's children. Speaking about one of her brothers who is closest to her in age, she said, "I feel a lot for him. It's such a weird feeling to have a sibling that you just really like. And I really care about him. He's very different than me in some ways, but then the characteristics we have are a lot the same. As for example, he doesn't follow like what everyone says you should do. He's a thinker. He thinks through things and does what he decides to do and he doesn't care what, like, if people think that's the normal thing to do or like academic or like . . . it's not so book smart. He's got a lot of common sense. And I see that. He can live off a certain amount of money just doing, working at an art museum or something. He likes creative things. We both like those creative things as far as just appreciating it and not trying to talk about people and stuff. So we really just get along really well. It's hard to explain."

Liz also feels close to her father's daughter. But to Liz's regret, her father's daughter has been affected by her mother. Liz explained, "Their mother has had more of an influence in their personality, I think, because they do have a different mom, so it's like, that's the thing with the siblings is that there is not that 100 percent or whatever, 50 percent . . . we're half-siblings so, I don't know what it is, but her mother's personality is somewhat strong in the girls" and different from Liz's. Liz observed, "With my siblings with my mother, I feel we have more personality traits in common than with my dad's kids and maybe because mom has a great deal of influence or the genes or something. I don't know what it is. We get along great. It's just her mother's personality, they're just like their mother."

When Liz met her mother's extended family, she immediately felt connected to them, despite the fact that they were aloof toward her. She reported, "Even though they don't want to be in my life, it's like I still feel like this is my history. These are where I come from. And when I talk about my nationality and everything, they are a part of it. They're part of where I came from. You know, when you look for birth, when you are searching for your roots, it's not just your parents, it's who came before them. How did they get into this country? Where did we come from? Where did I come from? I just didn't come from two people; it came from the people before them, so the genealogy and all that is very interesting to connect with the past, and I haven't been able to with them, but my birth mother and I are doing some genealogy, and my grandma is doing it, too, with her. And she knows I'm finding answers. And she's excited about what I find. But we don't have a relationship. What my mother did that was so bad they can't forgive. They hold onto it, you know. They hold on. They can't forgive her."

In contrast to Liz's mother's family, in her father's family everybody welcomed her. She commented, "My paternal grandmother accepts me a lot and knows the story and people talk about it openly, about where I came in — 'You're a part of the family.' And she'll look at my mole and she'll go, 'I knew when I saw you.' 'Cause that's one thing that the family has a lot of is moles on your body and birthmarks. I have them on my body as birthmarks and stuff and she saw my mole and she goes, 'That's a family mole. That's part of the family.' And then the cheekbones and just different features. She goes, 'I knew you were one of ours.' She just knew it. And she was like, um, never questioned it. But we got a DNA test anyway. Because remember, at the time, she [her birth mother] was saying two different people could be the father, and so it was good to. . . . But I didn't do the DNA until a year or so ago because I was sure, when I met him, he was my dad because we have so many different features and things that I could see that I got from him. I didn't have a doubt he was my birth father. I met the other one [the other man] because his daughter searched for me and found me and said, 'You know, my dad said he was for sure your father and he told me about you, that I have a sibling out there.' And she wanted to find me. So she found me and that's when I said, 'Listen, straight up, we need to have a blood, a DNA test, because I'm under the impression that I'm someone else's birth daughter.' You know, just to be sure. Because I want to know medically. I want to make sure, right? So I just said, 'Let's do a blood test.' So I did a blood test with the second father, who is not my birth father."

Liz needed to be certain which of the two men was her father because she wanted to know her family medical history. She stressed, "I was looking for medical information. I was so confused about stuff because doctors would say, 'Is this in your family?' or whatever, and I wouldn't know what to say." Liz noted that in the absence of such information, "they would never know if a symptom came, they wouldn't know because it runs in your family. And then, when they have you fill out forms they'll ask, 'What runs in your family?' It's always on their checklist. And before I met him, I didn't know what to say 'cause I didn't know if there was high cholesterol in the family or what, so it was always just kind of a confusion thing. And then I thought, also, if something happens to me medically and they need someone to match, like a donor or something for anything, they would look to family and it would have to match. I think there's different kidney or I don't know what it is, but I just knew I needed to know who was related to me. And so that's why I looked as well."

Liz arrived at the interview with two paternal cousins who live out of state. They had come to visit her, and she felt they had a great deal in common. Yet it was very clear that, compared to Liz, the two young women had a much lower level of education, which was immediately reflected in different speech patterns.[25] Liz noted, "I don't know if it's genetic or not, 'cause cousins it's like we keep getting further away, like the genes and how much we have in common, right? So I don't know, but we do happen to get along real well."

Liz's narrative adds another dimension to the tension between genetic inheritance ideologies and experience, specifically race. Her account accentuates the relationship between racism and biological inheritance ideologies, when she speaks of having been seen as a black person, despite the fact that her upbringing was "white," accentuating her difference from the rest of the community. Significantly, she recognized that while she lived with her adoptive parents her "skin changed colors," calling attention to how perception of color is actually contingent on context. Liz's case also points to a more conventional understanding of racism when she learns that her birth mother's family wishes to avoid her because they do not forgive the mother for having had relations with a black man.

Despite the color difference, Liz feels close to her white mother and her white siblings, who also share her common sense rather than bookish knowledge, suggesting that in her case kinship ideology overrides racism, even when the kinship ideology is buttressed on a biological model. Her father's family, too, is guided by biological determinism, recognizing that they share not only the same moles but also personality characteristics, such as salesmanship and humor.

Liz's account informs us how genetic inheritance ideologies mold her comprehension of her history that she views as being inscribed in her genealogical memory and anchored in her DNA. The DNA affirms who her true father is. No other information can be trusted to confer one's true identity. Furthermore, by reconstructing her genealogical past she gains access to what she defines as her nationality and her true origins by reason of her belief that the birth mother and father, of whom she knew little, transmitted to her all that she is now. Moreover, Liz, too, required a medical history to give her, like the other adoptees, a medical identity and a medical past, so that she would not be regarded, in Risa's words, "like an alien." Most significant, Liz's narrative reveals how medical historytaking reinforces racism when the physicians describe her in their records by her race.

Tara

Tara is a 30-year-old single graduate student and, like Liz, biracial. She too was adopted by an academic family, but her life experience, unlike Liz's, was satisfying. Tara loves her adopted family, which includes two sisters who are the biological children of her parents. Until she was 17 years old she felt very much a member of her adopted family. Tara began her search when she was 24 years old, and she had found her birth parents a year previous to our meeting.

Tara recalled that she had assumed she was adopted because she looked different from all the others in the family: she was brown and her family were not. But, she said, "there was never any public discussion of 'this is our adoptive daughter.' I never heard that, ever, coming from my parents or my sisters, at any time." When Tara was seventeen she read *The Autobiography of Malcolm X,* and she said, "my life kind of changed—I realized there was a whole world that I hadn't been privy to. But up to that point, I was very much a member of the family. I'm sure that people asked my parents or my sisters, but I didn't hear too much about it. I really didn't. And I just was not cognizant of being that different than my family members."

Malcolm X's autobiography taught her about the black community in a way she had never known before. She recalled, "I had never learned before, because it certainly wasn't taught in the public schools that I attended. So I really didn't see myself as different, because I was learning the same information everybody else was and didn't stick out as well. African people have been treated this way, or whatever. So I didn't think anything of it. So, when I did pick up that book, the world kind of opened up to me in a different way that it hadn't been before and I realized that I belonged to that group." Since that time, she has identified herself as black and has exclusively dated black men, "because it was my search to try and find authentic blackness when I read Malcolm X. I thought you had to be someone who was bad or rebelled against society or who was tough. It certainly couldn't be an intellectual or an academic like my dad. That didn't fit. You know, I had these binary . . . society presents black and white choices as binary opposites, and I accepted it wholeheartedly."

Tara searched for her birth parents in order to find her black ancestors because as an adult people never ceased to question her about her racial antecedents. Interestingly, Tara was the only person in the research group who made no mention of a desire to learn her medical history. She said, "I was most interested in wanting to know more about who I was because people constantly asked me that very specific question, 'What are you?' meaning, 'What ethnicity are you? What race are you? Where are you from? Who are your people?' That's the way the black community asks—'Where are you from? Who are your parents? Who are your kin?' And people ask me that all the time. And that's all I wanted to find out in my search for my birth parents was how I can better answer that question for others as well as myself. They want to know what I am, they want to know what is my ethnic background. Because I'll mess with people—and I'm using polite language for you. 'Cause people, I mean literally, when I'm downtown, when I'm busy, when I go anywhere, it happens to me on average about once a week if I'm out a lot shopping or whatever, and people will argue with me. If I say I'm black, they'll say, No. I had this one man who said he was sure I was Greek. And I'm not Greek. So people will say, they'll try to, and there's a variety of different ways that people will do it. Sometimes they'll say, 'Well, where are you from?' And I'll say, 'I'm from Oregon.' Well, that doesn't answer their questions. 'Well, where are your parents from?' 'Well, my dad's from California and my mom's from Montana.' Well, that doesn't answer that question. 'Well, uh, where are your parents' family from?' 'Well, my grandparents are from Tennessee and my mom's parents are from Montana.' And, you know . . . or they'll say, 'What nationality are you?' And I'll say, 'I'm American.' And I know what they're getting at 'cause they'll keep asking it. They'll say, 'No, that's not it. Come on. You know what I want to know.' And they want to know what race I am. They want to know who can explain why I look the way I look."

Until people questioned Tara about her racial background, she was not curious about her origins. She observed, "I didn't feel like I had any need to, and it's no problem because I felt so much a part of my family that there really wasn't a big push or need for me to do that. Then as I became more politically aware and politically active and started being in the black community more, I thought it might be interesting. And then questions of who I look like came up a lot, 'cause people, the more I would be active in the black community and be in the black community, it seemed as though more people would ask me what I was. Black people seemed to ask me what I was more than white people did. Black people would ask, 'What are you?' It happens at least once a week. The last time it happened was last week. This Indian man asked me if I was Indian. Indian Americans ask me if I'm Native American. Hispanics ask me if I'm Hispanic. But black people rarely ask me if I'm black, but they always want to know what I'm mixed with. And that became a pressing need to know, to answer these questions. I didn't seem to have very good explanations for it. I knew one of my parents was black and one of my parents was white, but I didn't even really know that precisely until I was 25."

After a long and difficult odyssey, Tara located both her birth parents, but neither one wished to meet with her at first. After they had met, her mother told her that when she gave birth to her, "she kept her eyes closed the entire time and that the nurse has asked her to hold me, to look at me and be able to bring peace to the situation and know that she was making the right decision in giving me away, and she couldn't do it, or decided that she wasn't going to do that and didn't do that. And so she had never seen me, never looked at me, even as she had me. She never told her parents who it was because she didn't want to disappoint them, and they would have been disappointed if they would have known he was black."

Tara feels no kinship to the woman. She said, "It's interesting to see what she looks like and see pictures of her kids, but there's nothing there. What's so bizarre and painful is that because I identify myself as a black female, African American female, I have wanted to feel more of a kinship to my biological father, and he is denying the whole thing ever happened, so that's very difficult for me right now, to make sense out of that. I don't have any anger for her at all, especially given the reality of what's played out, because I have romanticized this really wonderful black side that was rich in culture and all the greatness that is black culture, I had romanticized my father. I knew he was black, right? But it turned out she's the one that's dealing with me honestly and is proud of me and said things like, 'Wow, you're getting your Ph.D.' and those types of good things, whereas he's not acknowledging his responsibility in this whole thing. So the tables have turned. She was the bad white person, just being curious and wanting to know if it's true about black men, a racist who can't deal with a black woman, and now the tables have turned. She's the good, decent person now, because she's dealing with me honestly to the best that she can, which I will give is difficult to do after thirty years, after you've given a child up for adoption."

Despite the father's rejection, Tara feels connected to her father by race because of "the history of race in this country. I study race. I teach race. It would seem to me that I would have more in common with him than I would with her, because people react, the public, the general public reacts to people differently, right? They're going to react to me differently as a brown-skinned person than they would if I was not brown-skinned. Let's say if I was a very dark-skinned black person with short, kinky hair, people react differently. The world treats me differently because I have brown skin than they would if I didn't. There really isn't any closeness. I had this projection that there was . . . that we have more in common culturally because he's black and I identify myself as black. I don't identify myself as white. She's white."

For Tara it is ironic that, as she indicated, "I feel very much related to my [adoptive] parents and my sisters and my nieces and nephews. That's my family. And they're all white. But in terms of cultural aesthetic and how the world treats people, I felt like I would probably have more in common with my black biological father than my white biological mother because I have brown skin. Her kids are probably treated very differently in school than his kids are, and I figured, had this projection, that I would have more in common with his kids than hers culturally. But color has always played a huge role in the black community in this country."

Tara concluded, "If the racial analysis wasn't a part of my life because I had such a very comfortable life, I probably wouldn't have been that much more curious because I come from a home that's very, very politicized — and when I became politicized, it was over the issues of inequality and social injustice and apparently saw myself in a different category or culture than my family and I wanted an explanation for that. On the one hand, you're free to define it pretty much how you want to. People say that I've chosen to be black, that that was a choice that I made. It doesn't always feel like a choice to me, but fine, I'll accept that as a choice that I made and I made it in a way that I will affirm my identity as a black person with society, because it seems like you have to choose. That's the way I felt, that you did need to choose because people asked you."

Tara's remarkable insights into her life situation illuminate the fact that contrary to American cultural glorification of the existence in human life of individual choices, she lacked choice because she was constantly bombarded by questions regarding her physiological origins. The society and culture fashioned the choices for her. The choice was shaped by the ways in which American society and culture view her biological and genetic inheritance, rather than by her experience within her adopted white family. Her narrative clearly reveals how, ideologically, biology is culture, how her color defines her relationships. Moreover, biological determinism based on phenotypes pervades all segments of American society, including, as Tara makes clear, the black community. Both Tara's and Liz's accounts direct attention to the profound negative consequences of the cultural construction of genetic inheritance, which arguably surpasses even the belief in familial inheritance of medical disorders.

The adoptees we met thus far have tended to have various similarities, including the fact that they had searched for their birth mothers and found them, but found different degrees of comfort after having achieved their quest. I now turn to adoptees such as Bruce, who, unlike all the others, anchored his persona in his father; to June, whose birth mother found her; to Angela, whose birth relatives reject her completely; and to Mira, Karla, and Eric, who remain with unattained longings because they are still searching for their birth mothers. The latter four individuals are especially poignant because they exist not only in a state of conflict but also with a sense of being removed from their true selves. In the vocabulary of many adoptees, they have not achieved a "sense of wholeness" because they lack any knowledge of their "real heritage."

Bruce

Although for different reasons, Bruce like Loreta regards his biological father rather than mother as central to his persona. Bruce is a 26-year-old single college graduate, employed in public relations, who began the search three years earlier and found both his birth parents the same year I interviewed him.

Bruce initiated the search owing to a chance meeting with somebody who he believed resembled him, thinking that perhaps he was one of twins. He also wondered a great deal about his birth father, with whom he established a close relationship. Bruce noted that "in the beginning, I always thought that I could kind of keep a lid on the feelings that I had about it. I guess deep down inside there was more of a longing to know about this than I had let on. In the beginning it was strictly medical information — Who do I look like? How old were they? You know, just the basics." Later he thought he wished to initiate contact with his birth parents, especially his father, because "I needed to let him know that I was okay, that I turned out all right. It was never really an issue about my mother, but more my father. And it was really odd, when I finally found him. I have a good relationship with her. She's kind of shy about the whole thing. But with my dad, it just clicked and I found out that he had been wondering all these years what had happened to me. It's unusual, people never think the father . . . "

His father comes from a large family of siblings, and Bruce met most of them. Bruce, uniquely among adoptees we meet in this study, initially failed to recognize many similarities between himself and his father, but the family would, he said, "gasp and yell out that I did something like he did." But then he too noted that "we share little behavioral things. Personality quirks. I'm a procrastinator. And he is too. Kind of that scatterbrained disorganization like always losing the car keys or forgetting this little thing or that. I'm not really terrible at it and people have their own ways, but it was just amazing to see him walk through the house one morning yelling to his wife, 'Sue, where are my socks? I just had them here a minute ago. Are they in the dryer?' Whatever, just stuff like that I noticed. Characteristics I see in myself, including maybe some irreverence. He's a strong person mentally, and I definitely share that. And other physical things like, I don't know, we're double-jointed or something, a peculiar way that we stand up, the fact that all of us in the family are, I think, right-handed but we all have to bat left in baseball, the double cowlicks on my hair. Just all sorts of things like that. I really take after that side of the family. And I have some characteristics of my mother, too. A love of gardening and being outside and reading. She's a really big reader, and I love to read. You know, my dad, too, as far as the love of outdoors and being active and doing things and not just kind of vegetating; trying to be active and enjoy life and, gee, a lot of things. I'm really not a lot like my adoptive family in a lot of ways like that because I don't share a lot of that, the absolute independent thinking, the problem-solving nature, and all of that; I'm kind of analytical." Nevertheless, Bruce acknowledged that he shared with his adoptive family "a sense of stubbornness and things like that. There are some similarities, but I think, I do things like my biological family, but I believe it's kind of the way it manifests itself in a particular situation or kind of the way I express things" that may be more like his adoptive parents. Bruce, after having spent time with his birth father's family, became convinced that he had inherited all the behavioral characteristics rather than only diseases.

It was important to Bruce to obtain medical information. He observed, "All I had was that my maternal grandfather had a heart attack at age 55 and that was all. When I was a child, I had a heart murmur and I started thinking, 'What if I want to have kids. What am I going to pass on to these children? What if there's some horrible disease?' And I want kids one day, but I had it set in my mind that if I didn't get some answers and see what was going on genetically that I wouldn't have children. I didn't know that I would marry or anything else. I was very determined about that. It really worried me."

Actually, Bruce had learned that his grandfather's heart attack was "just an anomaly. Apparently he just walked in the woods and had a heart attack and keeled over. I don't know that there was anything genetically going on. I met my grandmother, who is in her late 80s. They all live to be way old and pretty happy unless they happen to smoke or do something ridiculous like that and die, then they all seem to be healthy people. No funny diseases or anything. That was a real relief to know that. I mean, to at least know that I should have a good life, a long life, if I take care of myself."

While Bruce became close to his birth father and his family, the person to whom he feels closest is his best friend. Bruce was one of the few who spoke openly against adoption, and his objections strike at the core of the American cultural definition of biogenetic kinship. "I think there's something that comes with adoption. It's kind of like — this may be a terrible thing to say, but I'm going to say it — it's almost like it's a setup, which I guess it is when you're put in this home and you're expected to love your adoptive parents, which I do. And they're expected to love you, which they do. *But there almost seems to be some artificial nature to it or something.* I'd say I'm so close to my best friend because that is a relationship that I built with him. We've grown up together like brothers, and he can read me like a book and I can do the same with him. And there's that natural closeness built, not a trust that's been forced there by the courts necessarily. It's a kind of natural thing."

Bruce perceives adoption as artificial because, according to him, "it's forced. It's forced. I mean they say adoptive parents get to pick out this child and they don't get to pick you out. They get whoever pops out at the time. And that's a bunch of bull, you know. In my case, they really didn't take the time to see that I matched or anything. I'm blond and blue-eyed, and everybody else on both sides of the family has dark hair, dark eyes, and stuff. And it was always funny when I was little, because I'd hear people say, 'Don't worry. His hair will darken up.' It never did. And I've still got these blue eyes. I think that it's all forced like that, and that is what gives it maybe an artificial quality. It's like it's not natural, it's manmade. The difference between real glass and then you've got plastic, sort of thing." Bruce believes that birth parents and their children "share so many similarities. I think a mother or father immediately knows their child and can understand their behaviors—when they cry, what they want, and all of this. I don't say that that doesn't come to an adoptive relationship, but it's just not there in the beginning."

Bruce had not anticipated that when he met his birth family he would care for them, but to his surprise he did, "because they're family. I can't really explain it. I found myself caring for them. I found myself thinking about them every day. And it's been a pleasant surprise," although admittedly, he did not have the same overwhelming feelings for his mother as he did for his father.

Bruce may have been correct when he said that most people think less about their fathers than about their mothers. He is indeed an exception that points to the emphasis American society places on genetic ties rather than on the bond between mother and child that may be established during pregnancy.[26] But Bruce conforms to the norms of other adoptees who believe that the person inherits from family and kin not only diseases but even the most trivial personality characteristics, revealing also the notion that a human being is but a receptacle for genes and blood to do their work.

Bruce's narrative reflects the separation in Western society between nature and culture. Blood and genetic ties are natural; adoption, as a cultural practice, is unnatural. Bruce's claim — that had he not found his birth family's medical history he would avoid having children — suggests how biogenetic ideology profoundly guides his experience. However, it also reassures him that he will have a long and healthy life, emphasizing the favorable consequences of this ideology.

Significantly also, while Bruce has internalized the ideology of genetic inheritance, his life adheres to the postmodern model of family that is defined, as for Roberta, by affection and friendship.

Angela

Angela, like Bruce and Loreta, believes that she inherited most of her attributes from her father. But, unlike Bruce, she had an excellent relationship with her adoptive parents. At 59 years of age, Angela, a college graduate, is divorced and lives by herself. She recently became an independently employed accountant after having worked for most of her life in a chemical and dye factory.

Angela, adopted by a minister and his wife, had been thinking about searching for 30 years but had not actually begun the search until two years earlier. She succeeded in finding a half sister, who refused to speak with her, and a first cousin, with whom she has had several telephone contacts. Angela was very saddened by her sister's rebuff, even after she explained that she was only seeking health information.

Angela stated, "I had a wonderful adoptive mother and father. And they lived to be old, really old people. My father died at age 80; he's been dead about seven years. And my mother is still living. She is 91 years old. And I always felt like that if I really looked for my mother, maybe mama and daddy wouldn't like it. And I just sort of put it off for years, even though I was grown. I was out on my own, making my own decisions, and I should have gone on with it, but I just sort of felt like they'd given me such a good life that why should I look for anybody else? But then I had developed some, uh, physical problems . . . Well, I had some kidney problems, for one thing. And also, I have always had bronchial problems, all my life, which is either bronchitis or asthmatic. I wondered if that was hereditary, but I had worked for a chemical company for 21 years and I worked with some beta naphthalene and I wondered if that might have caused my kidney problems. I just retired in July. So I feel like maybe the kidney problem may have come from that, but the asthma and bronchitis is genetic."

If Angela had any doubts about the cause of her diseases, they were dispelled after she spoke with her cousin. Angela established that her condition was genetic because the cousin told her it was all on that side of the family and, Angela said, "Quite frankly, right now I've got bronchitis. But my main concern was all these medical problems that I'm seeing. The medical problems. And I really didn't think too much about it until I got to my age and wondered, Why in the world am I having all this stuff, you know? I worked in the laboratories for, say, fifteen years, and I worked with all kinds of chemicals and dyes and, as a matter of fact, I worked on an infrared reflector. So I worked on that for maybe ten years before we ever got the patent on it. And, in making that stuff, it had the beta naph-thalene in it."

Notwithstanding her work history, Angela holds that her health problems are genetic because, she said, "I think a lot of things are genetic, because our whole makeup has to do with our background or our roots, because, you know, I was nothing. Well, in some ways I guess I was. When we start searching for birth parents, I think you wonder what is in the background. Like, am I susceptible to having heart attacks or strokes or cancer, or all these medical type things. And I think that's what you really want to know—what's in the background that I could possibly have that's going to take me out of here?" Angela had no doubt that her poor health resulted from her genetic inheritance. She noted, "I just have seen it in so many families that if you have, for instance, cancer, it may skip a generation and it may show up in the next generation or the next, you know."

To her regret, Angela was unable to acquire enough information about her family medical history. She learned that "there was some cancer that runs in the family. And some stroke victims, but other than that I haven't found out much else. You know, I don't know a whole bunch about genetics, I really don't, but I know enough to know that things do filter down over periods of time, including the color of the eyes, the color of your hair, the color of your skin. And your health situation." Other than having inherited her dark hair and olive skin, Angela believes that her birth daughter, who had twins, had inherited the twinning from Angela's birth mother's side of the family, who also gave birth to twins.

Unlike other adoptees, Angela believes that she acquired her business acumen and her desire for enjoying life from her adoptive father. She claimed to have inherited her character traits not from her birth mother but from her birth father, whom she had not yet met. She said, "And that's why I am going to try to pursue this thing with the father because I think I'm more like him. I think I look like my mother but I don't think I had any of her traits."

Angela's chief motive for searching was to obtain a health history. Her commitment to the ideology of genetic inheritance precludes her embracing other possibilities that could explain her health condition or her personality traits, even though she finds it feasible that her diseases might be associated with her exposure to toxic chemicals when she worked in the factory. Interestingly, too, like other adoptees, Angela assumes her persona is shaped by biological factors rather than by her vision of her own experience.

June

June was the only participant in the study whose birth mother initiated the search. June, a 38-year-old divorced mother of a 10-year-old girl, is a psychotherapist with an M.A. in counseling. June had not actively searched for her birth mother, although she placed her name on a list accessible to birth mothers who search for their children. She did so because people often asked her whether she was curious about her birth mother. June listed her name four years ago, and two years later her birth mother's husband contacted her. June recounted, "I was in denial, but then my adoptive parents did not take well to a search." June responded negatively to her birth mother's call, especially when she told June how much she loved her. June replied, " 'You don't know me.' She loved me without knowing me. How can this be?"

When June met her birth mother, she said, "I felt amazement and expected a more innate connection, that of a primal urge, that I didn't feel. There is a striking physical resemblance, but the woman is in terrible health, overweight, looks much older than her age. I don't want my life to be like this. What if it's in my genes to look like her? What if it's in my genes to have her health? She had breast cancer, colon cancer, diabetes, high blood pressure—every organ system was sick. June's birth mother knew very little about her father, who had been an alcoholic and a schizophrenic and had died in a mental institution, "and it's not fun to have DNA like that. Also there was hemophilia." June underscored that when she visits a doctor and is asked to fill out a medical history, she, unlike almost all the other adoptees, just fills in "no problems." While June believes her mother and father's health history can have an impact on her health, she nevertheless observed, "I have lived a different life; it will go better with me." She would have been upset about not knowing that there was a hemophilia line in her family if she had given birth to a boy, but fortunately she had a girl.

Nor does June feel connected to her adopted parents. Expressing sentiments similar to Bruce's about adoption, she indicated that, unlike with blood kin, adopted family could be disowned, whereas blood siblings cannot. "Adopted parent and sibling relationships are tied by word. The word made us a family, and we can undo it like a marriage. *In a biological family we cannot eradicate the way we are connected. I am walking around with your stuff in my body. You are part of my body and I am part of your body and that we cannot undo.*" In fact, according to June, adoptees have a choice: if things go wrong, one can say they are not real family. Significantly, June, like Pamela and Risa, became closer to her adopted parents after meeting her birth mother because she was astounded, she said, "that I came out of that woman's body."

Yet, she also felt she was different from the rest of her adopted family because she didn't come into the family through a birth ritual. She commented, "People usually talk about, you have father's nose, mother's chin, whereas this was not said about me." Her adoptive family was "very genealogically conscious, and they trace their ancestors to whoever, in the Revolution"; for this reason, too, she felt especially different from the rest of the family. June regards an adopted child as a replacement; in her case, she replaced a dead child, whose name she bears. She did feel close to her adoptive mother's parents, but in actuality she did not feel connected to any of them.

At the conclusion of our meeting, June observed that adoptees are not the first choice for an adoptive parent. In the majority of cases children are adopted, June claimed, because the couple is infertile, and thus the fact that adoption is a second choice ought to be discussed. In June's view, adoptees are second best. Her adoptive parents were "middle-class Protestants, and such parents are in a bind because they are judgmental. They are rearing a child whose mother lived a sordid life. They feel the shame of illegitimacy, that they were rearing a trashy parent's behavior. But, this is my DNA, and it should matter."

June, as a psychotherapist, is arguably more analytical about adoption than most of the other people in the study. However, she, like the others, displays a high degree of conflict between concepts of genetic inheritance and culture, as she conceives it. It could be said that June was a passive searcher; she only placed her name on a list. Yet, when she was found, she completely rejected the woman who gave birth to her. She claims she does not feel any ties to her birth mother. Paradoxically, as a member of American society, she holds that genetic-blood ties can never be severed, whereas ties established by culture, by "a word," as is the case with adoption, can, creating a profound conflict for her.

People Who Have Not Yet Found Their Birth Parents

Mira

Mira is 29 years old, a high school graduate, and a housewife with two young children. Mira had contemplated searching for her birth parents since she was 18 years old. She recalled, "I've always wanted to know, but the main thing that made me start looking, uh, I think it was 1988, my husband and I lost a child before it was born. We lost it to spina bifida which, I was told in the hospital, was one of the worst cases they had ever seen. They told me then I probably wouldn't have a normal child; that was wrong. He said the chances of me having a normal child were, my doctor told me this, slim to none." Mira ignored the hospital's advice, and she now is the mother of two healthy children. Although her children are well, she nevertheless wishes to secure her family medical history.

Mira continued, "But I got to thinking about all the different things, just like in my family — when I say 'my family' I mean my adoptive family, because they are my family — epilepsy runs in their family. My mother has it, my brother has it. A couple of other people in my mother's family have it. Uh, my dad's mother had diabetes and high blood pressure. He has diabetes and high blood pressure. She had a heart problem, and she died back in October; my dad has a heart problem. So many things run genetically down the line and it's not just me that I was thinking about anymore, so I'm more determined now. I've always wanted to know and always wondered, but with them [her children], I feel like there is no family history other than it stops with me. And I feel like that's not fair [to her children]. I wanted to know because of my children. That's one of the reasons that really pushes me. And basically I've always, like I said, I've always wanted to know. But because of them I push a little bit harder now. Once I find my birth mother, hopefully it will give a little bit of family medical history, that type of thing."

While Mira would like to know whom she resembles, more important to her is to trace her roots, in the same way as her husband had traced his antecedents to the *Mayflower*. Mira stressed, "I have no past. Everybody has a past. They can go back. My husband's family, they've traced their roots back to the *Mayflower*. My mother's sister did their genealogical tree back for years upon years upon years. Mine ends with me and begins with me. While my adopted family are a part of my past, there is a past that I don't know about. There are people out there that are blood-related to me whom I've never seen." When she finds her birth mother, she believes she will recapture that past.

Mira felt she lacked a past even in elementary school, when the children were asked to prepare genealogies that were displayed publicly along with the children's birth certificates. Mira's birth certificate lacked various kinds of information, and she felt very isolated.[27] When her classmates saw her birth certificate they asked her why hers was different, and she felt extremely uncomfortable.

Mira too stressed that she and her adoptive mother possessed very different personalities, and she had wondered how she acquired opposing characteristics from her adopted mother, including her love of horses and her desire to be a tomboy. Mira noted, "Well, like my mom has always been scared to death of horses. I have a love for them. I've loved them from the time I was old enough to say 'horse,' and mom was always scared to death of them. She'd say, 'They stink. They're nasty. They're this,' you know. When I got married my husband bought me a horse, and to this day I still shovel manure and still love the smell of hay. It came from somewhere. Just like my brother, my mother is inclined to like certain things. The reason they adopted is because they wanted a girl. Well, I wasn't exactly . . . I was a tomboy. 'Don't brush my hair. No, I don't want to wear that frilly dress.' You know, so it wasn't exactly the package she wanted, but she loves me anyway. She really does. I am not like my mother, personalitywise. The things I like. I like to go camping and do outdoor things, and mom is totally [different], she's an indoor . . . she's got to have her makeup on, she's got to have her hair just fixed right, even if she's just working around the house. That's not me. I mean that's just not me and never has been. I don't think it ever will be. When I was in high school I was hanging out with, I had more guy friends, and when my friends started dating and stuff, I'd be going to the football games or basketball games with the guys I played basketball with, you know. That was me, and mom would say 'What's wrong? Why are you doing this?' Most people can say, 'Well, I got this from my mom' or 'I got this from my dad.' Here I am, I have these certain ways and like these certain things and they don't follow anyone in the family. I don't understand what exactly makes up certain traits in people or that type of thing. But I know I don't have anything, I'm not anything like my mom."

Mira believes that she may have inherited these traits from her birth mother; otherwise, she cannot explain all those characteristics of her personality she enumerated. But while Mira is interested in knowing the origin of her personality traits, she stressed that she was mostly concerned about her genetic heritage because her adoptive family's history is not her history.

Mira maintains that a powerful bond is established during pregnancy with the infant, and she imagines that her birth mother, who was a college student at the time, must have been under tremendous pressure to give her away. Mira would like her birth mother to know that she shouldn't feel guilty about giving her away, that she made the right choice, because Mira was placed in a wonderful home and family. Mira would like to find her father as well, but her main concern now is to find her birth mother in order to discover her past, which she conceives in biological and genetic terms.

Biology and genetics will establish for Mira a permanence that her adoptive parents cannot give because they fail to share the same genes, the same blood. Only the same genes and the same blood can give Mira, and the others, her personhood. Biography and experience are of little importance. Mira cannot imagine that her interests originated in her own being. Mira's and the other adoptees' concerns flow from cultural conceptualizations of genealogical history reinforced by notions of genetics. Importantly too, in this instance, family medical history is a powerful incentive to search, to know that her children's health is not threatened.

Karla

Karla is a 21-year-old college student residing with her significant other. She was very unhappy with her adoptive parents. Her dissatisfaction and sadness are clearly registered in her facial expression. Unlike most of the other adoptees, a single and ill mother raised Karla because her adoptive father, a college professor, left the family.

Karla, who has not as yet found her birth mother, initiated the search a month before we met, because she desired to know, "Is there somebody that I look like? Somebody whose hands are similar to mine? Whose eyes are similar? There's a medical background issue, too. I know my paternal grandfather had high blood pressure, but it was controlled with medication. And that he wore glasses. And that my maternal grandmother was an alcoholic. But that's all I know. Now 20 years have passed, so is there cancer? heart disease? which would be relevant. Or like my mom, my adoptive family: migraines run in the family. High blood pressure runs in the family. Strokes run in the family. Cancer runs in the family. I'm glad I'm not biologically related to them. If you know that [the diseases], you can prepare. Maybe I could change my diet or exercise more, or if breast cancer runs in my family start having mammograms earlier. If cervical cancer runs in the family, have Pap smears more than once a year. Have physicals more often. If you are not adopted, you take that for granted."

Karla always knew that all these diseases were inherited. She claimed, "It's just like the type of ears you inherit: Why wouldn't you inherit the genes that make you have certain diseases? My mother's mom died in her late 50s of a stroke. My mom checks her high blood pressure. She knows that her great-aunt has diabetes because she stopped smoking and then gained lots of weight and then got diabetes so my mom knows to watch her weight so that she doesn't get diabetes. If I knew my biological parents, I would do things differently. If I had certain diseases in my background, like breast cancer or something, I'd start doing mammograms now. Because you know people say that cancer is rare in young people my age but I knew people in high school that died of cancer." Karla knows about diseases being inherited from observing her adoptive mother, whose father had prostate cancer and whose uncle now had it. She proclaimed, "So don't tell me that it's a coincidence, because I won't believe you."

Karla desires to know who she is. She has certain questions, including, "Why didn't you keep me? Why did you give me up? I have no baby pictures. What did I look like? What kind of baby was I?" Karla claimed she could trace her adoptive family to 1500, but that is not her biological family. She noted, "Like I could be the Daughter of the American Revolution, but I can't tell them I'm adopted."

Karla, too, claims to be completely different from her adoptive mother. They are "like total opposites. Her view of family is that I'm supposed to take care of her. It's my duty. She's taken care of me for this many years, so I have to take care of her. The way she looks at family is a little bit different than I do." From Karla's perspective, true, she is her mother and has taken care of her, but that "doesn't necessarily mean that now it's my turn and my duty to take care of you. I would do it because I love you, not because you took care of me for the amount of years. It's really weird when you sit down for a family portrait like with uncles, aunts, and cousins and you look nothing alike." In Karla's adopted family, people incessantly referred to the way they looked like other members of the ascending or contemporary generations, whereas Karla was left out of these discussions.

Wistfully, Karla noted how her boyfriend is like his father, whereas she is like neither her father nor her mother. "My mom has a dry sense of humor. I don't know if I'd call her ambitious, but she doesn't necessarily want to work or have a career, whereas I want to have a career, but not anything like my dad. Well, I'm stubborn. Both of my parents have that." Karla, however, concluded that stubbornness is learned rather than biological.

Karla is convinced that her learning disability was inherited. She learned that her biological mother wasn't very good at school. Her birth mother didn't like school, and Karla knew from the adoption record that the woman had learning disabilities, which Karla attributes either to genetic inheritance or to having been a premature baby. Karla's mother was very poor, and her father was ethnically Italian. She noted, "A person identifies with who they are. If they're Southern or their family has always been from the South of the U.S., they identify with being Southern. My father and my mother did this and my grandmother and grandfather did this and they came over here — there's a sense of pride, you know." Karla speculated that her birth family could be traced to colonial times.

Karla became desirous of knowing her birth family when she started college and did a paper on adoption laws. At present, she is concentrating on finding her birth mother, particularly since she desires children. She said, "There are certain genetic things that are passed down through the blood line . . . if you ever see those documentaries on TV. Or like if you have cancer and you need a bone marrow transplant and you need a match. Or like Alzheimer's. I'd really like to know if that runs in my family. You can be tested for the gene, and if you carry it it's 100 percent you're going to get it."

Karla is certain that when people in the same family do not look like their parents they must have been adopted. Her maxim is that all children look like their biological parents and that every aspect of one's physiognomy is inherited. While Karla also recognizes that a mother is the one who raises the child, she is alienated from her adoptive mother as well as from all other members of her adoptive family.

Several motives have moved Karla to search for her birth mother, not the least of which is her desire to obtain a medical history, which she, too, regards as a warning document controlling her health destiny. Concurrently, the same document may allay her fears of becoming afflicted by the diseases from which her adopted mother suffers, because her birth mother may have suffered from none of them. In addition to gaining a sense of certainty about her future health status, knowledge of her genetic inheritance will provide Karla with a sense of history and continuity, which she currently lacks. It may even demonstrate that she is a Daughter of the American Revolution, in which she could also take pride. Karla's persona is enveloped in her biological origins.

Karla's preoccupation with her body, her curiosity about whom she resembles physically, reflect her alienation and her feeling of isolation, as well as reflecting a postmodern absorption with the body. But she is also conflicted between her cultural understanding that her personhood was inherited from her biological parents and her experience of having been raised by her adoptive family, consistent with yet another postmodern sensibility — that family comprises those she chooses and loves, rather than those who raised her.

Eric

Eric is 51 years old, married with two children, a college graduate, and employed in a managerial position. He began the search eight months prior to our meeting, shortly after the death of both his adoptive parents, to whom he felt very close.

Sadly for Eric, the woman who, he is quite certain, is his birth mother has not responded to his several letters of introduction. Eric desires to meet her primarily because he wishes to obtain his medical history now that he is getting older so that he might learn what health problems to anticipate for himself and his children. Eric said that "the one thing that a lot of adoptees who are looking say when they go to the doctor's office and they take a medical history, and they are asked, 'Has there been any history of high blood pressure or heart disease or diabetes or glaucoma or whatever in your family?' And, of course, I, like them, always have had to say, 'I have no idea,' because I was adopted; I have no medical background. And heredity plays such a big part. I mean, I think it's become more evident every year as to how much heredity affects your genes, and DNA and all that affects your well-being throughout your whole life and what kind of diseases or whatever you are prone to possibly get. So, it was important for me from that perspective, the medical perspective, but not just for me, but for my children, because they have the same missing pieces in their medical background because I have them and I'm half of what they are. And as I matured and as I got older and, of course, the older you get, the more likely you are to come down with something or have something develop, whether it's your eyesight or whatever it is. And I've never liked doctors. I try to stay away as frequently as possible, not go, but the older I get the more I realize that it's an important thing that I need to be aware of and plan for the future and my children need it. And when and if they have children, that'll be something that — if I hand them that missing piece of the puzzle, or at least part of the missing piece of the puzzle, I would be able to pass along to them the knowledge that, yes, your maternal grandmother was prone to this problem or that or your great-grandmother or whatever."

Eric was also curious about his birth mother, because "it's a part of me that I don't know where it came from. I think the other part [not referring to the medical part] is just probably as much of a driving force in my search for beginning; it was just natural curiosity. I like to know, so many people compare, I mean, how many times have you gone and seen a new baby and heard people say, 'Oh, she looks just like so-and-so,' or 'He looks just like his dad,' or whatever. And I don't look like either one of my parents." Eric could not find any resemblance between himself and anyone in his adoptive family. Eric would like to find his birth father as well, but, in his words, "I am a novice in searching, and it has consumed enormous amounts of time on the Internet reading other people's thoughts and emotions and anger and guilt." Thus, he has lost the energy for the time being.

Eric believes that not only will he recapitulate his birth mother's medical history but that he inherited from his birth parents certain characteristics that he fails to share with his adoptive parents. He disclosed, "It used to amaze my parents with my ability to, or inquisitiveness about taking things apart, figuring out how they work, and putting them back together. Two of the things that I did a lot of as I was growing up and even into adulthood that my father would never do, my adoptive father, is if something broke, I'd try to fix it. He'd call a repairman. One of the things that I have oftentimes said, halfway in jest and halfway in reality is, 'I wish I could turn the clock back and say to hell with going to a university for four years.' I would have been a lot happier person, I think, if I had gone and taken six months' worth of community college courses in plumbing and another six months in [electrical work] and learned, because I admire very much the ability of someone to do things like that, to actually be able . . . not to just have to write a check and say, 'Come fix it.' And I get a real feeling of satisfaction about replacing the brakes on my car or repairing the television, not that I can repair televisions. The other thing that was so much different was my enjoyment of the outdoors from a sports standpoint. I love to fish and I did hunt a little bit. I haven't in years, but to the best of my knowledge my father never hunted, and about the only time he ever went fishing was when he took me out to a pond somewhere and watched me fish. And actually I went fishing with my mother's only brother, my uncle, on several occasions. I even camped out with him and went canoeing on the river down near my mother's hometown. I went deer hunting with him, and I've been on the river with him before, and that's just not something my father ever had any interest in. I think an awful lot of what a person is comes from their parents. From their birth parents, yeah. From the genes and the DNA and all of that; that's what made them up."

To Eric, kinship relations infer friendship as part of the relationship, of enjoying the same things but also being part of a biological unit. Eric stated, "Kinship is a feeling of togetherness or bonding or being part of . . . You know you enjoy the same things that I do, you love the same things that I love, whether it be the ocean or animals. I think that, to me, that's something else that you may have inherited. I mean your love of animals or your dislike for animals, you know—I hate cats, I love cats. My wife loves animals. My parents could have cared less. They always allowed me to have animals, but I never perceived any real affection to my dogs and my cats from them. I think you can be related by way of kinship and not be biologically related. Eric, like most of the adoptees we have met, conflates shared interest with blood ties. They cannot conceive themselves as agents of their own personhood. Their persona must have come from somewhere, if it did not have its roots in their adoptive families.

As with Kristen, the medical history was the chief reason Eric initiated the search for his birth mother, even though, as with the other adoptees, diverse motivations entered into his decisions. This calculus reflects his confusion about who is his real family—people for whom he feels affection and with whom he shares experiential commonalities or people with whom he shares a genetic inheritance that embodies medical and genealogical memory.

Ronold

I conclude this chapter with Ronold, who had contacted me when he learned of this research and volunteered to discuss why, as an adoptee, he has *not* searched for his birth parents.

Ronold, a 45-year-old single college graduate with a major in sociology, is employed in the real estate industry. Ronold explained, "I think the reason for not looking for my parents, my natural parents, for two reasons, I guess, is that my mom, my family made me feel as much like their natural child as I felt there was such a bond, and particularly with my grandma. My [paternal] grandmother, I think, made more of an impression familywise on me than my parents because it was such a small town and we knew everybody and everybody knew us and it was just a very tight-knit community and we were well connected in the church. My uncle was a minister, not there, but he was involved in the same denomination. We were all connected through the church as well as through the country club, and there was just a lot of social institutions that kept us all together. That would be number one. Number two would be that my grandmother made my family's life so real, so much like one of them."

Ronold was also concerned about the feelings of his birth mother, "because they have another life and they've put that whole thing behind them 40 — at that point it was 20 years ago — you know, they had built a life. I had built a life and my parents were still living and there was really no need, and then when I saw several pictures of natural parents and their child reuniting and it's almost always that the natural mother is in tears, that the father or the child will either have a blank or smiling expression, but the mother is almost always crying. Would I want, had I sired a child 20 years ago, would I want them ringing the doorbell in their second year at the university and they need $20,000 for tuition? And that kind of solidified with me not getting in touch with them. So that's kind of the way I've rationalized it. Probably 50 percent of the people that I've talked to in the last 25 years that have been adopted have made the effort to find out who their natural parents are," including Ronold's adopted sister.

Nevertheless, Ronold's questions are similar to those of other adoptees we met in this chapter. He is curious about whom he resembles, and, he said, "If I had a blood disease, for instance, and needed a transfusion, I would have no qualms whatsoever in contacting them. If I needed a liver or a kidney, I would definitely — then I wouldn't have a problem at all. And if I thought they had a problem and needed blood from me, I wouldn't have a problem there at all."

Significantly, Ronold believes he would have nothing in common with his birth parents. He stated, "I've always thought that my environment basically dictated the way . . . I mean, when I lose my temper, I sound just like my father. My sister has told me that several times. I'll hear it. Now that she's pointed it out to me, I'll hear it. I'll get mad and I'll say something that sounds just like dad. And then I'm over that and my temper's gone. My temper's gone real quickly. I guess he had such a bad temper and it was, we don't want to be like daddy. I didn't go to all this trouble to end up like my dad. I wouldn't change a thing. The only reason I would get in touch with my parents would be a medical emergency."

Ronold's physician had obtained his birth family's medical history, and he informed Ronold that there was no family history of any disease.[28] Ultimately, however, Ronold too seemed to believe that a child and its natural mother bond more closely than a child and its adoptive mother, when he said, "To be perfectly honest with you, I've seen the natural bond between my mother and her siblings; we didn't have that. But then, my cousins did. My cousins, uh, my cousins had a mama that was just as close as any mom I've ever seen to her children and just as understanding and forgiving and loving and would do anything for them. There was never that forgiveness, that loving forgiveness that 'no matter what you do, I'll still love you.' I've seen natural parents that have a much more solid connection. My girlfriend at this point has a daughter, and I see how they are; no matter what they say to each other, they still come back and they're still just as fond as they can be. And I don't see that, I never felt that with our parents, and my sister didn't have it either." Ronold attributes this special bond to the birth process, "that kind of spirituality," he said.

It is noteworthy that Ronold was not motivated to search for his birth parents because of a need for his family medical history, although the medical domain still impinges on his consciousness when he refers to kinship and the need for transfusions. He also has embodied the understanding, perhaps attributable to his sociological training, that genetic inheritance, to the exclusion of a person's life experience and biography, fails to influence a person's being, yet he, like Risa and Loreta, imbues biology and the relations it fosters with spirituality.

In this chapter we have met fifteen adoptees, thirteen of whom had actively searched for their birth parents. Each embarked on the search for different reasons, but with the exception of Tara and Ronold they shared an overarching concern for their medical histories, illuminating the ways in which biomedical conceptualizations mold people's understanding of health and disease, reinforcing people's sense of kinship established by reproduction and genetics. This leads me to propose the notion of the medicalization of kinship which is brought into bold relief not only by cancer patients and those who come from families with cancer, but especially by the adoptees' narratives. For the majority of adoptees, perhaps even more than any other segment of the population, their family medical histories are the histories of the people whom they consider genetically related, and this also defines them as people.

From these narratives we also glean other important themes that flow from the adoptees' conceptualization of genetic inheritance that bear on the nature of family and kinship in modern life; on the nature of truth and fiction, as June and Bruce make us aware, on issues of class, ethnicity and race, when we hear Loreta, Tara and Liz; on a desire for memory and continuity that we encounter in most of their accounts, and on a yearning for what adoptees identify as wholeness, in light of their fragmentation. In fact, these narratives also reveal the degree to which the adoptees are fragmented people torn between their idealization of kinship based on genetic ties, some even elevated to spiritual heights, and their experience of having been raised and cared for by people to whom they are tied only by what June called "a word," or by love. Are this fragmentation and its resulting tensions culturally constructed and unique to American society, or are they existential concerns experienced universally by all humans? Can we then separate reproduction and birth from kinship and genetics, as the Schneider school is wont to do? As I noted previously, in order to address this issue we require empirical data from societies such as the Navajo and others where kinship ties are not based on concepts of genetic ties. Do individuals there still long to learn who gave birth to them, irrespective of cultural indifference to birth ties? Are the Schneiderians correct in stating that what are seemingly existential issues are ultimately culturally molded dilemmas?

Adoptees direct our attention to the fact that conceptualizations developed by sociobiology are manifested in their quest for birth parents. Sociobiological theories, a variant of nineteenth-century Social Darwinism, form part of these individuals' consciousness, whether they have formally studied them or not. The adoptees in this study, for the most part, hold that not only do their bodies recapitulate histories of their genealogical kin but also their personas—behavior, personality, and all aspects of existence—are carried in the DNA, that human beings are inactive repositories stamped by DNA, independent of their lived experience.

Whereas the questions raised by the adoptees' materials cannot be theorized but can best be addressed empirically by cross-cultural research, we can question and meditate on the role the ideology of genetic inheritance plays in contemporary life in broader terms. This is the subject of the next chapter.

Part III
Implications

Chapter 8
The Ideology of Genetic Inheritance in Contemporary Life

The Medicalization of Kinship

In the previous three chapters, individuals with family histories of cancer, breast cancer patients, and adoptees illuminated the ways in which the concept of genetic inheritance variously influences day-to-day experience. In this chapter I propose that one important consequence of contemporary genetic conceptualizations has been the medicalization of family and kinship, which came into bold relief in the preceding three chapters. I begin by exploring the notion of medicalization and its ramifications for contemporary understandings of kinship and family.

The Concept of Medicalization

The concept of medicalization is not a twentieth-century phenomenon, of course. Promoted by a growing secularization, in the eighteenth and nineteenth centuries, for example, suicide and homosexuality came to be viewed in England as diseases rather than moral transgressions.[1] It is, however, difficult to establish precisely when the term *medicalization* acquired cultural currency and became part of our routine vocabulary. Broom and Woodward suggest that the notion of medicalization first appeared in 1968 when it was identified as a tendency for medical institutions to deal with nonconforming behaviors by labeling them as sickness.[2] Surprisingly, there is considerable agreement concerning the definition of medicalization: it usually involves both expansion of medical jurisdiction to cover forms of deviant behavior and surveillance of nondeviant behavioral phenomena, which I will discuss shortly.[3]

Medicalization refers to the drawing into the biomedical domain of physical aspects and behaviors such as antisocial conduct that could be understood alternatively as a sin, a crime, a moral fault, or a disease.[4]

Alcoholism, domestic violence, criminal behavior, child abuse, personality characteristics, learning disabilities, and even gambling — formerly considered religious, ethical, or moral transgressions or matters of character — have been reinterpreted as diseases.[5] Bauman suggests that even death has been medicalized, owing to fears of it in contemporary society, as evidenced by the search for its causes in degenerative or defective genes, rather than acknowledging that humans are mortal beings and that death is merely part of the human condition.[6]

Although men have not escaped the grip of medicalization, as with, for example, impotency and male pattern baldness,[7] it is women's natural bodily processes that have been most subject to medicalization. Menstruation, menopause, birthing, and reproduction have been brought under medical scrutiny.[8] Women are treated medically for even slight discomfort during menstruation, but especially when it is labeled as premenstrual syndrome (PMS). Menopause and of course birthing require close medical supervision.[9] Aesthetic sensibilities, too, have been medicalized with the emphasis on a thin body and youthful appearance requiring maintenance through cosmetic surgery.[10] New technology has extended the medical gaze to the fetus, making it visible: with this direct visualization through sonography, even the unborn is treated like a patient.[11] Lastly, as Witzig points out, race, characterized in American culture by three major racial groupings, is medicalized every time an association is made between such groupings and specific diseases.[12]

Medicalization changes people's perspectives on reality, on their being, and on how they experience the world. In Englehardt's view, this new perspective translates sets of problems into medical terms that mold the ways in which the world of experience takes shape; it conditions people's reality. When seen as medical problems, behaviors are usually characterized as circumstances that deviate from physiological or psychological ideas regarding proper levels of functioning, freedom from pain, and achievement of expected human form.[13] For example, in his discussion of the medicalization of homosexuality in the nineteenth century, Hansen points out that a new type of person was created and a new core identity given to such persons: now a homosexual was regarded as having a particular genetic makeup.[14] Previously, homosexuality had been viewed as a type of behavior, albeit an aberrant one; now, with its medicalization, the homosexual became a new "species" of person.

When we accept a phenomenon as a medical problem, we also seek its causes by describing them, in Englehardt's words, as "genetic, infectious, or environmental diseases,"[15] caused by an alteration of chemical processes in the DNA, by pathogens, or by the mechanics of the body having broken down. By doing so, we create a different kind of reality from that of, for instance, the traditional Mexican belief that sickness is caused by witchcraft, evil spirits, transgressions against God, or emotional discharges.[16] In the Mexican example, people's understanding of reality — and most important, their relationship to the world and to other human beings — is shaped by these explanations, including the fact that other human beings can do harm to one another by manipulating evil forces, that the cosmos is composed of disincarnated spirits, that a punishing deity exists, and that human feelings such as anger provoked by others can cause sickness. The latter is especially interesting because the attribution of sickness to anger crystallizes a human's sense of morality, a sense of what ought to be, an outrage at injustice.[17] The medicalization process, on the other hand, focuses on the physicality of human existence to the exclusion of other dimensions of being human, including social relations and moral evaluations, or even the recognition of evil.

Medicalization restructures reality by intruding on the world people take for granted, on their tacit understanding of what is normal, by transforming the taken-for-granted state into an abnormal, disconcerting state, separating the individual from the larger whole. Contemporarily, the view is that human beings are constituted of myriad genes that describe the whole organism, and the genetic system in all humans is the same; variation is abnormal. Deviations among people are expressed chiefly in anomalies or defects. If people differ from their kin, or from what is construed to be the ideal in their kin map, they are considered abnormal.[18]

Consider three examples from Mexico that are especially instructive of the ways in which the medicalization process changes one's view of oneself and reality. In the first instance, we see a person resisting medicalization. A peasant woman gave birth to two Down's syndrome children in succession. She was counseled to avoid having any more children; however, she refused to regard these children as suffering from an affliction. In fact, she claimed that she preferred such children because they were more docile and more manageable than her other children. The Down's syndrome children were also better field hands than the rest. For this peasant woman, her Down's syndrome children were an asset and unproblematic. By medicalizing their beings, the woman began to perceive her children adversely rather than as positive contributors to the household's welfare.[19]

The second example is of three sisters diagnosed with oculopharyngeal muscular dystrophy.[20] Two of the sisters, on referral by their physicians, had surgery performed to correct the condition, even though they failed to comprehend why their situation was considered a disease, since their mother, sister, and several other family members experienced the same condition. These women unwittingly became patients and viewed themselves as abnormal only after their physicians referred them to the hospital.

The last example is of a woman who, having been diagnosed with neurofibromatosis Type 1,[21] failed to comprehend that she had a disease. Although she regarded the brown spots on her body as aesthetically unattractive, even repulsive, and she feared that it might make her less attractive to her husband when he returned from the United States, where he had been working for several years, she attributed the ugly spots to witchcraft and not to disease. When this 37-year-old woman learned that she was suffering from a hereditary disorder, her one concern was that her only child, a 10-year-old girl, would blame her for transmitting the condition. In this case, the woman's aesthetic reality was transformed into a medical actuality that provoked terror in her life.

As with all human actions, medicalization can be a double-edged sword. On the one hand, it standardizes aspects of human life to fit into a medical norm so that anyone who fails to fit that norm is considered to suffer from a disease. While medicalizing a set of problems may relieve afflicted individuals of one set of devaluing labels, they become burdened with another. Thus, in all three Mexican cases, the normal and the taken-for-granted became transformed into the abnormal and the evil, for which the family became culpable.

On the other hand, when cases of drug addiction, crime, and alcoholism become converted from moral transgressions to diseases,[22] the person is absolved from responsibility and blame for specific acts. What is more, medicalization may provide people with a sense of coherence and meaning, such as when a diagnosis of chronic fatigue syndrome helps explain the unexplainable, the unaccounted-for painful sensations, by giving a label to an incoherent and disorderly experience.[23] Still, the medicalization process turns the person into a deviant, sometimes stigmatizing him or her while ignoring the underlying causes of the problem. In the case of people suffering from chronic fatigue syndrome, for example, they may be experiencing a sense of meaninglessness in their lives, which medicalization fails to address.

There is yet another dimension to the dual aspect of the medicalization process. Consider, for example, contraceptive technologies, which have given women greater freedom by enabling them to control conception, thus relieving them of the fear of an unwanted pregnancy. Simultaneously, these technologies have made women dependent on the medical profession and have often adversely affected women's health.[24] Take birthing as another example. While medical technology has been instrumental in saving difficult or abnormal cases, the majority of women experiencing uncomplicated births have forfeited, wittingly or unwittingly, participation in the birthing process, which is a normal human experience, and have become patients.[25]

It has long been recognized that the medicalization process had become a form of social control.[26] In much the same way that women came under surveillance with the medicalization of their reproductive capacities, Szasz noted some four decades ago, socially undesirable behaviors were medicalized in order for society to deal with socially defined deviance. If Szasz is correct concerning the medicalization of antisocial behavior, then, from a political standpoint, it can be argued that medicalization is a form of internalized control, doing the job of the state. As I suggest elsewhere, in a democratic society, where the state must eschew the use of overt force, people's internalized self-controls and biomedicine's designation of deviant behavior as disease may act as a type of police force in lieu of the state.[27]

I must stress that not all individuals in our society and elsewhere (e.g., Mexico) embrace the notion of medicalization.[28] In fact, some scholars have questioned the degree to which the concept of medicalization has penetrated the popular consciousness, since in the late twentieth century the medical profession began to lose its dominance. One measure of this loss is that increasingly people have turned to alternative treatments.[29] Nevertheless, because of biomedicine's hegemony, medicalization has continued to be a powerful force in contemporary society by extending its reach to domains such as infertility and kinship.

The Medicalization of Infertility: The New Reproductive Technologies

In Chapter 3 I called attention to the ways in which the new reproductive technologies have required us to reconsider our kinship relations. Here, I will consider how infertility has been affected by the medicalization process. Infertility, of course, has been a dilemma for women cross-culturally and has been attributed to numerous supernatural causes, including the will of God, punishment by God, or witchcraft.

In Western society, in the same way that fertility became controlled by biomedicine, so, too, has infertility.[30] Whereas contraceptive technologies have medicalized fertility, the new reproductive technologies have medicalized infertility and pronounced it to be a disease. Women without children are frequently regarded as abnormal, even though many contemporary women opt to remain childless.[31]

Raymond describes how surrogacy and the new reproductive technologies have been glorified in the press and how they have created areas for new research and new industries, even though many infertile women may not be as desperate to have children as is being represented by the media and biomedicine.[32] Infertility among all women of childbearing age in the United States, as of 1988, affected only 7.9 percent of the population,[33] but its medicalization has numerous social and cultural ramifications in addition to those I discussed in Chapter 3 within the context of kinship relations.

Underlying the medicalization of infertility is the cultural conviction that motherhood is an important aspiration for all women. In fact, infertility is regarded as a form of failed motherhood because the woman has failed to produce an offspring. The very identity of the woman is threatened. Franklin found that infertility gives women "the feeling that their bodies had 'let them down' [and] made many women feel unnatural and excluded from normality as well as womanhood."[34]

In much the same way that the medicalization of fertility and conception has created dilemmas for women, including the loss of control over their bodies to the medical profession, the medicalization of infertility has created its own set of dilemmas. On the one hand, surrogacy frees women from what Raymond has called "reproductive bondage" by liberating and debiologizing motherhood. As we have seen, the new reproductive technologies separate the child bearer from the child rearer and enable women to become mothers without having to experience the pain and inconvenience associated with pregnancy and parturition.[35] From this perspective, biology is not destiny for individual women, who can be freed from giving birth to children and for whom motherhood is a social rather than a biological experience rooted in a notion of maternal instinct. By contrast, the medicalization of infertility resulting in in vitro fertilization and surrogacy has raised myriad ethical concerns. The fertility industry has declared a "new age," when people can design their own children, and when "parents will not only be able to correct chromosomal abnormalities but also choose from a list of 'hereditary options' such as blue eyes, blond hair, high intelligence, physical strength and even delayed aging."[36] Supporters of the new in vitro fertilization techniques promise, in Franklin's words, an "eventual elimination of genetic impairments."[37]

On an individual level, for women who seek to have a family, the medicalization of infertility by means of in vitro fertilization holds out extraordinary hope and promise for a fulfilling future. Yet, from a broader societal perspective, these techniques alarm numerous critics who see the potential link between genetic engineering and reproductive technologies as a new form of eugenics.[38] Women with genetic deficiencies may be dissuaded from reproducing, or women who may not like their own genetic makeup might commission another woman's ova to produce an offspring. The possibility thus arises of creating humans to one's personal taste and, in the extreme case, the technologies could lead to creating a master race.[39] Yet another obvious ethical concern is that the medicalization of infertility through the new reproductive technologies will lead to a commodification of humans, to "baby shopping" and to the violation of the sacredness of life.[40]

We must also not overlook the fact that while the medicalization of infertility may assist some women in producing infants, the medical procedures may have an iatrogenic effect that is hazardous to women's health while providing a low rate of success. In fact, some have claimed that in vitro fertilization success rates are minimal but that we only hear about the spectacular successes, perhaps because they are so sensational.[41]

In sum, the medicalization of infertility has created profound concerns from the perspective of both the individual and the society and has led to a reexamination of traditional understandings of kinship.

The Medicalization of Kinship and Family

To the array of human experiences that have become medicalized, I propose that we must now add kinship and family. As we saw from the people we have met, especially the adoptees, family and kinship relations are being defined in terms of the genetic inheritance transmitted through reproduction. American kinship, understood as biogenetic, has come under medical scrutiny through the prevailing explanatory biomedical model of disease etiology. Our kinship relations have been given a new dimension that stresses faulty genes. As we saw in Chapter 3, in earlier times and in premodern American society, people inherited their status, their rights and duties, and their property and power, as well as their poverty, from their kin. In contemporary times, however, kinship relations are usually not expected to confer on people any particular status among most of the population.[42] In a democratic society, a person's class status is denied or effaced. In fact, the majority of middle- and lower-class families may have little property to transmit to their descendants other than ephemeral moral values.[43] Instead, genetic transmission, for better or for worse, is arguably of greater cultural significance than are class boundaries. As we saw, people may take pride in the genetic inheritance of favorable characteristics, but they can also presumably inherit defective genes that transform them into patients and perpetually sick persons.

Giddens proposes the notion of "toxic parents," parents who can harm their children by damaging their sense of personal worth and causing them to deal with memories and figures from their childhood that harm them as adults. Following Giddens, "toxic" refers to parents who are emotionally inadequate, who have abdicated their responsibilities to their children, or who control them. Alcoholic parents and verbal, physical, or sexual abusers are examples of people who are considered to cripple their children's personal development. Giddens comments that those who wish to rework their involvement with toxic parents can do so through therapy and realize that "you are not responsible for what was done to you as a defenseless child."[44]

One could, of course, sever one's ties with toxic parents, but following the biomedical model of genetic inheritance, one cannot declare independence from one's genetic parents, as some of the adoptees also recognize. If Schneider is correct, as I believe he is, love cements bio-genetic kinship relations in American society and allows for a degree of choice in deciding whom a person will love within the family and kinship group. With the medicalization of kinship, a connection is established irrespective of love and choice. While people may fragment family and kinship ties by selecting whom they will love among those in their bio-genetic group, biomedicine unites those who may not feel connected or have chosen to be united, as for example, with Karen and Alice, whom we met in Chapter 5. Family and kin connections are framed in terms of genetic inheritance from parents, grandparents, and other relatives. We saw earlier that there are now over 5,000 medical conditions attributable to genetic inheritance,[45] and with the work of the genome project we learn each day of another disorder that is traceable to genetic transmission. As Bobinski observed, "Information about genetic makeup is gotten from examination of a person's medical record and analysis of his or her family genetic history. A family history of a particular disorder, for example, would mean that there was an elevated risk that the individual might be a carrier who could pass the condition on to a new generation."[46]

As we so clearly learned from adoptees' accounts, as well as the healthy and recovered women, physicians prompt people to remember their genetic heritage. Invariably, people become conscious of their family and kinship connections and the potential harm they may inflict when their physician first asks for a family medical history. Every time doctors take a family medical history, they reinforce the notion that there is an association between kinship and health, as Loreta and others clearly recognize. Good medical procedure requires physicians to do a physical examination, laboratory tests, and other technical diagnostic procedures and to take a patient's personal and family medical history. A physician failing to do so would be judged remiss.[47] But not only physicians reinforce the medicalization of family and kinship. The popular press, as I noted in the Introduction, reminds us of it frequently, and by so doing tends to validate physicians' insistence on the importance of genetic inheritance. We saw various examples of how people were urged to search for their family's faulty genes, and how doctors recommended that every family find its genealogy. Both the mass media and the doctor-patient encounter imprint on people's consciousness the notion that families and kin pass on disease.[48]

This is not to say that Americans universally accept the genetic model of disease. In fact, as we saw in Chapter 6, Tina, Jana, Leah, and Dina (see also Chapter 6, n. 1) tend to reject genetic inheritance explanations. To what extent such explanations are accepted in American society remains an empirical question that awaits further study on a large population sample. One can assume that mainstream Americans, especially middle-class Americans, are more likely to accept genetic etiological theories. Important too, the vignettes illustrate the tension between hegemonic biomedical ideologies and an individual's evaluation of received knowledge, a point I make in the Introduction. The tension we encounter among these women may reflect a broader trend in the larger society that may vary by class and experience. Yet, concurrently, we saw in Chapter 7 that the adoptees in search of their birth parents do not doubt for a moment that their persona and disease are genetically determined; they exhibit no such tensions. In actuality, their total acceptance of the model contributes to their conflicts as adoptees.

As we saw in Chapters 5 and 7, in the lived experience of those related to people afflicted with breast cancer, or of healthy adoptees who learn their birth parents' medical history, the medicalization of kinship leads healthy members in the afflicted family to redefine their reality by experiencing a new vulnerability that draws them into the biomedical domain. People like Eve become perpetual patients, despite the fact that they are perfectly healthy women. Still, they exist with an ongoing fear of a disease because a member of the family has suffered from it. Also, we saw that some women we met in Chapters 5 and 6, both healthy and sick, acted on the basis of the medicalization of their family and kinship connections by resorting to treatments such as prophylactic surgery.

People may no longer need to present complaints to be regarded as sick. They may be considered sick prior to having any symptomatology, other than originating from a family of people with a particular disease. Those people who have a member in the family or kinship group who has suffered from breast cancer, colon cancer, or Alzheimer's disease will be assumed to have inherited it in an autosomal-dominant fashion. Jonsen anticipates that

persons could be designated patients in an anticipatory sense. Some with monogenic disorders will be patients without symptoms, but sure to have them in the future. Others, with the genetic patterns associated with polygenic or multifactorial disorders, will be known as a schizophrenic or cardiac or cancer patient long before any illness is felt or any pathology damages the organism; indeed, they may never be affected at all, yet still be marked. Persons will become patients before their time: They will be described in disease terms but 'feel fine' and 'be fine' for years, perhaps always.[49]

People's realities will encompass a future that is incessantly punctuated by worry. Indeed, the medicalization of kinship alters people's perceptions from "if I get breast or colon cancer" to "*when* I get breast or colon cancer" or any one of a hundred diseases believed to be inherited from family and kin, as the people we met in Chapter 5, and also some of the adoptees in Chapter 7, clearly illustrate. The notion of genetic risk for a disease has now become almost a disease in and of itself as has the notion of predisposition.[50] The concept of the genetic inheritance of predisposition extends even more the medicalization of kinship to encompass almost everybody, converting most people to potential patients.

We have already seen that both adoptees who have learned about their diseased genetic history and the healthy patients we met in Chapter 5 live with these fears. Granted, as we saw, belief in genetic inheritance alerts individuals to take charge and take preventive measures, such as mammograms and blood tests in anticipation of potentially falling ill[51] and also helps explain the fortuitousness of the affliction. Ultimately, however, as could be seen in Chapter 6, various women afflicted with breast cancer may employ gambling metaphors to make sense of their condition. This results from the unpredictability and randomness that accompany present-day risk assessment, which gnaws at one's being. Jonsen foresees that while "today these risks are written in abstract numbers that have but remote impact on the way in which persons see themselves, tomorrow these risks will be written in each one's genome, an indelible part of themselves."[52] Knowing that one is at risk, as I noted before, merges one's experience of the present with the future and, as we saw, may, for example, influence one not to bear children, aggravating further a woman's identity as a potential mother.

The medicalization of family and kinship creates a new dynamic within the family. Some have suggested that it may lead to parental guilt and resentment by the offspring.[53] It may split families and tear them up because one member inherited a disease and another did not. It may stigmatize them, as we saw in Lydia's case, whose family became estranged from her when they learned she had developed breast cancer. Or, as in Eliza's case, her husband became perturbed because he feared that her breast cancer may have been transmitted to his daughter. Healthy members of a family or kin group may resent being told that they are potentially at a high risk for developing a disease.[54] But Wexler, in discussing Huntington's disease, observes that "remarkably few interviewees expressed conscious anger toward the parent who had given them this legacy. Compassion and grief were by far the most common feelings. It was considered in particularly bad taste to harbor hostility toward a parent who was already broken and ill."[55] However, Lynch, Lynch, and Lynch found that "family members manifest anxiety, fatalism, denial and even accusation directed toward the spouse, parents, or to her family members who have '*caused the disease among us*'" (emphasis added).[56]

Conversely, Wexler was surprised that people failed to express anger toward their families for having passed down a lethal disease, as I too had hypothesized they would, but for which I had not found support. As we saw in Chapters 5 and 6, none of the women with breast cancer or family histories of cancer expressed anger at their families or the ancestors who may have transmitted the disease to them. Instead, the interviewees reasoned that their ancestors were unaware of having the disease and had transmitted it unwittingly.[57]

With the medicalization of kinship, the individual is no longer the sole patient, able to choose the course of treatment. Contrary to the broader societal process, in which individualism and freedom of choice are emphasized, the medicalization of kinship creates a tension between the stress on individualism and choice in a democratic society and an orientation to family and kin. Individualism insists on an autonomous person, standing outside any one socially defined unit and selecting his or her life course,[58] whereas kinship relationships based on genetic inheritance call for connectedness and circumscription of choice. The ideology of genetic inheritance unites, often unwillingly, the individual with his or her family and kin, over and above the nuclear family. Whereas individuals may choose kin on the basis of affective ties, as is the case in modern society,[59] the new genetics prescribes one's kin relations on the basis of birth rather than choice, as we saw, for example, in Karen's case, or among adoptees. The medicalization of kinship thus subverts the ideology of choice regarding the people one selects as one's kin. According to genetic theory, genes may act at random, but once they have been transmitted to the individual and the individual is formed by them, the selection of individual members of family and kin becomes determined by biomedical definitions as much as by choice. In an interesting contradiction, with the medicalization of kinship, freedom and choice, so profoundly embedded in mainstream American consciousness, must confront determinism, and predestination.

Against this background, the traditional biomedical model is based on a physician-patient dyad. With the HGP and the increasing expansion of attributions to genetic inheritance, leading to the medicalization of kinship, the individual may no longer make medical decisions independent of his or her family.[60] We saw in Chapter 5, for instance, that Kelly was not permitted to make her own decision independent of her mother and sister on whether to have a genetic test. As in Alice's case, especially within the domain of genetic testing for disease, family members must cooperate in order for a physician and a geneticist to assess the patient's condition. Family and kin of different generations must be drawn into the diagnostic process.[61] It can even be said that the medicine of the future will not be the medicine of the individual but of the family. Wexler goes so far as to say that "anybody in a family with a genetic disease — this probably includes everybody — should think about storing samples of DNA from relatives whose genotype would be essential to know for a diagnostic testing. The most important relatives to you are those in the family with the illness and those clearly unaffected, parents of these individuals and your own parents. If you have a genetic disorder, banking your own DNA could be critical for your descendants. Each family might have its own genetic variation, its own 'genetic fingerprinting' of the gene in question, and it is best to preserve a sample of the particular gene that plagues your family rather than extrapolate from the genes from other families." Tests are currently being prepared for breast cancer, colon cancer, heart disease, Alzheimer's, manic depression and schizophrenia.[62]

The medicalization of kinship may not necessarily affect all people adversely. Undoubtedly it reassures some people that, if no one in the family past or present has suffered from a particular disease, they too are protected from becoming afflicted. It may furnish the person with a feeling of security, even though this sense of protection may be nothing more than an illusion. It also may give meaning to the randomness of an affliction for which biomedicine lacks an explanation by shedding light on familial origin of a senseless disease and by addressing the issue of "why me" and not someone else. Most important, as we saw in Chapter 6, by medicalizing kinship relationships through concepts of genetic inheritance, the senselessness and randomness of breast cancer can become meaningful by establishing for a woman a connection with her family and ancestors.

Additionally, too, we saw that, through the medicalization of kinship, people are brought together with kin with whom they may have lost contact; it may even lead to reestablishing relationships among family members, as for most of the people we met.[63] Family members may become closer to one another, not only because they share the same disease, but also because they develop a new sense of sharing the same genetic heritage. Eve made it very clear that she began to think about her family and her ancestors when she fell ill. In fact, family and kin become closer not only to the living but also to the dead, whom they must recall to account for their genetic heritage. This may promote a sense of continuity with the past, even if it is based on adversity.

The family medical history recapitulates by means of genetic inheritance the kinship history for people whose kinship memories may lack depth. In contemporary American society, where memory is shallow, the DNA remembers the past in ways that people's living memories may have forgotten. The medicalization of kinship binds the person to the past as well as to the future — even though, ironically, the tie is mediated by suffering — propelling people to search for ancestors and also to anticipate future afflicted descendants, as we saw among adoptees as well as among women who have recovered from breast cancer. Human beings may well be the sole animals in the cosmos that contemplate a past and a future, and our genetic conceptualizations emphasize that aspect of our humanity. Lamentably, the DNA harboring memory of ancestors is devoid of morality or affect, the hallmark of family and kinship relations.[64] DNA molecules are inherently impersonal: they do not impose, express, or insist on responsibilities, obligations, or love, other than requiring living relatives to furnish blood samples in order to establish genetic markers on chromosomes.

From a familial and socio-political perspective, the medicalization of kinship can be construed as an equalizing and democratizing process. On a familial level, all members of the family possess the same chance to inherit a disease, even though it is never known who has until tests are done. Genetic testing therefore may contribute to the divisiveness of a family. But we also saw in Chapter 3 that, from the seventeenth to the nineteenth centuries liberal theorists regarded the family as natural. In the words of Minow and Shanley "like slaves, children born out of wedlock, widows, and abandoned wives and their children as well as those who explicitly rejected conventional family life and instead pursued solitary or communal households fell outside the legal norms of the patriarchal family in nineteenth-century U.S. law."[65] Viewed from the perspective of genetic inheritance, all those unfortunate individuals at the margins form part of family and kin, equalizing their status with the dominant family members. The DNA will not permit this kinship to be denied. On a societal level, the DNA conceals differences produced by class rather than genetics. As we saw among adoptees, genetic connections are often mistaken for class differences,[66] obviating the necessity to address such differences, although a few of the adoptees are well aware of their class privileges.

My introduction to the notion of the medicalization of kinship and family has attempted to highlight both the benefits and the drawbacks of this process for the individual and society. Various social scientists and biologists, however, have vigorously criticized the ideology of genetic inheritance within the context of the new genetics. I turn to these critiques in the next chapter and the extent to which such critiques reflect the day-to-day realities of the people we met in Chapters 5, 6, and 7.

Chapter 9
A Multidimensional Critique of Genetic Determinism

In the previous chapter I explored the concept of medicalization. I argued that kinship became medicalized as a result of the prominence of molecular biology and genetics associated with inheritance of disease. In this chapter I examine some consequences of the ideology of genetic inheritance on both macro and micro levels of analysis. Paradoxically, the regnant ideology of genetic inheritance produces differing consequences on these two levels of experience. On the level of the broader society, the ideology of genetic inheritance forebodes a return to the era of eugenics. On the level of the individual, the medicalization of kinship may, as we saw in previous chapters, be both comforting and troubling, contingent on that person's life situation and experience.

From a societal perspective and within the broader context of biological determinism, criticisms have been launched at genetic determinism, as manifested in the HGP. Moreover, notions such as genetic predisposition and practices such as genetic testing that flow from this ideology have been questioned. These critiques merit consideration.

As we learned in Chapter 4, the basic assumption of the HGP is that the essence of being human resides in the gene, and that since some of its secrets have been unlocked already, all that comprises our humanity will soon become visible.[1] The HGP has been criticized for many reasons, including the fact that it is big business, creating a new industry of better living through genetics. A growing number of new commercial laboratories are marketing genetic tests for more and more gene-related disorders.[2] Given the current claim that there are about 5,600–5,700 known genetic disorders, it is likely that everyone in the population will carry some "faulty" gene; eventually, everybody may need to be tested for a genetic disease.[3] Tests now exist for about thirty disorders or their predispositions, including Alzheimer's, cancer, and alcoholism,[4] and these tests may influence whether people have children, as we saw in some of the narratives in Chapters 5 and 7.[5]

On a more profound level, scholars have questioned the ethics of this project, which may ultimately result in manipulating the biological makeup, not of groups, as the eugenics movement had advocated, but of individuals. In this modern counterpart to eugenics, families may be able to select the children they desire.[6] The HGP promotes a biochemical causal model of human affliction and, given its aim of therapeutic management, may lead to designing individualized therapies to replace bad genes with good ones. The project can lead to a program of genetic engineering that will substitute the manipulation of an individual's genes for a social program, as eugenics had advocated. Nelkin notes that "it has been argued that compelling social interests call for compulsory genetic testing of people at risk of genetic disease and for informing family members about the biological status of their relatives,"[7] which may lead to a form of eugenics. For some, this project smacks of Germany before and during World War II.[8]

Genetic testing for susceptibility to certain types of cancer, such as ovarian and breast cancer, is currently part of clinical management for families with histories of such a disease, as shown in Chapter 6, or even for women whose family history includes "one first or second degree relative diagnosed with breast cancer below the age of 40 or two relatives diagnosed below the age of 50."[9] The perils of such testing are, however, recognized, including the fact that a person may lose his or her insurance or become stigmatized by family members if, for example, they have a breast cancer gene,[10] even though such tests may lack reliability.[11] In response to those concerned about the adverse potential of human genetic engineering, one can contend that the individual is given a choice whether to be tested or not, as discussed in Chapter 6. However, if, indeed, human beings are programmed genetically, then of course, they are left with no abilities to choose, unless a gene is found for making choices.

Importantly, also, from the perspective of the individual, the HGP offers the power to label persons as diseased.[12] Anyone who fails to conform exactly to the norm of the kinship map may be designated as diseased or predisposed to disease, thereby converting an asymptomatic, healthy person into a patient, leading to profound changes in the doctor-patient relationship. No longer will physicians be concerned with symptoms, but rather with the genomic information and disease susceptibility or risk. As Jonsen notes, the modern physician will treat not the patient, nor just the disease, but a minuscule part of the person's DNA mutations and nucleotide sequences. A patient's pains may be ignored unless the genome map marks a disease location. Jonsen characterizes modern medicine as predominantly a collection of diagnostic and therapeutic actions that start in the logic of clinical judgment and terminate in interventions that are often admitted to be unsuccessful. Jonsen fails to foresee cures for the diseases the genome will identify because "as the mapped genome opens up broad vistas of information, it will in a strange sense, return to medicine's impotent past." He predicts that the genome will convert biomedicine to soothsaying when he observes that "prognosis, the ancient art of predicting the natural course of disease, is likely to be the principal clinical beneficiary of genomic information, at least for the foreseeable future."[13] Jonsen's assertion that to know the existence of genetic impairment fails to guarantee the development of new treatments is supported by the example of sickle cell anemia. As Wexler points out, this disease has been known for over a quarter of a century, yet no effective cure has been found. Knowing a disease at the genetic level and diagnosing a disorder presymptomatically places individuals and families in danger of losing health and life insurance and may also lead to discrimination, stigmatization, and ostracism.[14]

Ultimately, Lewontin emphasizes, every human genome differs from every other, and there is never an absolutely clear replication of the DNA. For this geneticist, the problem of using genetic causality is "that we do not know even in principle all of the functions of the different nucleotides in a gene, or how the specific context in which a nucleotide appears may affect the way in which the cell machinery interprets the DNA . . . because there is no single, standard, 'normal' DNA sequence that we all share, observed sequence differences between sick and well people cannot, in themselves, reveal the genetic cause of a disorder."[15]

In contrast, Hamer and Copeland claim that the HGP can no longer be stopped. In their view, the HGP will help produce new drugs, reduce birth defects, and allow us to live longer and healthier lives. They even predict that the HGP will provide science with the ability to change and manipulate human behavior through genetics for the good of mankind.[16]

Other scholars, however, have questioned the basic claim that diseases are caused genetically, and their objections merit consideration. Granted, genes are undoubtedly the raw material of heredity and play a crucial role in new species formation.[17] Furthermore, studies of genetic diseases have contributed to biomedical advances as, for example, in unraveling sickle cell anemia, PKU (phenylketonuria), cystic fibrosis, Tay-Sachs, Huntington's chorea, and hemophilia, to note the most well-known inherited diseases.[18] Besides, contemporary understanding of genetic diseases may have even dispelled earlier prejudices as, for instance, in the case of porphyria, which propagated the myth of vampires.[19] But critics of the genetic ideology note that such inherited disorders are produced by random genetic mutations of DNA sequences and are exceptional diseases: the majority of diseases require a particular environment.[20] Most of the diseases that are claimed to be genetically transmitted are responses to environmental conditions and environmentally induced mutations as much as to genetic inheritance. What can be said with greater certainty is that there exists an interplay between the environment and the genes.[21] In his classic paper on sickle cell anemia, a disease that is unequivocally genetically determined, Livingston demonstrated that a genetic mutation became prevalent as a result of ecological changes brought on by cultural practices associated with the development of agriculture. In the absence of an agricultural environment, the sickle cell gene failed to flourish.[22] Current scientific assessments suggest that genetic factors by themselves explain only about 5 percent of all cancers, with the rest attributable to behavioral factors associated with class, ethnicity or race,[23] or age, gender, and environmental conditions,[24] especially radiation and environmental toxins, which may induce mutations.[25]

Cancer is, certainly, not a single disease, even when it arises in the same site within an organ. It is a collection of numerous diseases, some of which are common and some rare.[26] Environmental carcinogens such as chemicals and radiation and, probably, viruses may be responsible for 70–90 percent of cancers by increasing probabilities of mutations.[27] Cumulative exposure to estrogen, including that contained in birth control pills, may cause cancer, because "the longer that birth control pills are used, the greater a woman's total exposure to estradiol and the greater her risk of acquiring breast cancer."[28] Lloyd furnishes the example of liver cancer, regarded as hereditary. The gene that causes this disease is especially sensitive to toxin-induced mutations, which prevent the gene from carrying out its usual physiological role.[29] Similar arguments can be advanced for cancers of the breast, brain, bladder, and colon, as well as insulin-dependent diabetes. In all these disorders the role of environmental toxins is usually ignored by researchers or at best minimized.[30] The reason such diseases run in families may be explained by the fact that family members usually live in the same environment and are exposed to the same toxic chemicals found in that environment and may therefore be exposed to the same mutations.[31] Krieger and Fee summarize the issue best when they observe that after "researchers turned to sex chromosomes and hormones to understand cancers of the uterus and breast and a host of other sex-linked diseases, they no longer saw the need to worry about environmental influences."[32] Carcinogens in the environment increase the likelihood that cancer-initiating mutations will happen. Hubbard and Wald argue persuasively against the genetic basis of disease: "Relatively few diseases or disabilities are genetic, even fewer can be predicted, and most of the risks we and our families encounter are not biological at all."[33]

According to Lewontin, genetic etiological explanations isolate, for example, "an alteration in a so-called cancer gene as *the* cause of cancer, whereas the alteration in the gene may in turn have been caused by ingesting a pollutant, which in turn was produced by an industrial process," which, according to Lewontin, may be associated with investment decisions (emphasis in the original).[34] Thus, Lewontin adds a politico-economic dimension to the argument against the ideology of genetic inheritance.

Hubbard and Hubbard and Wald argue convincingly against any kind of reductionism that gives exaggerated power to particles and ignores the internal and external environments in which they are embedded.[35] They point out that the same impulse which led physicists to describe matter in terms of atoms and later subatomic particles led biologists to presuppose that inheritance is mediated by intracellular, hereditary particles — that changes flow from the genes to the organism.[36] Hubbard proposes the converse, a transformational model of biology whereby organisms in which particles are embedded influence the structure and function of these particles. She states, "We would not be entitled to conclude that DNA controls or programmes the many different ways in which proteins participate in the structure and function of organisms, not to speak of controlling or programming the complex characteristics of individuals and species." She continues, "All traits are polygenic in the sense that they are produced by many interacting and often mutually regulating processes that involve many enzymes and substrates, and therefore many genes.[37]

Additionally, Hubbard and Wald contend on both empirical and logical grounds that behaviors such as alcoholism cannot be genetically determined. They reason that since there are more nonalcoholic parents than alcoholic parents, most people who become alcoholic have nonalcoholic parents.[38] Moreover, as Griesemer points out, recessive genes produce most genetic diseases, and there are always more carriers in a population who are healthy than afflicted.[39]

Lewontin is, arguably, the scientist who most vociferously critiques notions of genetic determinism in general.[40] He, like Hubbard and Wald and others,[41] questions any explanation that is based on a single unitary cause of disease. Every organism is the outcome of unique interaction between genes and environmental sequences modulated by the random chance of cell growth and division. Hence, for Lewontin, the separation between biology and environment is spurious: they simply cannot be separated in the same way as human cultural efforts cannot be separated from their biology. He notes, "The interaction between them [genes and environment] is indissoluble. When an environment changes, all bets are off." Lewontin asserts that "turning off and on of the production of the body's constituents is itself sensitive to external conditions. For example, if the sugar lactose is provided to the coliform facterium, the presence of the sugar will signal the bacterial machinery to start making a protein that will break down the lactose and use it as a source of energy. The signal to start translating the gene code into a protein is, in fact, determined by part of the gene itself. The signaling system is a mechanism by which environment interacts with genes in creating organisms."[42]

In sum, scientists such as Hubbard and Wald and Lewontin argue forcefully against genetic reductionism on the grounds that genes do not stand independent of and cannot be isolated from the internal and external environments in which they are embedded, including political and economic forces. Spanier, as well, calls attention to the wrongful focus on genetic etiologies of cancer rather than on cancer-promoting chemicals and radiation in the air, water, and food, produced in good measure by industrial processes and societal conditions and habits.[43] The environmental argument is one we have heard several of the women with breast cancer make, for example, Leah, Jana, or Betty but, because of the hegemony of the gene they may dismiss it, as Jana and Betty had done. The obvious consequence of concentrating on genetic causality rather than on environmental phenomena is that there is no incentive to institute environmental changes.[44]

It is not uncommon to exonerate the environment by labeling the individual as possessing a "genetic predisposition." Not only does this label convert most humans into potential patients, as I noted in the last chapter, but also, as Nelkin persuasively advances, "the idea of genetic predisposition encourages a passive attitude towards social injustice, an apathy about continuing social problems, and a reason to preserve the status quo."[45] The notion of genetic predisposition is powerful because it is not easily refutable. If one says a person has a drug addiction because he or she is predisposed to addictive behavior, it cannot be disproved. The outcome is the proof, exculpating the individual and the environment from responsibility. The construal of genetic causality or predisposition in diagnosing disease may absolve the environment and the individual from blame, but in the end the onus falls on the family, kin group, and ancestors. The ideology of genetic inheritance converts people's specific ancestors into diseased ancestors, into malevolent ghosts. Whereas Mendelian principles follow laws of probabilities governed by random chance,[46] the ideology of genetic determinism tends to instill in people a fear of and a certainty concerning the inheritance of specific disordered characteristics, removing the objective reality of the very randomness inherent in genetic transmission. Even when geneticists discuss diseases in terms of their multifactorial aspects, people tend to regard their diseases as genetically determined, as can be seen in the case vignettes discussed in Chapters 5 and 6.[47] What is more, it is noteworthy that after it is announced with a great deal of fanfare that a gene has been found for a given disorder, not infrequently the discovery is later retracted with very little publicity, as in the cases of schizophrenia, manic depression, or mental illness in general among the Amish.[48]

Stephen Jay Gould is a prominent critic of genetic determinism as a broad theory of human behavior, although he appears to accept the notion of the heritability of genetic diseases. Gould rightly recognizes that human behavior is adaptive and that adaptations occur through cultural change, which occurs at a much more rapid pace than biological changes. Whereas human biological ranges are narrow, human behavioral repertoires are very broad, marked by a great flexibility that is not dictated by genes. Gould rightly notes that just as Freud's theories of human behavior, and dysfunctional psychosexual states, and neurosis arising from suppressed or misdirected development were erroneous, so too are contemporary theories of genetic determinism. He states, "If insightful non-genetic theories could be so egregiously exaggerated in the past, should we be surprised that we are now repeating this error by overextending the genuine excitement we feel about genetic explanations?"[49] In Gould's view, normal variation cannot be equated with pathological causality.[50] But Gould does find a biological explanation for disease a relief. Referring to his autistic child, he states, "I celebrate the humane and liberating value of identifying inborn biological bases for conditions once deemed purely psychogenic, i.e., autism, that were previously blamed on parents," cautioning that "we should not move from this style of explanation to the resolution of behavioral variation in our general population."[51]

Gould's expression of relief at knowing that autism is rooted in biology explains in part why the ideology is easily accepted on an experiential level. In fact, as we saw, similar reactions were voiced by the breast cancer patients and adoptees whom I interviewed, because it removes the responsibility from the individual. It will be recalled how relieved Roberta and her adopted mother had been when they could attribute Roberta's gayness to heredity. However, for the most part, the available literature identifies the negative experiential consequences of the ideology of genetic inheritance. For example, we read that people with a "genetic illness" often "respond with depression, attitudes of learned helplessness, alienation, or fatalism" and may feel that nothing can be done — that they are doomed. Cullinan notes that "an angry 'why me?' or 'why us?' often accompanies the response, and a sense of victimization and depression can ensue,"[52] while Forstenzer and Roye comment that "the fact that the child has an inherited flaw represents a reinjury on two levels. The parent reexperiences the original sense of her own imperfection and then has to relive these feelings through and with her daughter." The most obvious source of resentment is "Why did I get it?"[53] Or, as Wexler notes when speaking of Huntington's (HD), "When one person in a family is tested, the entire family is tested and all must live with the outcomes. Many parents of persons at risk feel guilty about and responsible for their children's risk status, even though they may have known nothing about HD when the children were born."[54]

From a phenomenological perspective, the ideology of genetic inheritance depersonalizes medical diagnosis by ignoring the environment and other factors associated with adverse health status such as poverty, poor nutrition, lower birth weight, deprivation in the womb, as well as a person's biography, or what I have identified as a person's *life's lesions*.[55] I was struck by Fox Keller's reference to Delbruck's claim that molecular biology unraveled the secret of life.[56] By claiming to solve the riddle of life, genetic ideology removes the mystery and complexities of existence, making life seemingly uncomplicated. In the same manner that genetic determinism effaces the environment, it obliterates the person's biography. Once the secret of life has been unlocked through genetics, we need no longer concern ourselves with the person's motivations, actions, and, most important, his or her suffering, any or all of which may have contributed to the onset of the disorder and the adverse effect on the person's sickness.[57]

Genetic etiological explanations meet the primary criterion of biomedicine by supposedly measuring an individual's disorder objectively. The person's symptomatology may even be ignored, as we saw was the case with Connie and Dorothy, whose symptoms were largely overlooked by physicians. Likewise, as we saw with adoptees, genetic reductionism joins and condenses the person, the person's individual experiences, the person as agent of his or her own behaviors, and class differences to a mere gene. The person's being is discarded; what remains is a person's character, which is confirmed by that which was transmitted by familial DNA.

As came into view in Chapter 7, the ideology of genetic determinism creates numerous dilemmas for adoptees. Yet when we consider the women with breast cancer, the satisfying aspects of genetic ideologies outweigh the negative fallout. For most of the people in this study, knowing that their disease was rooted in their genetic heritage gave meaning to the randomness of the disease. It explained why it happened to the individual, even to the women who had "done everything right" and who, in some measure, felt morally aggrieved because, despite minding all the risk factors, they were nevertheless afflicted by the disease. Otherwise, how could they have explained it to themselves, if the disease was not genetically caused? An individual from another culture, say, like Maya, could contemplate that her family was bewitched, but for all the others who lack alternative explanations in their cultural pool of understandings, a genetic explanation is satisfying and reasonable. Additionally, as Betty pointed out, a genetic explanation is simple, elegant in its parsimony. The fact that it eschews multifactorial considerations — its very simplicity — may even be a consolation at a time of great suffering.

We saw, in addition, that to know that one's disease was rooted in one's inheritance is to remember the past and one's foremothers and forefathers, even if it is only in the DNA, a knowledge that allows a person to unite with his or her ancestors. In Eliza's case, for example, she discovered that the ancestor with cancer was also renowned, a source of pride to her, despite the fact that the ancestor may be reduced to the level of a DNA strand. Remembering the person by the strands of their DNA at once separates the individual from the ancestor's being but may also facilitate memories of ancestral existence and deeds.

For healthy individuals genetically presumably predisposed to disease because of the medicalization of kinship, and for adoptees, to know that the disease was in the family is, paradoxically, to have some control. On the one hand, there is a sense of inevitability, a sense of fatalism, as we saw earlier among so many of the women in the study. Conversely, to Americans, who feel a need for a sense of control, as for example Melanie or Eve, the ideology allows people to believe that they can do something about their potential disorder, including many of the women we met. They can change their lifestyle, as Melanie had done after she fell ill, which gives her the feeling of control that she yearned for. Eve set up an oncology team to prepare herself for what she regards as the inevitable, giving her a modicum of control over what she is convinced is her "destiny." Paradoxically, while the ideology provides the illusion of control by guiding people to avoid risk factors, it runs contrary to the Enlightenment notion that one can dominate nature. Genetic inheritance ideology embraces a belief in predestination, since the person's genetic heritage, diseases, or even quirks in behavior are destiny encoded in their DNA. It is reminiscent of the seventeenth-century theory of preformation. While the individual may have a "toxic" family with faulty genes, the family is not responsible for what befalls generations to come because of its genetic destiny. Arguably, more than any other scientific belief, the ideology of genetic inheritance brings us closest to a Christian (Catholic) theology of being born with original sin (read disease)[59] and returns us to a state of passivity as mere recipients of genes that control our fate. At the same time, it denies our capacities as thinking, feeling, and acting beings, as adoptees clearly bring into view.

Chapter 10
Conclusion

My goal in this book has been to deepen our understanding of the way in which biomedical ideologies are played out in people's day-to-day experiences. Specifically, my focus has been on the ideology of genetic inheritance and the ways in which it shapes current understandings of family and kinship in contemporary American society and influences people's notions of normality and abnormality, agency and memory, while concurrently enmeshing them in numerous paradoxes. We saw that family and kinship relations were, until recently, conceived in terms of blood ties. Within the past several decades, however, the meaning and practices of family and kinship have changed, having become fluid in response to dynamic social processes and economic transformations. Individuals who constitute a "significant same" circle may be recruited by choice rather than by reproduction, and the criteria for membership may not necessarily hinge on genetic links.

In the same way that the everyday experiences of family and kinship relations have been gradually transformed in the past centuries, so, too, have notions of heritability. Conceptualizations have moved from the belief in the inheritance of acquired characteristics to the inheritance of DNA molecules that influence behavior and health. We saw, however, that the same ideology has different impacts on people with dissimilar life experiences. For women suffering from breast cancer, the ideology of genetic inheritance may lucidly address profound concerns of ultimate causality, adding a temporal dimension to the person's experience of family and kin by recalling ancestors and by establishing a continuity and closeness with the dead, living kin, and the unborn. Concurrently, memory embedded in the family and kin's DNA may turn healthy individuals into a new category of the sick: people who suffer from neither an acute nor a chronic disease but who are asymptomatic perpetual patients. Such individuals, subject to the authority of biomedicine and its practitioners, may exist with a ceaseless anxiety about their future health state.

Ideologies frequently lead to action. Human beings act upon received knowledge, especially when under duress. Women's fears and anxieties may lead to frequent mammograms, and at an earlier than prescribed age, biomedical tests, and even prophylactic surgery.[1] In this manner, kinship, like other aspects of human existence, becomes drawn into an ongoing process of medicalization. By the very fact that a person is genetically related to others who have experienced an unexplained disease, he or she is potentially diseased as well.

As we saw, the ideology of genetic inheritance and the medicalization of kinship create special dilemmas for adoptees that do not affect individuals who have been raised by blood kin. Their experience illuminates the complexities of inheritance ideologies, or what I have called the hegemony of the gene. The medicalization of kinship in part impels adoptees to search for blood kin in order to learn the medical history of their genetic relations, in the absence of any shared experience. Whereas contemporary American societal concepts of relatedness may no longer be contingent on biogenetic ties, the ideology is nevertheless sufficiently pervasive, especially because of biomedicine's authority, that many adoptees fail to accept the fiction of being related "as if" by blood to their adoptive families. The power of the ideology of genetic inheritance, pitted against their experience of love and solidarity with their adoptive families, often leads to the search for birth parents, resulting in conflict and pathos and placing the person in profound contradiction. Let us recall Pamela, who firmly internalized the belief in genetic inheritance but had difficulty reconciling it with her experience of having learned all she knew from her adoptive family and resembling its members, especially her father. What is more, it is significant, if also puzzling, that adoptees who find their birth parents recognize not only physical but also behavioral similarities to such people, whom they have met so late in life. While Lewontin is not concerned with adoptees, he anticipates the questionable reasons for searching when he notes that the "resemblance of parents and children is the observation to be explained. It is not evidence for genes. For example, the two social traits that have the highest resemblance between parents and children in North America are religious sect and political party. Yet even the most ardent biological determinist would not seriously argue that there is a gene for Episcopalianism or voting Social Credit."[2] Adoptees, in fact, take on new personas, create a past with new ancestors, and become transformed by their newly formed relationships and knowledge of biogenetic kinship. In all likelihood the ideology of genetic inheritance guides adoptees' perceptions of similarities with social and cultural strangers.

Genetic inheritance has gained a new meaning, not simply that "like begets like," but also that families beget the abnormal individual, not owing to parental bad behavior before their child was born, which was purportedly transmitted to their offspring (as Lamarckians believed in the nineteenth century),[3] but because of random chance. Contemporary genetics presupposes that all humans are composed of like DNA molecules except for the rearrangement of some molecules, which results in "abnormality." Abnormality becomes defined by deviation from the family's standard genetic map, which then may become manifested in aberrant behavior or disease. Invisible connections are now being made visible, comparable to social and economic positions of the past. It could be said that the HGP, taking genetic reductionism to its logical conclusion, echoes back on North American democratic ideals of equality and conformity, that all humans are created equal, obliterating all social differences. Yet, paradoxically, the same egalitarianism promoted by the notion that all people are composed of identical DNA molecules masks the hierarchy that is reinforced by notions of ontological predestination, even if determined by random chance. In the words of one interviewee, the inheritance of DNA that specifies each person's essence "is a crapshoot." Yet the genes people inherit determine their being, thereby fixing them in a status quo, for no one is accountable for the genes inherited by any one individual.

Contemporary humans are no longer Aristotle's political, Descartes's rational, or the anthropologist's cultural animal: humans are just animals comprising specific sequences of DNA that distinguish them from other animals by an ever so slight molecular arrangement.[4] Granted that the human evolutionary heritage is shared with all other animal species; nevertheless, we evolved as cultural and social beings. But, in the present day, the scientific and biomedical view of humans is moving toward our being genetically programmed animals, independent of culture and morality: priority is being given to genetic rather than cultural inheritance.[5] This view is but a logical extension of the biomedical conceptualization that the body is a machine. The machine has now been reduced to its ultimate components: the gene, even though, as I pointed out in the Introduction, tensions exist in contemporary society between scientific reductionism and a holistic view of human beings.

The ideology of genetic inheritance deprives the person of agency: the genetic vision of humanity is that their genes predetermine people. Paradoxically, while the hegemony of the gene diminishes humans as actors, the individual is nevertheless moved to act to avoid risk, even though such actions may prove futile; it simultaneously provides a sense of control and frustrates it. One might have anticipated a degree of fatalism among the sick, but curiously the ideology becomes reinterpreted in such a way that it moves people to act on the belief that to comprehend the reason for one's affliction is to prevent it. As we learned from many of the women in Chapters 5 and 6 and from the adoptees, they tend to believe that if one knows one's predisposition to inherit a disorder, something can be done to prevent the inevitable, if only by avoiding identified risk factors. In the case of adoptees, the very consciousness of genetic inheritance moves them to act by searching for their birth parents.

Yet various scholars have questioned the validity of notions of genetic determinism in general and of biomedicine's tenet of genetic inheritance in particular by suggesting that diseases characterized as genetically transmitted are, in actuality, influenced by numerous mutation-causing environmental toxins. In fact, the majority of women with breast cancer do not have relatives with the same affliction. The validity of genetic inheritance can also be questioned on theoretical grounds. Thus, while the most ardent critics will accept the reality of the DNA molecules and the incontrovertible evidence that a handful of diseases are inherited,[6] it must also be recognized that the meanings we give are subject to social and cultural interpretation.

Whereas diseases such as breast cancer are palpable realities, as are DNA molecules, notions advanced by the HGP project — that eventually all diseases are genetically produced and genetically transmitted, or that individuals are genetically predisposed to diseases because they originate from certain families — are arguably social and cultural constructions. The ideology of genetic inheritance establishes a continuity with the past and incorporates future generations in physical terms; it may even substitute for people's nostalgia for past ancestors who may have been embellished by myths, longing, and affect. Ancestors coming on the *Mayflower* may no longer form part of one's persona. We saw that in ancient times, and in non-Western traditions, people's existence was embedded in family and kinship relations: a human being was defined as a social person, legitimized by the inheritance of status, power, goods, poverty, or other aspects associated wtih personhood. A small elite may still transmit status, power, and wealth to its descendants, but, by and large, in contemporary times, increasingly the biomedical vision of family and kinship is established by DNA inheritance rather than by a sense of morality embodied in solidarity, responsibility, obligation, and affect. Concurrently, the ideology of genetic inheritance expands the circle of people that comprise the significant same group by incorporating many more persons than are usually considered part of the kindred. The expansion of the significant same circle may, as we saw, establish a sense of unity, albeit even if unwittingly with those sharing the same genes, despite the new definitions of family and kin, which are based on a sense of socially defined sameness. In spite of this unity, people's personhood becomes encapsulated in their DNA and what it foresees for their future health status, around which people's lives tend to center more and more.[7] The physical body and genetic identity tend to characterize the individual rather than the so-cially and culturally acquired aspects of his or her being.

Formerly, whatever their social or economic status, people could take pride in the fact that their families and ancestors had bequeathed to them what they considered positive aspects of their person such as blue eyes, a lanky body, and other culturally valued aspects of their being, even when these might be offset by unfavorable characteristics such as heavy thighs or other deprecated physical attributes, as in Betty's and Kate's cases. But it is often overlooked that such disesteemed aspects of the person do not draw the individual into the medical domain in the same way as conceptualizations of genetic inheritance of disease have done.[8]

In contemporary times, the medical family history forms part of the person's identity and memory. Family and kinship relations may be defined more by the heritability of disorders and pain and less by the inheritance of status and social attributes. Unmindfully the DNA records and remembers a person's ancestors better than does the person's fragile memory. Ancestors may be recalled less for their achievements or beliefs, more for their physicality and dysfunction.[9] Although the DNA establishes continuity with the dead, it is a continuity comprising hollow particles that lack the feeling tones that normally accompany memories. Even if a person wishes to forget her antecedents and to reinvent herself, the physician will remind her of her "true" biological ancestors, as adoptees become painfully aware every time they visit a doctor. Within the biomedical domain, the medical history and biological antecedents confer upon the adoptee his or her personhood; knowing one's genetic ties is even raised by some to a spiritual state, a transcendent experience.

The objective of my empirical research was to explore how people negotiate contemporary scientific and biomedical beliefs that have stamped on their consciousness that biological inheritance shapes their existence.[10] During the course of my fieldwork, I was led to examine the phenomenological consequences of genetic inheritance ideology and its various implications for individual experience and family relations. My more theoretical concern when I embarked on this project was to determine why the notion of genetic inheritance and genetic reductionism has become the regnant biomedical ideology, as evidenced in the mass media, by the HGP, and by people's preoccupation. What are the social processes that have led to these conceptualizations, given their serious political implications?[10] Given that scientific ideas are nurtured within a specific societal environment, to which the rediscovery of Mendel's work, for one, clearly attests, the problem still remains. Why has the pendulum swung so drastically toward genetics, particularly in American society since the 1970s?

Indubitably, there are numerous explanations for the hegemony of the gene — and indeed, other scholars have addressed this question. Bowler, for one, suggests that biological determinism has been perpetuated because genetics developed into molecular biology, which claims to unlock the secrets of life and is represented as the great wonder of modern science with biotechnology as its new frontier.[12]

Yoxen points out that the science of genetics was uninterested in disease because of its perceived lack of relevance to treatment until recently, when genetics and medicine became wedded to each other and the notion of genetic diseases was invented. He was one of the earliest scholars to call attention to the construction of genetic diseases and to question why genetic diseases have been singled out. His response revolves around an analysis of the role of status and power plays within different biomedical disciplines by claiming that genetic diseases were identified as those that were not in competition with established specialties.[13] Whereas Yoxen was right on target in posing the question, and his response may have been valid in the 1980s; his explanation is currently wanting because the concept of genetic diseases is being appropriated by all biomedical specialties.

Likewise, Fox Keller has examined the predominance of beliefs in genetic inheritance. According to this scholar, the development of molecular genetics and genetic determinism are the ultimate forms of reductionism because of their assertion that to comprehend the behavior of an organism, its cells and molecules must be known. We exist in an age of materialist reductionism, a biologism that touches all spheres of medicine and psychiatry, and geneticization is but a logical extension of biologism.[14]

Lewontin tends to reduce his response to economics when he attributes the development of the HGP to "what are said to be fundamental discoveries about the nature of life [which] often mask simple commercial relations that provide a powerful impetus for the direction and subject of research." From Lewontin's perspective, commerce is the driving force behind the ideology of genetic predominance. He describes how billions of dollars have been invested with few results and rhetorically wonders why the biotechnology equipment manufacturers envision genes for alcoholism, unemployment, domestic and social violence, and drug addiction. He responds that "what we had previously imagined to be messy moral, political, and economic issues turn out, after all, to be simply a matter of an occasional nucleotide substitution. While the notion that the war on drugs will be won by genetic engineering belongs to Cloud-CuckooLand, it is a manifestation of a serious ideology that is continuous with the eugenics of an earlier time."[15] The economic motive cannot be excluded in societies, including the United States, that are driven by a market economy and that are based on the assumption that "human nature" is founded in selfish interests, even genetically determined, to maximize profits.[16] Granted, even if we accept that these ideologies are nurtured by an economic motive — and the argument is compelling — the economic motive fails to explain why people readily accept genetic explanations, unless they are also consonant with profound cultural conceptualizations that assist people to make sense of disordered, random events.

Biologism and economics may have laid down the templates in order for the ideology of genetic inheritance to prevail in modern society, as the scholars I cite persuasively argue. Indeed, genetic determinism not only nurtures industry but also tends to preserve the status quo by justifying the socioeconomic inequalities pervading modern society. The reasoning is that social and economic conditions cannot be changed, if such conditions are genetically determined, any more than if they had been determined by the gods. As in the nineteenth century, the reductionist view advanced by the ideology of genetic inheritance inclines people to ignore social ills by removing the responsibility from society for the prevalence of life-threatening diseases such as cancer.[17] Only the individual needs to change through genetic engineering; the environmentally induced mutations can be overlooked, if each person's destiny is written in the DNA molecule transmitted by kin rather than by his or her individual social and economic situation and position in society. Not surprisingly, for some people the ideology fosters a sense of fatalism by removing the sense of mastery, even though at the same time it may move them to act.

Whereas Yoxen, Fox Keller, Bowler, and Lewontin have advanced our understanding of the hegemony of the gene, their explanations need to be carried farther. Although there is no one overarching rationale that elucidates the prominence assumed by the ideology of genetic inheritance and genetic determinism in contemporary society, I will submit several interrelated reasons for the medicalization of kinship and the hegemony of the gene. These revolve around the current state of biomedical knowledge, American kinship conceptualizations, contemporary family structure, and the nature of memory in postmodern society. I am aware that in developing these lines of argument I may have tended to set aside other factors of importance, or given some factors more importance than they merit.

While biomedicine has achieved an exquisite knowledge of anatomy, physiology, and the pathophysiology of most diseases, it lacks etiological explanations for the most common chronic currently understood as non-infectious diseases afflicting individuals in developed nations, including such life-threatening afflictions as cancer and heart disease. The decrease in the prevalence of acute diseases and the exceptional rise in American society of chronic diseases that lack any recognized and definitive causes beg for explanations that assure a degree of measurable certainty and even predictability. Some diseases, including AIDS, cancer of the cervix, or even lung cancer, possess known etiologies, if not cures. The majority of afflictions for which biomedicine lacks a definitive etiology are relegated to the hereditary causal bin.[18] In this manner biomedicine and its practitioners are absolved from any further explanation and from any responsibility to attempt to alter aspects of a person's ecological and social environment that may be implicated in the etiology of a disease. Neither viruses nor genes have lobbies in Congress. They cannot stand up in righteous indignation to declare that they have been falsely maligned, as many environmental polluters or cigarette companies have done successfully until recently. In developing nations such as Mexico, biomedicine's hereditarian ideology may help exculpate the state from failing to address the abominable public health conditions that cause so much suffering and affliction.

My argument parallels Rosenberg's discussion of the prevalence of hereditarian concepts during the nineteenth century,[19] which illuminates the present situation. At that time medicine failed to explain the causes of almost all diseases and viewed those it could not explain as hereditary. Indeed, the predominant diseases in the nineteenth century, such as tuberculosis, hysteria, rickets, and pellagra, were considered hereditary until other etiologies were found, including pathogens and vitamin deficiencies, or in the case of hysteria were largely eliminated from biomedical nosology.[20]

Related to the proposition that the current state of biomedical knowledge fails to explain the causes of most chronic diseases is the fact that biomedicine also fails to address the most profound and oft-stated question human beings pose when afflicted with a life-threatening disease: "Why me?" Biomedicine masterfully elucidates the proximate causes of the "how" and the "what" of a disease, but it fails to shed light on the ultimate cause of "why" any *one specific individual* becomes afflicted.[21] Understandably, when struck by affliction and suffering, human beings often desire to know why, rather than what the pathophysiology is of the disease: people may be less concerned with theoretical knowledge about how a disease happens than they are with why it happened to *them*. Biomedicine is based upon a norm of generalized knowledge about disease and its course.[22] But when a patient seeks to understand why *he* or *she* fell ill, biomedicine is silent.[23] By attributing a disease to faulty genes inherited from one's family, genetic reductionism purports to explain the ultimate cause. For people suffering from an unexplainable condition, genetic inheritance provides a plausible and eloquently succinct answer that is easy to grasp, especially when the patient is confronted with the complex how and what of her condition. She can easily fall back on the genetic ideology in light of experiential evidence that other members of the family have similarly been afflicted. Genetic explanations can make even death itself reasonable. Bauman asserts correctly that human recognition of death has been rationalized in modern times. Mortality is no longer accepted as an existential fact but construed in many ways, including as a result of "defective genetic stock."[24] Moreover, by anchoring its diagnoses in molecular biology and genetics, biomedicine becomes unquestionably a science rather than an art, naturalizing completely its beliefs and furthering its validation.

Unlike patients, adoptees may not find answers to profound existential issues of abandonment and rejection, questions such as "Why was I given away?" which may be the deepest reason for searching for their biological mother. Their cultural comprehension of kinship in biological terms allows them, however, to attempt to deal with such dilemmas by reestablishing contact with their birth mother and by creating for themselves a history, even if it is only a medical family history. By becoming reunited with their birth families, the fragmented adoptees, phenomenologically torn between cultural ideologies and lived experience, become, in the words of many, "whole," arguably masking the fragmentation people may feel more generally in contemporary capitalist society.

The prevalence of the ideology of genetic inheritance is facilitated by mainstream American conceptualizations of kinship. In fact, to attribute disorders to genetic inheritance, which makes them comprehensible to people, is not only to gracefully and simply address ultimate causality but also to build on American cultural understandings of kinship, which are put in biogenetic terms. It is noteworthy to recall Schneider's argument, alluded to in Chapter 2 that "kinship has been defined by European social scientists, and European social scientists use their own folk culture as the source of many, if not all, of their ways of formulating and understanding the world about them."[25] Schneider recognized that social scientists impose their folk knowledge on non-Western kinship, but he erroneously distinguishes scientific knowledge from Western folk knowledge and fails to discern that scientific claims frequently follow a similar pattern.[26] I propose that the emphasis given to genetic transmission elaborates the mainstream American folk category of bilateral kinship, which has its roots in the early modern period of Europe. Not surprisingly, then, the fact that American kinship builds on a biogenetic template facilitates the wide popular acceptance of the hegemony of the gene. Folk notions of family as a biogenetic entity allow for an effortless embrace of the scientific and biomedical notion of genetic determinism, which creates a sense of naturalness precisely because it mimics cultural conceptualizations of kinship.

In keeping with this point, genetic determinism weaves into a mantle of science the historical and cultural grasp of kinship and reaffirms the family and kinship cohesion that has been lost in the lived world. Returning to Schneider's observation that I cited in Chapter 3, he emphasized that biological unity was the symbol of the relationships of solidarity in American society.[27] Whichever solidarity may exist, it rests in genetic unity. We saw in Chapter 3 that while the American family has not disappeared, it lacks unifying forces, a phenomenon that even Tocqueville had recognized when he stated in the mid-nineteenth century that "not only does democracy make men forget their ancestors but also clouds their view of their descendants and isolates them from their contemporaries."[28] In contemporary society people have tended to become separated from kin, if not from their immediate family, and family and kinship have taken on an amorphous cast, for multiple reasons, the most obvious perhaps being geographic dispersal.[29]

I suggest that biomedicine, by means of concepts of the genetic inheritance of disease and genetic determinism in general, pins down and defines the family in precise terms by uniting, wittingly or unwittingly, individuals with their families and kin. The more social processes (including, if Tocqueville is correct, democracy itself) tend to distance people from family and kin, the more biomedicine tends to move it closer to consanguinity, creating new forms of interaction that may be embedded in the *very absence* of interaction. People are compelled to recognize consanguinity even when in the lived world they define family by a sense of sameness that may be grounded in friendship or sharing of affect and interest, rather than genes. With the ideology of genetic inheritance and the medicalization of kinship, interaction with family and kin may no longer be required in order for people to recognize relatedness and connection. A point I noted before merits repeating: in the past, the family was identified by honor, status, power, or even poverty, whereas in contemporary times family and kin tend to be stabilized and bounded by the sharing of DNA molecules, which lack the moral responsibilities associated with relatedness.

Phenomenologically there is a distinction between experiencing oneself as a member of a significant same group, which feels a sense of unity and relatedness associated with shared experiences from the beginning of life, and experiencing oneself as a member of a group that shares DNA molecules, which are not easily discernible. The notion of shared experiences suggests being in the world and interacting with others, whereas being part of the same DNA circle requires no social interaction. Bauman points out what Merleau-Ponty knew: that the only way we can comprehend ourselves and know that we are alive is because we know that life means being with others. To sense that one forms part of a family chiefly because one shares the same genes, requiring no social participation nor sense of responsibility to those who are related except to provide blood

samples for testing purposes, removes the moral context of family relations. Lévinas, as quoted by Bauman, observes that humans are beings
with meaning and that meaning comes out of our responsibility for others. He asserts that "being reduced to the 'is' being without the 'ought'
equals solitude."[30] To be human is to be a moral being, to insist on the
"ought" and the "should" even against all odds, and the sense of responsibility to others that ensues from the "ought" is initially experienced in
one's significant same group. Relations between family and kin, however
defined, are governed by a special morality arising out of the recognition
of commonality,[31] whereas relations established on the basis of the new
genetics lack moral imperatives.

Kinship and family relations established on the basis of sharing DNA
molecules carry no moral load and require little or no responsibility.
Genes are amoral physical entities. For this reason, my initial hypothesis
that people would blame their ancestors for their afflictions had to be
rejected because I had not initially realized that genes, indeed, are blame-
less. Therefore, breast cancer patients do not hold their ancestors responsible for transmitting "faulty" genes. Uniformly, the women I interviewed said that their ancestors and family were not accountable for their
affliction and thus were inculpable. Indeed, how can genes be blamed for
anything? Concurrently, and significantly, the ideology of genetic inheritance gives meaning to the randomness inherent in genetics, to the "luck
of the draw," by supplying a reason for suffering and thereby making it
more bearable. Ironically, it may even bring people back to the religious
notion of original sin and bearing the burden of the sins of the fathers.
Not, surprisingly, as we saw in Chapter 6, for many women, including
Jana, Dina, and Katherine, the disease is redemptive, almost uplifting,
furnishing a new meaning to the person's life. In fact, McCarthy and
Loren suggest that breast cancer leads to a heightened spirituality.[32]

Yet, ironically, the contemporary individual, solitary, independent,
and autonomous, willingly or not becomes unified with genetic family
and kin by the very fact of having shared asocial and amoral DNA. Bauman correctly observes that "the *sociality* of the post-modern community
does not require *sociability*. Its togetherness does not require interaction.
Its unity does not require integration" (emphasis in the original).[33] The
individual can enjoy traditional kinship and family relations without obligation, responsibility, or sociability. At the same time, the ideology of
genetic inheritance expands the recognition of family and kin and gives
them new importance for the individual, which they may have lacked
before. Paradoxically, molecular biology and the genetic model of family
and kinship bridge the essentialism of modern science with postmodern
ideologies and experience. It could even be said that the ideology of
genetic inheritance promises contemporary humans immortality within

the flux of the postmodern world. The individual exists in a transient world but is fastened biologically to the past and the future.

Genetic determinism substitutes for memories lost. Kinship is not only a relationship of the present; kinship relations are repositories of and connections with the past, sustained in the genealogical memories of one's forbears. Memories are usually embedded in sounds, smells, affect, and tales of past ancestors and kinship ties. Memory through DNA never forgets and leaves nothing to mystery[34] and is embedded in *the absence* of experience and feelings. The DNA remembers what has long been forgotten. Nor does it permit reinvention of the self or the embellishment of past ancestors: it only recollects that person's physicality. People cannot invent or appropriate ancestors because the DNA will reveal the truth.

Tocqueville noted that in a democracy, "those who have gone before are easily forgotten."[35] Indeed, in postmodern times more than ever, memories may be depthless, but genetic inheritance establishes depth and continuity with previous generations and unifies people with their past. It reinforces, or arguably reintroduces, the experience of chronology, of time passing. But, in characteristic postmodern fashion, when time and space have become compressed,[36] memory is reduced to an exquisite simplicity of DNA molecules. While the postmodern individual may chiefly know the present, genetic inheritance ideologies remind people that there was a past to which the individual is connected, thus defining an intergenerational space. In day-to-day experience, aunts, uncles, and even grandparents may not be recalled, whereas they must be remembered, especially when one's body is in disorder, when one is asked for a family medical history.

Building on biologism, the medicalization of kinship reinforces contemporary humans' physicality and postmodern emphasis on the body by assigning shared identities to people who may have little in common in the past or in the present, particularly as adults, people with whom they have shared few experiences. By doing so, the hegemony of the gene reinforces consanguineal ties to the exclusion of affinal ties established by marriage. As marriage ties loosen, it is the order of nature that connects us, rather than culture, the order of law, or shared experience.[37]

The ideology of genetic inheritance adds a new dimension to memory while distancing the person from his or her being by erasing the complexity of living, if not of life. Drawing on concepts in phenomenology, I discuss the notion of *life's lesions,* referring to embodied adversity and moral contradictions captured in our biographies, which become inscribed on the body and expressed in non-life-threatening symptomatologies.[38] Within the context of genetic inheritance beliefs, people's lives and experience become irrelevant to their disorder. Chemical construction of the gene is registered on the family and kin body, overlooking people's biographies.

The responsibility for a person's disorder rests with the individual, or more precisely with the individual's family and kin. Ironically, while the person's biography becomes inconsequential, the person is simultaneously both blamed for and absolved from his or her afflictions. It is not the individual but the family and kin from whom the person inherited the disorder that was instrumental in causing the disease.[39] In a profound contradiction, on the one hand, the medicalization of kinship compels people to remember their relatives and ancestors who, in actuality, bewitch their descendants by bestowing defective genes. On the other hand, North American culture glorifies the freedom to choose, including one's kinfolk. But it removes the possibility of choice in selecting one's family and relatives,[40] as becomes evident with adoptees. What is being allotted to choice is the possibility of genetic engineering. The prevailing vocabulary of choice incorporates technological control, which presumably is left to personal choice. Potentially, genetic engineering promises to create faultless individuals, bringing us back full circle to eugenics' goals enacted through technological management. But whereas eugenics promoted a form of social control through enforced selected breeding, genetic engineering creates medical control through technology.[41] Discourse on race is out of fashion. We no longer speak of racial difference, but we can speak of its individual counterpart based on differences among families produced by the continuity of genetic inheritance.

Curiously, the focus on the genetic basis of family and kinship is contrary to people's contemporary social experience of a significant same group comprising individuals who are recruited by choice. As we are informed by Dolgin's analysis, until the 1990s the American legal and biomedical systems tended to move in opposite directions regarding the role of genetics in defining the family. The courts favored contractual arrangements over those of genetic ties. But more recently, legal and medical interpretations have tended to become coterminous, following the genetic model of family and kinship.[42]

One final point merits consideration. I expect that irrespective of class differences, the compartmentalized postmodern, fragmented individual has become joined to his or her ancestors by DNA and to living relatives by the ideology of genetic inheritance. While given the small sample size of this study we cannot draw any conclusions about class differences, I hypothesize that belief in genetic inheritance cuts across gender and class lines. This supposition is based on the fact that the ideology is unceasingly promoted not only in the biomedical but in the popular literature as well,[43] and by family medical historytaking, to which most people are exposed if they resort to a biomedical initial consultation.

Whereas the people we met in Chapters 5, 6, and 7 include high school and college graduates and differ in economic position, generally speaking, they can be classified as belonging to that giant American sea identified as the middle class. Whether they form part of the lower, middle, or upper middle class, as we saw, with a few exceptions they generally accepted genetic inheritance ideology. We lack comparable data dealing with working-class Americans such as, for example, Jana. I postulate that people's responses will differ depending upon their family experience and kin interactions, their expectations, and their definition of their significant same. It thus remains an empirical question as to what extent various social groups reinterpret the biomedical and mass media messages and codes concerning genetic inheritance. How does it influence their actions, including their relationship to family and kin? To what degree might the ideology influence mate selection? I cannot stress enough the importance of studying in the future the ways in which this ideology is interpreted across class lines.

To conclude, an observation I made previously requires reiteration. I do not question the truth or falsity of the ideology of genetic inheritance. I have argued that kinship and family have become medicalized in contemporary society, with the hegemony of the gene attributable to contemporary American societal and cultural sensibilities. While we saw that some biological and social scientists have furnished empirical evidence and compelling arguments against genetic reductionism,[44] I contend that if we accept that medical systems are embedded in culture, then the hegemony of genetic inheritance becomes less puzzling. The medicalization of kinship is but an extension of an ongoing process of the expansion of the medical gaze to our deepest relationships, building on the cultural template of bilateral and biogenetic kinship, which historically forms part of American cultural beliefs and practice. This process is further fostered by the economic, political, and social order. With the medicalization of kinship and family, dispersed and loosely connected family and kin tend to become linked by inexorable genetic ties that in part reestablish their continuity beyond parental relations. With the medicalization of kinship, uprooted families become reunited and, desirous or not, they must recognize a connectedness, even if it is mediated by disorders. Some predict that the significance of blood bonds may wane if marriage as an institution weakens.[45] This prediction may have had some plausibility if kinship and family ties had not become medicalized in contemporary times.

My concern in the present work has been with North American society, where kinship practices are rapidly changing. But it is important to call attention to developing nations such as Mexico, where the family and not the individual is still the primary unit of existence, and where the person is embedded in a network of family and kin.[46] The biomedical notion that one's family may be harmful to one's health may be disorienting. How can one's family be the pillar of one's existence and yet transmit sickness? While in Mexico breast cancer may not as yet be regarded as genetically inherited, with the diffusion of biomedicine, accompanied by the practice of family medical historytaking, the ideology of genetic inheritance may well prevail the world over in the near future, with globalization in full force.[47] We need to attend to the phenomenology of the medicalization of kinship in such societies.[48] It will be especially important to examine how people in kinship-oriented societies such as Africa, Melanesia, the Middle East, and India interpret the belief in the genetic inheritance of disorders when confronted by biomedical explanations of disease etiology. This issue has not been explored cross-culturally, yet it is of crucial importance not only for academic purposes but also for practical reasons to understand how people respond to biomedicine and ultimately to its treatment modes. For example, Dumars and Chea discuss the high frequency of alpha and beta thalassemia and E hemoglobin among the Cham (an ethnic group originating from Southeast Asia), and how the medical personnel explained the reasons for the "neurodegenerative disease in their offspring that resulted in many newborn deaths. However, this *did not alter their reproductive behavior*"[49] (emphasis added) because, according to the authors, the people were not concerned about the fact that this was a genetic disease, any more than was the woman in Mexico who bore a child with oculopharyngeal muscular dystrophy, or Down syndrome.

I have analyzed the current ideology of genetic inheritance from various dimensions of individual and societal levels of experience. No one is a sufficient soothsayer to be able to predict how the ideology of genetic inheritance will play itself out in the future. History teaches us, and we know from the study of the history of scientific epistemology, that scientific knowledge is discontinuous,[50] even if scientists are reluctant to overthrow existing paradigms for new ones.[51] Postmodern scholarship brought into bold relief the culturally contingent nature of biomedical knowledge, refuting scientific claims of objectivity. If the totalizing postmodern assertions are correct, can it be assumed that notions of genetic determinism and ideologies of genetic inheritance will be eventually discarded for "new" ideas that will recognize that the secret to human life, if there is one, is that human beings are thinking, not always rational, usually ambivalent, feeling and moral beings who seek meaning and purpose? Notwithstanding the elegance of genetic explanations, DNA molecules cannot stand in for human existence. They may symbolize it and contribute to it, but humans cannot be reduced to DNA molecules — or can they? This question, however, will have to be answered by future scholars in the new millennium.

Notes

Preface

1. Finkler 1974.
2. Finkler 1994a, b; 1991.
3. In an extensive study of biomedical practice, patient response, and management of illness, I explored in depth the sickness attributions of all patients. Folk etiological explanations included sudden fright, anger, environmental assaults, nerves, witchcraft, and heredity. See Finkler 1991.
4. Finkler 1991.
5. I regard myself as a social critic who uses my moral imagination to, in Rosaldo's words, "move from the world as it actually is to a locally persuasive vision of how it ought to be" (Rosaldo 1994: 183).
6. Finkler 1994a.
7. I carried out a two-year study of medical practice in one of these hospitals (Finkler 1991, 1996).
8. This hospital is part of the Mexican Social Security System, IMSS.
9. In these hospitals cancer is not managed as a genetic disease, even though I hasten to add that all the genetic specialists I interviewed adhere to McKusick's (1998) classification of genetic diseases. One genetic counselor indicated that their unit could not deal with breast cancer as a genetic disease because they would have too many patients to attend to. They attend and treat congenital malformations, mental retardation, Turner's syndrome, Klinefelter's syndrome (boys with XXY chromosomes instead of the normal XY), muscular dystrophy, neurofibromatosis Type I and II, oculopharyngeal muscular dystrophy, spinal muscular atrophy, and other classical genetic conditions. They do not attend to diabetes, cancer, or rheumatic disorder, for example.
10. Finkler 1991.
11. Finkler 1994a.
12. Finkler 1994a.
13. My notion of structuration builds on the work of Giddens 1984.
14. Hood 1992; Nelkin and Lindee 1995.
15. Allen 1996; Hubbard 1997; Lewontin 1984.

Chapter 1. Introduction

1. *Science* 267 (March 17, 1995) and in the new biology curricula; Spanier 1995: 150.

2. Angell 1997: 44.

3. Turner 1997.

4. Bodmer and McKie 1994; Hood 1992; Jonsen 1996; Richards 1996. In a recent keynote address Francis Collins, director of the National Human Genome Research Institute, hailed the Genome Project as the "Book of Life" that will be opened by the year 2002 and that will explain, cure, and predict most all human disease (Collins 1999a). For a popular portrayal of Collins and his goals for the GNP see Nash (1994).

5. Hubbard and Wald 1997; Jonsen 1996; Nelkin and Lindee 1995.

6. There were numerous television programs such as *Turning Point* (ABC) and *Dateline* (NBC) featuring issues related to genetic inheritance. Radio programs on National Public Radio's *Fresh Air, Morning Edition* (1997a) and *Talk of the Nation Science Friday* (1997b) have presented recent developments in genetic inheritance. National Public Radio's *All Things Considered* (1998a) discussed the usefulness of mastectomies to save lives for women "who've seen their mothers or sisters die an early death from breast cancer" (National Public Radio 1997). A program presented on CNN, *Your Money,* instructed its viewers to track down their family history to "provide useful hereditary information" (Brooke and Metaxas 1997). Films such as *Gattaca* have dealt with the dangerous consequences of genetic engineering. I collected articles appearing in the popular press from 1996 to 1998 that deal with genetic inheritance and related topics. I also consulted the Periodical Literature Data Base and the World Wide Web, and I have identified several categories of articles according to whether they are questioning and critical or what I call "gaga" about the achievements of contemporary genetics. My sample suggests that those critical of genetic inheritance are in a minority (e.g., Begley 1996, 1997; *Economist* 1995; Marty 1996; *Turning Point* 1996), although some present the issues from both a positive and a negative perspective (Herbert 1997; Turner 1997). The majority of the articles report on the extraordinary achievements of genetics, genetic testing, and genetic engineering (e.g., Blakeslee 1997; Brownlee and Silberner 1991; Brownlee et al. 1994; Carey 1997; Carey and Flynn 1997; Elmer Dewit 1994; Freundlich 1997; Glausiusz 1995a, b, 1996; Grady 1994; Higgins 1997; Jaroff 1989, 1994, 1996; Nash 1997; Rubin 1996; Seligman 1994; Sack 1997; Wade 1997). These articles speak about the "wisdom of genes." Some may show, for example, that the priestly line in Judaism can be traced genetically to 3,330 years in the past. Others may demarcate ethnic groups, including Ashkenazi Jewish women for their high risk of breast cancer and, for the Ashkenazis in general, colon cancer (Bluman 1998), although some writers are concerned that delineating ethnic groups may lead to discrimination against that group (Wade 1997:5; Feldman 1998). In a broadcast on National Public Radio on May 6, 1999, Joe Palka reported the recent controversy regarding a new study of the genetic basis of schizophrenia among Ashkenazi Jewish families. One of the commentators vehemently objected to the study because of the stigmatization of Ashkenazi Jews. Still other articles discuss how DNA is being used to learn who is related and who is not, and to "sort out family members' kinship issues, and the number of such tests is on the rise nationally" (Ostrom 1997). The *Chattanooga Times* (Associated Press 1996) reports that people are searching vigorously for family trees to learn "their ancestors' causes of death to clue them in on genetic

diseases" (p. 5). Finch (1996) reports in *Health* that "Tracing your roots to learn your family's health history may be the single most important thing you ever do to bolster your well-being" (p. 92) and instructs the reader on how to go about doing a family tree. Monmaney (1995) in the same magazine observes that genetic testing may be "kids' latest rite of passage" (p. 22) to avert breast cancer. See also SerVaas 1995. Rather than adopt children, infertile couples may harvest their own eggs or sperm to assure genetic continuity, while sperm banks seek intelligent donors for women (usually without partners) who wish to be inseminated. Kolata (1998) reports on sperm or egg banks seeking individuals with higher education and prestigious occupations that assiduously screen for physical and mental characteristics and personality traits. The article does point out that genetics experts caution that such selections can provide only limited assurances. But Kolata also observes that one psychologist noted that despite her reluctance, she would, nonetheless, if she were seeking a sperm or egg donor, "check the person's scores on the SAT and intelligence tests and personality traits" (p. 12). This article also calls attention to what I call the globalization of genomania by finding women "who are extremely bright, attractive and kindhearted" in places such as Australia (p. 12). There are numerous articles in the popular press that report on the genetic inheritance of behavior, including infidelity, crime, and addiction (Hawley 1997; Metzler 1994; Morrow 1997). Health newsletters and the press report on numerous genetic diseases (Alter 1998) and predispositions, including obesity, Alzheimer's (*Johns Hopkins Medical Letter* 1997), taste, anxiety, alcoholism, and attention deficit disorder (Morrow 1997). The *Johns Hopkins Medical Letter* reporting on surgery to prevent breast cancer states: "Indeed, individual risk increases for every first- and second-degree relative (mother, sister, grandmother, or aunt) who has had the disease, especially if they had it before age 50" (1999: 1).

Uncritical reports suggest that women undergo prophylactic mastectomies if they have a family history of breast cancer (Ziv 1997). Some articles suggest that those who have "faulty families" trace their family trees. One especially interesting article from the *Wall Street Journal* (Bounds 1996) stresses that "mapping family medical histories is at the heart of genetics research" (p. B1) and that "doctors recommend every family make its own medical tree" (p. B5), instructing its readers on how to produce a family tree. The family medical history is touted as a lifesaver (Adato 1995). Conflicts with insurance companies are cited in most articles, primarily associated with genetic testing (e.g., Carlton 1997). Some articles focus on adoption, especially how adoptees seek access to their genetic history (Park 1997), and how, for an adoptee, "Finding My Parents Saved My Life" (Cool 1994) because she was able to learn her genetic history. Such articles advocate open adoptions and open medical records. In a rebroadcast, the television program *60 Minutes* reported on adoptees clamoring for open adoption records. Various reasons were given for their desire to know their birth parents, including the medical history (1999). In an article in the *New York Times* on how an adoption agency never mentioned an adoptee's genetic legacy of schizophrenia, Belkin asserts, "The growing recognition that schizophrenia had a genetic element *paralleled an awareness that most disease in general has a genetic element. That in turn led to a change in how adoption agencies viewed a child's medical history*" (1999: 47, emphasis added).

Occasionally one can find an objection to the mainstream view, as for example in Ruth Hubbard's (1998) letter to the editor in response to what she describes appropriately as the "current genomania" that is reflected in Groopman's (1998) article in the *New Yorker.* When a book written by Hamer and Copeland (1998) about how genes determine human behavior was published, the first author was interviewed twice in the same week on National Public Radio. Nelkin (1992) describes how *Business Week* heralded "The Genetic Defense of the Free Market." DNA is even touted as teaching history. See Rothstein (1998), who says that the "new history is inscribed in strands of DNA" (p. 5).

7. Siebert 1995: 74, 94.

8. *Dateline* 1998; Nelkin 1992: 181.

9. Hubbard and Wald 1997.

10. Carey et al. 1997; also Hamilton and Flynn 1999; Freundlich 1997.

11. Nelkin and Lindee 1995; Kass 1998.

12. Fox Keller 1992; Nelkin and Lindee 1995: 198; Petersen 1998; Collins 1999a.

13. L. Turner 1997.

14. Bounds 1996: B1.

15. *Wall Street Journal,* 1996: B5. Milunsky (1992) similarly advises his readers to keep track of their pedigrees. In an extensive cover story in *Time* on the contemporary "mania" for learning about family trees, one segment is entitled "Genealogy Saves Lives"; it displays a picture of three sisters, one of whom is quoted as saying, "knowing my family's health history saved my life" (Hornblower 1999: 57).

16. *Consumer Reports* 1996: 97.

17. Siebert 1995.

18. Matthews 1999; also Brownlee et al. 1994.

19. Herbert 1997.

20. Conrad 1997.

21. By "ideology" I mean a dominant system of beliefs, an authoritative intellectual current, that in Geertz's phrase provides "maps of problematic social reality and matrices for the creating of collective conscience" (1973: 220) that move people to action. More recently, Wolf defined ideology as "unified schemes or configurations developed to underwrite or manifest power" (1999: 5): in the instance of ideologies of genetic inheritance, power is lodged in biomedical hegemony. I am not concerned with the truth or falsity of the ideology but rather with the ways in which these beliefs shape people's lives.

22. Hubbard and Wald 1997 refer to the same phenomenon as geneticization. I prefer the "hegemony of the gene" only because the concept of hegemony embodies the ability of power to impose the ideology on others. I employ the Gramscian notion of hegemony, which not only rests on the use of force or the power of the state but also permeates the social and cultural fabric of daily life. The Gramscian conceptualization suggests how a dominant ideology becomes internalized in the general population by consensus rather than by coercion. See Gramsci 1971.

23. Brandt 1997; Finkler 1994a.

24. Dolgin 1997; Franklin 1993, 1997a, 1997b; Hubbard and Wald 1997; M. Strathern 1992a, b, 1995.

25. Yoxen (1986) also posed this question, but the answer incorporates many more dimensions than those he offered.

26. Cranor 1994; Dolgin 1997; Franklin 1997b; Hubbard and Wald 1997; Kevles 1992b; Lewontin 1992; Nelkin and Lindee 1995; M. Strathern 1992b.

27. Chiefly Pembrey 1996; Richards 1996.

28. Richards 1996.

29. Pembrey 1996: 76.

30. Richards 1996: 265.

31. Yoxen 1986: 4.

32. See Green et al. 1993, who emphasize that this information is needed by genetic counselors but is unavailable.

33. Dewey 1929: 8.

34. Allen 1996; Cranor 1994 (entire volume); Duster 1990; Fox Keller 1992; Nelkin and Tancredi 1989.

35. Griesemer 1994.

36. Finkler 1994a.

37. Wexler 1992.

38. Fox Keller 1992; Hubbard and Wald 1997; Lewontin, Rose, and Kamin 1984; Lewontin 1996; Nelkin and Lindee 1995; Spanier 1995; and others.

39. Berliner 1975; Englehardt 1986; Martin 1987; Osherson and Amara Singham 1981.

40. Significantly, in a lecture titled "Genetics and Faith," Francis Collins, head of the HGP, advanced the notion that he sees no conflict between religion and genetics and that uncovering the genome is a "religious experience" (Collins 1999b).

41. Angell 1997. Unquestionably a different conceptualization of "risk" exists among professionals and lay people. For example, Shiloh observes that in the literature on genetic counseling the "risk" is restricted to "the probability of occurrence of a negative genetic outcome" (p. 91). Those who are counseled tend to regard "risk" in personal terms and ignore the ambiguities of the concept of "risk," and the fact that it is based on statistical data alone.

42. Giddens 1991.

43. Bernstein 1996. See also Hacking 1975, who designates the year 1660 as the birth of probability in Western society.

44. Brandt 1997.

45. Petersen and Lupton 1996.

46. Berner (1996: 291), e.g., reports that among asymptomatic women 17 percent intended to have mastectomies and 33 percent to have oophorectomies, as prophylactic measures.

47. Collins (1999a) suggested that clinical genetics explains certainty. In an especially telling article, Meyer (1997:58) states, "Knowing which diseases run in your family—whether they're gleaned from genetic tests or from charting your medical past—help you live longer. The power of knowledge" provides that certainty. See also Veciana-Suarez 1996.

48. See Finkler 1996.

49. Boyarin 1994: 27.

50. Connerton 1989: 77.

51. See the very moving meditation on memory by Bourguignon 1996.

52. Connerton 1989.

53. Gottlieb 1993.

54. See Marcus and Hall 1992 and discussion in Chapter 3.

55. Durkheim 1964: 320.

56. Similarly, DNA may also exonerate an individual of false accusations of fatherhood with its attendant obligations, or of rape, for example (Herbert 1999; Willing 1999); it has created havoc for some and a boon for others. DNA testing, of course, confirms fatherhood, as it has for Liz, in Chapter 7. But see also Kristen's case in Chapter 7. In this instance the presumed father overlooked the fact that his and Kristen's DNA did not match, and he insisted on assuming the responsibility of being her father.

57. To use a simplistic example, can genetic determinism have an objective reality in light of, for example, Nelkin and Lindee's report (1995) that the Ernest Gallo Clinic and Research Center, founded in 1984, had identified biological causes of alcohol abuse? In 1993 this center's scientists found what they believed to be a gene for alcoholism, suggesting, of course, that the drinking habits of an individual are the faults of the person's genetic makeup. See also Hubbard and Wald 1997 for discussion of the vested interests of scientists in biotechnology.

58. Bowler 1989: 12, 13, 17.

59. Hahn and Kleinman 1983; Finkler 1991; Ingleby 1982; Krieger and Fee 1994; Lock 1980; Lock and Gordon 1988; Martin 1997; Wright and Treacher 1982; Young 1981.

60. Brandt 1997; Fujimura 1996; Haraway 1991; Kuhn 1970; Latour and Woolgar 1979; Martin 1997; Richter 1972; Bowler 1989 for genetics.

61. Berliner 1975; Osherson and Amara Singham 1981; Turner 1992. See especially Douglas 1970/1992 on how our comprehension of the body reflects broader societal themes; see also Martin 1987.

62. Finkler 1991; Wright and Treacher 1982; Turner 1987, 1992.

63. Johnson 1987; Martin 1997; Petchesky 1987; Ritenbaugh 1982; Rodin 1992; Yanagisako and Collier 1990.

64. Granner 1988.

65. *Consumer Reports* 1996; Nelkin 1992; Nelkin and Lindee 1995; Nelkin and Tancredi 1989.

66. See, however, Rosser (1994), who argues that genetic theories reflect social and sexual hierarchies. It is noteworthy, if paradoxical, that the current focus on the bilateral transmission of genetic disorders gives mothers and fathers equal status. At the same time, the X-chromosome, which bears the major burden for defective genetic transmission, is associated with the female, even though it is also transmitted by males, thus placing women in a contradictory position. See Finkler, 1994a. Also a study done in Britain of cognitive functioning of women with Turner's syndrome who had received their X-chromosome from either their mother or father. The study found that the women who had inherited the X-chromosome from their father had better social and cognitive skills than those who inherited the X-chromosome from their mother (Skuse et al. 1997). See also Chapter 7.

67. Fujimura 1996: 1.

68. Latour and Wolgar 1979.

69. Haraway 1991: 184.

70. Ibid., 187, 191.

71. E.g., ibid.

72. Fujimura (1996) describes how the oncogene became the final explanation of cancer at this time, resulting from a process of social negotiation.

73. Finkler 1991, 1985/1994; Foster and Anderson 1978; Kleinman 1980.

74. See Finkler 1991, 1994a. By this I mean that each culture has its own cultural pool of (etiological) understanding that people draw upon when experiencing an illness. Normally they may not be aware of an illness attribution until they fall ill and the *experience* impels them to search for an explanation, at which point they turn to their cultural pool of understanding. For example, a middle-class American's cultural pool of understanding does not usually include witchcraft as a sickness attribution, as it does in Mexico, where people nevertheless do not necessarily believe in witchcraft until they begin to search for an explanation of their affliction. In complex societies there exist competing pools, which are

historically contingent, and people will draw upon them differentially depending on gender and class and experience. The notion of the genetic basis of disease flowed into the Western pool of cultural understanding in the nineteenth century and took firm root in North America in the twentieth century. See Chapter 3.

75. Finkler 1994a.

76. Wexler 1992.

77. Fox Keller 1992. An article in *Time* (1962: 37) refers to "the *baby* science of 'molecular medicine,' " (emphasis added).

78. Allen 1996; Billings et al. 1992. Nelkin (1992) even cites an article from *Business Week* defending the free market on genetic grounds.

79. Wertz 1992.

80. *Merck Manual* 1977, 1997.

81. Franklin 1995. Yoxen provides the example of an embryo created by fertilization outside the woman's body and donated by another man and woman and then transferred to the womb of an infertile woman's sister, who carries the developing fetus to term. With this example, he shows that it is possible for the new baby to have three "fathers and three possible mothers." Yoxen 1986: 8–9.

82. McKeown 1985.

83. Richards 1996 notes that genealogical charts used by geneticists are the same as those learned by every anthropology student from the time of Rivers, the founder of the genealogical method in anthropology. See Rivers 1900. According to a genetic counselor (Cecile Skrzynia, personal communication), the family history includes both sets of parents, grandparents, aunts and uncles and first and second cousins.

84. M. Turner 1987.

85. Because of the spiritual ties, godparents are regarded by some as kinfolk, whereas others regard this relationship as pseudokinship. See Parkin 1997.

86. See also Finch and Mason 1993; M. Turner 1987; Witherspoon 1975.

87. Dolgin 1997.

Chapter 2. The Role of Kinship in Human Life

1. Lévi-Strauss, quoted in Lowie 1948: 57.

2. Morgan 1971: 13.

3. Lowie 1948: 57.

4. Gross 1992: 364.

5. Fortes 1970: 281–82, 290–91.

6. There are exceptions, as for example in the Arab world, where parallel cousin marriage (between offspring from the same descent group) is encouraged. See Mair 1971.

7. Holy 1996.

8. Holy 1996; Harris 1990; Peletz 1995; Parkin 1997; Sahlins 1968; Stone 1997. See also any introductory text in anthropology (e.g., Gross 1992, Graburn 1970). The foremost earlier scholars in kinship studies include Malinowski 1970, Radcliffe-Brown 1952, Lévi-Strauss 1969, and Schneider 1965, 1972, 1984.

9. Delaney 1986, 1991.

10. A. Strathern 1972: 13.

11. M. Strathern 1992b: 61.

12. Evans-Pritchard 1962: 247–48.

13. Parkin 1997: 38; see also Inhorn 1994, who provides a fine discussion of

various Egyptian beliefs of procreation associated historically with different medical traditions. The prevailing conviction, however, is that the man through spermatogenesis actually creates the fetus, which is deposited in the woman's womb through intercourse and housed there until birth.

14. See Leach 1961 for an interesting discussion of these phenomena.

15. Carsten 1995.

16. Parkin 1997: 138.

17. Malinowski 1922: 71.

18. Parkin 1997.

19. Schneider 1965, 1972, 1984.

20. Holy 1996: 3.

21. Schneider 1972: 37.

22. Schneider 1965: 95.

23. Not unlike Bourdieu (1977) later.

24. Lévi-Strauss 1969; Radcliffe-Brown 1952.

25. Schneider 1972: 37.

26. Schneider 1984: 193.

27. Schneider 1984, quotation on 79.

28. Veyne 1987: 11, 12.

29. Witherspoon 1975: 15.

30. Ibid., 43.

31. Ibid., 53.

32. See Finch and Mason 1993; M. Turner 1987. I will return to this point in Chapter 7 and the Conclusion.

33. Witherspoon 1975: 12.

34. Weismantel 1995: 695, 697.

35. Trawick 1992: 135.

36. See Gough 1968.

37. Collier and Yanagisako 1987; Delaney 1986; Peletz 1995.

38. Peletz 1995.

39. See Keesing 1975; Evens 1989; Scheffler 1991.

40. Keesing 1975: 13.

41. Scheffler 1991: 372.

42. Carsten 1995: 224, 235.

43. See Hubbard 1995a.

44. Holy 1996: 9.

45. See also Evens, who similarly argues persuasively that the notion of relatedness is the foundation of kinship.

46. Bourdieu 1977.

Chapter 3. Family and Kinship in American Society

1. "American" refers to the dominant culture of the United States, brought by settlers from England and northern Europe.

2. Pomata 1996: 59. I must, however, quote Herlihy (1985: 6), who states that "scholars may argue as to how the early Romans reckoned kinship, but no one doubts that in the Republican and Imperial periods they discerned blood relationships as running through both males and females. The domain of kinship was, in sum, cognatic."

3. Pomata 1996.

4. Ibid., 47, 50, 51.

5. Veyne 1987.

6. Gold 1994.

7. Schwartz 1996: 28; also Delaney 1986.

8. Graburn 1970: 11; see also Maine 1861/1931.

9. Sahlins 1968, 1976a; Fortes 1970.

10. Giddens (1990: 101). He refers to "premodern" societies, while anthropologists have used "primitive" or "simple" to describe stateless societies.

11. M. Strathern 1992a.

12. Durkheim 1964: 239.

13. Duby 1987 notes that a genealogical literature flourished in France in the twelfth century, testifying to the interest that had emerged in extended kinship relations. According to Herlihy (1985: 82), the transformation took place in Europe between the eleventh and twelfth centuries.

14. Stone 1975; Gottlieb 1993; Jordanova 1980; Klapisch-Zuber 1996; Dolgin 1997.

15. Stone 1975.

16. Gottlieb 1993.

17. Ibid., 253.

18. Gottlieb detects an ambivalence between blood and kin by marriage in this definition, an ambiguity that had its roots in the fourteenth century and persisted until the eighteenth century.

19. Gottlieb 1993; see also Jordanova 1980.

20. Goode 1970, 1977; see also Domhoff 1983; Marcus and Hall 1992.

21. Gottlieb 1993: 181.

22. Stone 1997.

23. Gottlieb 1993: 183.

24. Stone 1997.

25. Minow and Shanley 1996, quotation on 6.

26. Mintz and Kellogg 1988.

27. Mintz and Kellogg 1988; Dolgin 1997; Stacey 1990.

28. Mintz and Kellogg 1988.

29. Dolgin 1997.

30. Wallace 1980: 65.

31. Ibid. Historians differ regarding the changes that took place in nineteenth-century America. For example, Mintz and Kellogg (1988: 101) claim that in farm families the commercial revolution and migration westward, far from weakening family ties, actually strengthened family bonds and obligations. Also, people relied on kinship ties for financial assistance during the Depression of the 1930s (138). Others deemphasize the role of the large family unit in colonial life. Demos 1977, for example, claims that among the settlers of North America the nuclear family was always of central importance; by the end of the eighteenth century, the extended family had become even more dispersed and had given way to the individualism we know today. At this time family life was transformed, including a break in the tight web of connection between the family and the larger community, with young people leaving the household (Demos 1977; Stone 1997). Significantly, Demos's view is reflected in Tocqueville's 1840 observation on the American family, a point to which I will return in the Conclusion.

32. Although from a social evolutionary perspective human society may have moved from status to contract, using Maine's terms, or from kinship to state-organized society.

33. Dolgin 1997; Stacey 1990.

34. Gottlieb 1993: 189.

35. Giddens 1991; Sahlins 1976a.

36. Sahlins 1976a.

37. Giddens 1990: 102.

38. Giddens 1992.

39. Schneider 1980: 25. It is noteworthy that according to *Black's Law Dictionary* (Black 1990: 604), family is defined as "A group of blood-relatives; all the relations who descend from a common ancestor, who spring from a common root. All descendants of a common progenitor."

40. Schneider 1980: 53.

41. Thorne 1992. Schneider is less concerned with love between spouses than, for example, are Bellah et al. 1985, but it is interesting that the notion that love and marriage are linked is relatively new, having come into Western society with industrialization. See Cancian 1985; Finkler 1994a; Taylor 1989.

42. Giddens 1992.

43. M. Strathern 1992a: 29.

44. M. Strathern 1992a; also Finch and Mason 1993.

45. Cancian 1985; Dolgin 1997; Minow and Shanley 1996.

46. Dolgin 1997; Stacey 1990.

47. Stacey 1990: 6. See also Dolgin 1997; Popenoe 1993.

48. Stacey 1990: 17.

49. Gottlieb 1993; Stacey 1990; Thorne 1992.

50. Giddens 1992.

51. Mintz and Kellogg 1988; Giddens 1992.

52. Gottlieb 1993: 200. It is important to note, however, that not all scholars agree that family and kinship relations have become diluted in contemporary times. See, e.g., Shorter 1977 and Segalen 1986. Based on European data, Segalen argues against the view that family and kin ties have been greatly weakened by industrialization; in fact, she suggests that they may have become more powerful than before. She does, however, recognize that in traditional societies kinship was the basis of all social relations, whereas in modern society family and kinship are in competition with other social institutions, especially the state (p. 6). Having said that, Segalen nevertheless argues that while family relations may have narrowed, they have not disintegrated or disappeared. Instead, the family today is "powerful, a refuge and the special focus for our feeling" (p. 2). Relationships with the nuclear family and among close kinfolk have become intensified. From Segalen's perspective, the crisis rests with society and not the family. There seems to be a tendency among American scholars to claim that the family is taking on new forms, whereas European scholars such as Segalen and Finch and Mason 1993 regard family and kin relations as continuing to be based on genealogical ties, reflecting a somewhat different pattern in Europe and America. See Hacke's (1997) review of a series of publications on the changing nature of the family in America.

53. Redfield 1941; Giddens 1990; Bellah et al. 1985; Taylor 1989.

54. Bellah et al. 1985: 89.

55. Giddens 1990; Gottlieb 1993; Stacey 1990.

56. Finch and Mason 1993.

57. Witherspoon 1975.

58. Finch and Mason 1993: 170. Significantly, Black (1990: 604) also defines family as "a collection of persons living together under one head, under such

circumstances or conditions that the head is under a legal or *moral* obligation to support the other members, and the other members are dependent upon him or her for support" (emphasis added). Black's assessment supports Finch and Mason's contention of the moral underpinnings of family relations.

59. Finch and Mason 1993: 164–65. On the other hand, Rapp 1992 claims that whereas kinship relations predominate in the working class, in the middle class friendship has superseded kinship relations, seemingly reversing the historical relationships where kinship was emphasized more among the upper class. See also Fischer 1982. Rapp has less to say about the upper class, although it is known that historically, as well as at present, extended kinship relations have prevailed among upper-class families (Domhoff 1983; Marcus and Hall 1992), even at a psychological cost to their members, because family unity militates against individuality. It is difficult to assess whether the different perceptions among scholars concerning the role that family and kin play along class lines are associated with different research venues or with ideological presuppositions. There is a tendency to idealize the working class, including notions that it retains family values, in contrast to the middle class. It is true that the middle class has access to societal institutions that provide economic support that the working class lacks. Under these circumstances, kinship may become an important resource for the working class. See Fischer (1982), who points out that among the middle class "the extended kinship system is genealogically contracted, spatially expanded, functionally specialized, voluntaristic, and largely latent" (pp. 364–65). This pattern is attributed to spatial dispersion and economic mobility. However, based on the data from women with cancer, which I will discuss in Chapters 5 and 6, the variability discussed by Finch and Mason (1993) and others (M. Strathern 1992a) transcends class disparities. It can be said with greater certainty that kinship ties and kinship relations are maintained more by women than by men, not because women have a greater propensity for social interaction but because women are placed in situations that propel them to maintain their kinship relationships. For example, Finch and Mason demonstrate how women are locked into sets of responsibilities with relatives because they are in greater need for assistance with child care and financially. If unemployed, women may also have time to do kinwork (Leonardo 1992) by keeping up contacts with a kin network. The notion that kinship must be "worked at" in modern American life is also suggested by Cherlin and Furstenberg (1994).

60. Marcus and Hall 1992: 167.

61. See Franklin 1993: 128.

62. Strathern 1995.

63. Becker and Nachtigall 1994. It could be argued that the skewed relationship in fertility priorities between economically developed and developing nations reflects political relations that aim at containing population growth in developing nations while enhancing it in nations with advanced economies.

64. Schmidt and Moore 1998.

65. A great variety of in vitro fertilization techniques have been developed, including embryo transfer (when one woman gestates a fetus from another women's fertilized ovum), cryopreservation (when fertilized eggs are frozen for years), and fertilization of eggs from aborted fetuses for gestation in the bodies of women who do not themselves produce ova that can be fertilized (Dolgin 1997: 3). Also, it is now possible to remove a woman's ovum, fertilize it outside her body, and reinsert it into her womb; or remove the ovum, fertilize it outside her body, and implant it into the womb of another woman. There is also zygote interfallo-

pian transfer, where the embryo is placed into the fallopian tube, travels downward, and implants itself in the uterus, thereby mimicking the "natural" process. In gamete interfallopian transfer, an unfertilized ovum is placed in the fallopian tube and semen is injected into the tube so that fertilization takes place in the woman's body (Ragoné 1994: 32–33). These various techniques lead to two types of surrogacies, traditional and gestational. In the former, the woman carries her own biogenetic child; in the latter, the mother does not contribute her own ovum to the formation of the offspring (Ragoné 1994: 73).

66. Franklin 1997b.

67. See Cherlin and Furstenberg, who suggest that with the proliferation of stepparenthood in contemporary America, concepts of blood kinship ties may lose their relevance completely.

68. This is also prescribed by the Old Testament: see Deuteronomy 25: 5–10.

69. Paige and Paige 1981: 171.

70. Parkin 1997.

71. See Evans-Pritchard 1990. Evans-Pritchard reports that once the marriage rites between the two women were completed, the husband sought a male kinsman, friend, or neighbor to beget children by the wife-husband.

72. Parkin 1997.

73. Ibid.

74. Thorne 1992; Shore 1992. But see Schneider (1992: 308), who argues that these technologies do not alter our basic categories of biogenetic kinship; rather, they revise our notions of whom to assign to the traditional categories we know as parents and kin.

75. Hartouni 1997: 69.

76. Dolgin 1997; Ragoné 1994; M. Strathern 1995.

77. Ortner 1974; Jordanova 1980.

78. See also Edwards 1993; Hartouni 1997; Hirsch 1993: 68.

79. Dolgin 1997: 121, 122. Dolgin's analysis of the *Baby M* case reveals the struggle faced by the courts regarding concepts of motherhood that are claimed to be inherent in the mammalian species. See, e.g., Fox (1992: 304), who claims that a woman who has gone through gestational parturition will be "primed" to bond with her child, unlike a man who is easily recognized as the father because the sperm is the carrier of the genetic makeup. He asserts that there is an instinctual drive to parenthood, and that infertile women are desperate to have children because motherhood is a natural drive and infertility is a disease (Fox 1993). See Chapter 8 on the medicalization of infertility.

80. The *Johnson* case is especially interesting in this regard. Following Dolgin 1997, the Calverts contracted with a woman (Ms. Johnson) to produce a baby for them by implanting Johnson's uterus with an embryo produced from the Calverts' gametes. As the result of a dispute between the two parties that could have prevented the Calverts from receiving the contracted baby, the Calverts sued Johnson, seeking a declaration of their parental rights. The California court upheld the Calverts' right to the child on a new basis: that Johnson may have been the gestational carrier, but she was a genetic hereditary stranger to the child. At this time, an earlier ambivalence exhibited by the courts regarding the parentage of a contracted baby was replaced by the court's declaration that the family unit was defined uniquely on the basis of shared genes between the baby and the pair that had contracted it. In her discussion of the Calvert case, Hartouni states that the judge "found the genetic connection alone both made and sustained a family unit and that gestation was merely incidental in this case" (1997: 93). This also

comes into view in discussions with surrogate mothers. Rarely does a day pass by without a report on some matter associated with surrogacy. For example, on March 25, 1998, the National Public Radio program *All Things Considered* interviewed egg donors about their feelings as donors. Significantly, one young woman claimed that her mother was upset because she did not know what had happened to the "baby" who possessed her genetic materials. Another young woman claimed that she knew nothing about the child floating out there that is made up of half of her. Viewed from the perspective of genetic motherhood and the fact that our genes make us the people we are, it is not surprising that these young women regarded their eggs as their children.

81. Dolgin 1997: 129. She adds, "The Calverts, said the court, were 'desperate and longing for their *own genetic product*' " (1997: 130, emphasis in the original).

82. She delivered a baby for an Australian couple, revealing the globalization of surrogacy.

83. MSNBC, 4/21/98: 3, 6. Significantly, there has been a shift from adoption to in vitro fertilization for this very reason, in order that couples may have genetically related children (see Ragoné 1997).

84. Dolgin 1997; also Hartouni 1997.

85. Dolgin 1997.

86. Shore 1992; Parkin 1997.

87. Shore 1992.

88. On March 10, 1998, the California Court of Appeals ruled on the case of a couple (the Buzzancas) who had commissioned a child but had not contributed to its biological makeup. Shortly after the child was commissioned, the couple dissolved their marriage and the Orange County trial judge held that the child had no legal parents. The Court of Appeals reversed this judgment, arguing that, although Mr. Buzzanca refused to accept responsibility for the child, he was the actual father, and that the gestational surrogate was not its genetic mother because the child was formed from unknown gametes. The appeals court finally ruled that Mr. Buzzanca was still responsible for the resulting offspring, reinforcing the contract made with the gestational and social mother (MSNBC 4/21/98: 5).

89. Gottlieb 1993.

90. Finch and Mason 1993, for example.

Chapter 4. Concepts of Heredity in Western Society

1. Gottlieb 1993; Wailoo 1996.

2. Durkheim 1964: 308.

3. Gottlieb 1993: 201.

4. Ibid., 210.

5. Dolgin 1997: 21.

6. Durkheim 1964: 313.

7. Rosenberg 1976.

8. Malinowski (1929/1962) found that the Trobriand Islanders recognized only likeness to their father. They were, in fact, insulted when he pointed out a person's resemblance to the mother or her relatives, despite the fact that the Trobrianders believe that they inherit their substance from the mother (see Chapter 2). For an interesting analysis of this paradox, see Leach 1961. Malinowski's observation in the current context is significant because it stresses the degree to which human perceptions, even of resemblance to oneself, are filtered

through our cultural screen. A similar view — that children resembled only their father — was held in Europe prior to the eighteenth century. See Jacob 1973; Pomata 1996. I have been told in village Mexico that an *unwed* mother's offspring usually resembles only its father.

9. Bowler 1989.

10. Bowler 1989; Pinto-Correia 1997.

11. Jacob 1973: 28.

12. Jacob 1973; Pomata 1996.

13. López-Beltrán 1994: 213.

14. During the early part of the nineteenth century modern medicine took hold in Europe, displacing Galenic and medieval medicine. During this period new theories swept in, including those of Marie François Xavier Bichat, considered by many to be the founder of the new medicine. Using cadavers, Bichat had demonstrated that disease was found not in organs but in tissues (Reiser 1978, Shryock 1979). He advanced the theory that in the absence of investigations of organs and tissues, the study of patients' symptomatologies would fail to yield a coherent understanding of disease. New disease paradigms emanated from Claude Bernard, whose goal was to develop a medicine without the sick and who promoted the mechanistic paradigm that to this day constitutes the scientific foundation of medical education (Reiser 1978). Bernard reduced the entirety of the organism to its constituent parts (Jacob 1973: 127). As described by Reiser and Rosen, the new medicine sought "a single, unchanging cause or set of causes that could be known with certainty. Second, it sought to discover causal relationships by means of decisive experiments in which the observer had no effects on the observed other than those intended in the context of experimental manipulations. Third, it insists on the separation of objective and subjective knowledge and excludes the latter from Science" (1984: 188–89). See also Finkler 1991.

15. López-Beltrán 1994: 233.

16. Ibid., 211.

17. Rosenberg 1976: 34.

18. Ibid., 41.

19. Ibid., 27.

20. Ibid., 30.

21. Jacob 1973. The notion that pregnant women's thoughts and acts in general terms could influence the nature of the embryo goes back to the Greeks and was not new to the nineteenth century (Pinto-Correia 1997).

22. Lubinsky 1993.

23. Rosenberg 1976: 43; Lubinsky 1993.

24. Lubinsky 1993.

25. Haller 1984.

26. Zihlman 1995.

27. The rediscovery of Mendel's work on peas, recognized 50 years after he had performed the initial experiments, complemented Weismann's germ plasm hypothesis. Mendel's theories asserted genetic assortment and stated that hereditary information was passed on in discrete units in accordance with specified mathematical probabilities (Zihlman 1995). Mendelism was not preoccupied with disease: its major concern was with statistical probabilities of the transmission of normal characteristics, including color, shape, and size, and their variations. Mendel's work moved the study of the visible (phenotype) to the invisible (the genotype). With his work, the science of heredity acquired the rigor of mathematics based upon laws of probability.

Especially significant was Weismann's theory of inheritance, introduced between 1892–1902, which destroyed the concept of acquired characteristics. He advanced the notion that the germ cells contain the hereditary substances and that the somatoplasm does not influence the germinal material within its host, so therefore the body cannot alter the germ plasm. Any characteristics the body acquires that are not stored in the germ plasm cannot influence new hereditary units; variation can only occur through changes in the germ plasm. Importantly, too, Weismann declared that male and female parents contribute equally to the heredity of the offspring and that sexual reproduction generates new combinations of hereditary factors. It is noteworthy that Weismann's theory was initially rejected because of its implications for human progress. If acquired traits, even if improved, were not transmissible, then human beings could not be enhanced. Social reforms were therefore useless. The first demonstration that a particular gene had a locus — that it could be assigned to a particular chromosome — was published in 1910, in effect creating the first genetic map, one showing the relative locations of six genes on one chromosome. See Bowler 1989; Gros 1989; Judson 1992. For an excellent and lucid discussion of modern genetics, see Hubbard and Wald 1997.

28. Avery showed in the 1940s that bacteria could be changed from an active to a passive form, predating the discoveries made by Watson and Crick, who developed the model of genetic material including DNA and RNA in 1953, for which they received the Nobel Prize.

29. Gros 1989: 34.

30. Griesemer 1994: 75.

31. It is important to emphasize that in a strict sense "DNA does not replicate itself. Their reproduction or replication happens as part of the metabolism of living cells. Even if we understand in detail how DNA is synthesized and replicated in cells, this information cannot tell us how the replication of genes is translated into the transmission of traits from one generation to the next." Hubbard 1990: 81.

32. Granner 1988: 374.

33. Judson 1992: 48. I must stress that an important distinction exists between genetic diseases attributed to mutations, either induced or occurring at random, and genetic diseases regarded as familial, inherited from a family member. In the popular mind the distinction is often lost. In this book my focus is on genetic diseases attributed to familial inheritance.

34. Granner 1988.

35. Bowler 1989: 179; Hubbard 1995a. In fact, reverse transcriptions pass from RNA to DNA (Hubbard 1995a).

36. Jacob 1973: 1.

37. Ibid., 2, 10.

38. Fox Keller 1994: 89.

39. Fox Keller 1986.

40. Yoxen 1984, 1986.

41. Fox Keller 1992.

42. Fox Keller 1994.

43. Judson 1992.

44. Begleiter et al. 1995; Doria 1995; But see Holden who relates the various disputes among scientists regarding the genetic basis of alcoholism. An extensive study funded by NIH was undertaken to search for a "susceptibility gene" for alcoholism and also for drug abuse, types of psychopathology that "may be genetically related" (1991: 163). Also Cloninger et al. 1996.

45. Cullinan 1989; Gros 1989.

46. Griesemer 1994: 97; see also *Diagnostic and Statistical Manual of Mental Disorders*, 4th ed. (American Psychiatric Association 1994) for the many disorders that are regarded as having a familial hereditary components classified as "predisposing factors." For an incisive discussion of the implications of the notion of "predisposition" see Nelkin 1996a.

47. Milunsky 1992: 94–95.

48. For an excellent example, see Martin 1997.

49. Cranor 1994: 125; Hubbard and Wald 1997.

50. National Human Genome Research Institute 1998. See also the special January 11, 1999 issue of *Time*, which heralds the Future of Medicine as resting in genetics and genetic engineering.

51. Hood 1992: 158. At the time of its inception in 1988, the HGP had a budget of $27.9 million, which progressively increased till its budget in 1998 was $302.6 million. See National Human Genome Research Institute 1998. Collins (1999a) similarly reported on the alliance between the HGP and the pharmaceutical industry.

52. Over 6,000 genes have now been mapped to particular chromosomes; or 12.5 percent of the human genome has been sequenced so far (see National Human Genome Research Institute 1998). It is believed that the sequencing will be completed by 2001 at a cost of $3 billion (Wade 1998).

53. Richards 1993.

54. Wertz 1992.

55. Kevles 1985: ix.

56. Haller 1984: 59.

57. Kevles and Hood 1992a: 7.

58. Marks 1995: 80; Haller 1984. Eugenics was practiced until recently. For example, Buchanan 1997 reports that a Canadian woman was unbeknownst to her sterilized in 1955 because she was assessed as a "mentally defective moron."

59. Stepan 1991.

60. Haller 1984.

61. Hubbard and Wald 1997. The eugenics movement led to the enactment of the Immigration and Restriction Act of 1924 in the United States, which prohibited the entry of people from southern and eastern Europe. Beginning in 1917, laws were passed in two dozen American states favoring sterilization; California was in the vanguard of this zealotry. Eugenics became institutionalized in Germany beginning in 1918, with the establishment of what became the Kaiser Wilhelm Institute for Research in Psychiatry. The institutionalization continued with the creation of a chair for race hygiene in 1923. See Kevles 1985; Ludmerer 1972.

62. Gould 1998.

63. It must, however, not be overlooked that Freudian theories were permeated by biological determinism — for example, Freud regarded the postulated stages of development and the differences between men and women as rooted in biology.

64. Fox Keller 1992.

65. Thom and Jennings 1996.

66. Cited in Kevles 1985: 272.

67. Kevles 1985: 272.

68. Kevles 1985: 274.

69. Kin selection refers to a notion that natural selection was ordered by kinship

groups consisting of some individuals willing to sacrifice themselves for the good of the group. Here the assumption is made that kinship is a genetically determined behavior universal in all human groups. See Sahlins 1976b, who persuasively rebuts the sociobiological notion of kin selection; also Kevles 1985. According to Lieberman et al. (1992), within the academic professions these basic tenets of sociobiology are most widely accepted by biologists, biological anthropologists, and developmental psychologists. As we will see in Chapter 7, the adoptees' narratives suggest that laypeople accept the genetic basis of human behavior.

70. Ridley 1997.
71. Hamer and Copeland 1998.
72. Ibid., 65.
73. Ridley (1997: 252), quoting Marx from a letter Marx wrote to Friedrich Engels in June 1862.
74. Haraway 1991: 65.
75. Foucault 1975.
76. For example, PKU could be largely avoided by control of diet, especially in early childhood (Paul Leslie, personal communication, 1999).

Chapter 5. People with a Genetic History I: Patients Without Symptoms

1. The names are pseudonyms. The women were referred to me by a genetic counselor who forms part of a treatment team consisting of a radiologist, oncologist, surgeon, psychologist, and social worker. The counselor explained to all interviewees that the study would focus on the meaning of experiencing a familial disease. I met the majority of interviewees at their homes and a few at a coffee shop. Aside from asking each patient about her age, education, occupation, and the people she considered closest to her, the interviews were open-ended. The central focus of our discussion revolved around the person's understanding of family and kinship and her relationship to family members from whom presumably she may have inherited the disease or a predisposition to it. Did the woman's knowledge of having inherited a genetic disease or a predisposition influence her family and kin relationships? Other issues were raised during the discussion, including a history of the interviewee's affliction, other members in the family who suffer or had suffered from the disease, to what the individual attributed the disease, and what guided her management of the disease. Each interview, lasting between one and three hours, was tape-recorded with the person's permission and transcribed. For the most part, the observations I present here were offered spontaneously by the women. I identified the recurrent themes presented in these interviews. For further discussion of the methodology, see Finkler 1994a.
2. Rather 1978.
3. The ancient Greek humoral theory of disease attributed most illnesses to an imbalance of the "humors," which consisted of blood, black and yellow bile, and phlegm (Foster and Anderson 1978).
4. Rather 1978.
5. For a full account of the transition, see Finkler 1991, also Chapter 3, n. 14. For a history of views of cancer, see Rather 1978.
6. Fujimura 1996; Kevles and Hood 1992a: 21; Fearon 1997; Weinberg 1996.
7. Weinberg 1996: 62.
8. According to a review in *Science* (1993: 623), 45 percent of breast cancer cases

appeared to be linked to the BRCA-1 gene. But "high cancer rates in families not linked are probably caused by other susceptibility genes or chance." The press has reported on recent studies that have questioned the degree to which the BRCA-1 and BRCA-2 actually raise the risk for breast cancer (Coleman 1998).

9. Cited in McCarthy and Loren 1997: 153.

10. Jim Evans and Cecile Skrzynia, personal communication.

11. Spanier 1995: 107. In a *Science* (1993) article, cancer is attributed to either genetics or chance; but the environment is not mentioned at all.

12. Richards 1993: 573.

13. See Finkler 1991 for the consequences of believing in witchcraft in Mexico.

14. Cousin marriages are widely practiced cross-culturally, and there seems to be no evidence that these types of marriages have adverse health effects in the offspring. See Ottenheimer 1996.

15. Her mother had suffered from familial adenomatous polypsosis, believed to be a genetically caused colon cancer.

16. To establish a genetic profile of a healthy individual, it is necessary to have the genetic makeup of the sick lineal or collateral relatives. Cecile Skrzynia, personal communication.

17. Kaufert 1996.

Chapter 6. People with a Genetic History II: Recovered Patients

1. But see Martin 1987 and Rapp 1992, who argue for class differences in response to biomedicine and its knowledge. On the one hand, it could be argued that, because the women in the study had been exposed to genetic counseling, their views about their disease were influenced by the counselor. In my previous study of doctor patient relationships, I found that patients changed their etiological beliefs after having seen the doctor (Finkler 1991). Nevertheless, three of the women (Tina, Jana, Leah, and Dina) originating from different class strata tend to reject genetic inheritance ideology, suggesting that even in mainstream American society not everyone accepts the hegemony of the gene. On the other hand, none of the adoptees had been exposed to genetic counselors, yet they strongly believe in genetic determinism, as we will see in the next chapter.

2. She referred to books by Bernie Siegel.

3. I never inquired of any of the women or the genetic counselor whether a patient had been tested for the BRCA-1 and BRCA-2 gene, or what the result may have been. Eliza was the only one in the study to volunteer that she had tested positive for the cancer gene. Eliza asked why an adverse result is always termed "positive," a question I had always asked myself.

4. The fact that her disease was genetic was also confirmed for her by the television program *48 Hours,* which she had seen.

5. The epidemiology of breast cancer is the same in the area of the country in which Carol grew up and still resides as in the rest of the country.

6. The state of North Carolina, where Chris lives, passed Senate Bill 254 in August 1997, prohibiting insurance companies and employers from discriminating against people with genetic conditions.

7. Interestingly, injury was a common explanation for breast cancer in the nineteenth century as well as currently, in Mexico, for example (see Preface), and among some people in the United States. See Wardlow and Curry 1996.

8. See Finkler 1994c.

9. Tamoxifen is a hormone-blocking drug that may be given as a follow-up treatment after a woman has had surgery for breast cancer (*Merck Manual* 1997: 1106; see also Begley 1998).

10. The formally recognized risk factors for breast cancer are being female, being older than 65 years of age, having a parent or sibling with breast or ovarian cancer, breast biopsies (even if benign), no children or being over age 30 when the first child was born, menarche before age 12, and atypical hyperplasia on biopsy (Cecile Skrzynia, personal communication). Breast-feeding is included in the popular mind, as we can see in these narratives. It is noteworthy that risk factors for breast cancer include not having children or having them at a later age, which revolve around issues relating to motherhood — as, for example, in the cases of Lydia, Tina, and Betty. In one way, contemporary medicine is not unlike its nineteenth-century predecessor, when women's behavior was believed to influence the outcome of a pregnancy and the health of the child. In this case, women's avoidance of motherhood also suggests dire repercussions, such as breast cancer. See also Chapter 4.

11. Lucie's mother participated in an experimental group where she received extra chemotherapy rather than bone marrow transplants. As it turned out, according to Lucie, "most of the people in her study that had bone marrow didn't make it." Lucie's mother had one month less of life than the five years she was promised by the program.

12. Lucie frequently referred to this point. It is a not uncommon popular belief, although an incorrect one, that the father's side of the family has little influence on the development of breast cancer. In fact, one healthy woman mentioned, like Lucie, that her physician too informed her that because breast cancer was only in her father's family, she didn't need to be concerned.

13. Neotrophils are a type of white blood cell.

14. The current thinking is that prophylactic mastectomies reduce the risk of developing cancer by 90 percent, based on 1,000 women followed for an average of 17 years by the Mayo Clinic (personal communication, Cecile Skrzynia). In a more recent study published in the *New England Journal of Medicine*, it was reported that the procedure is highly effective in reducing the risk of breast cancer, by about 90 percent (Hartman et al. 1999). These findings were immediately reported in the popular press.

15. This refers to a transverse rectus abdominus muscle flap. Tissue from the lower abdomen is moved up to the place where the breast was and is attached to and supplied with blood by the muscle. A new breast is made from this tissue.

Chapter 7. People Without a Medical History: Adoptees

1. Bartholet 1993.

2. Veyne 1987: 17.

3. Minow and Shanley 1996: 8.

4. Dolgin 1997: 39.

5. I interviewed each of the 15 adoptees individually, most in their homes, a few in a restaurant, and four by telephone. Each of the interviews lasted between one and three hours.

6. Importantly, one of the group's major functions is to promote open-record adoption by changing the current laws to permit each adoptee to have access to the name and medical history of his or her birth mother.

7. See Andersen 1993; Bartholet 1993; Modell 1994. There is also an extensive network on the World Wide Web about adoption and how to help people search. See ⟨www.highfiber.com/leninger/internet.html⟩, which encourages searches in order that the person learn "where you came from, who you look like, where you got a special talent or strange oddity in your personality. Your medical information, though maybe not important to you now, will be in the future when you have children" (1997: 1). Also ⟨www.ibar.com//TIES/mission.html⟩.

8. For ethical reasons, I had not attempted to recruit adoptees who had *not* searched for their birth parents. I believe that to have broached the subject with an individual who had not searched would suggest to them that perhaps they ought to do so.

9. Andersen 1993: 105. To understand adoptees' psyches and actions, Andersen's book is considered by some as the "bible."

10. Because Andersen was what is known as a "black market baby," infants presumably offered for adoption by prostitutes, there were no official records of his birth (quotations 106 and 138).

11. Bartholet 1993: 166, 167, 172.

12. Ibid., 227–28. Dolgin (1997) in fact reports that donor-inseminated offspring seek their genetic fathers.

13. Bartholet 1993: 113.

14. Lynn Giddens (Coordinator of the Center for Advancement of Adoption Education of North Carolina), personal communication. In the United States, 2.5 percent of the population is adopted; of these, about 300,000 are said to be searching for their birth parents (⟨www.highfiber.com/leninger/internet.html⟩ 1997).

15. As we saw in Chapter 2, even Schneider asserts that in societies where biogenetic relations are not recognized, there is still a strong bond between mother and child.

16. Bartholet 1993; Belkin 1999; Modell 1994.

17. In addition to eliciting basic demographic data from each participant, including age, birth date, marital status, and number of children, the interviews were open-ended. I posed only one question to each of the adoptees: why they searched for their birth mother and father. If they had not searched for the birth father, I asked why. The interviews were recorded with each person's permission and transcribed.

18. The consensus is that the ratio of women to men seeking their birth parents is 9:1 (Lynn Giddens, personal communication). The reasons for the disparity along gender lines are not clear. According to Giddens, the gender disparity is due to the fact that "women are more sensitive to birth and pregnancy issues than men" and to "men's lesser abilities to connect to the birth process."

19. The underlying cause of Raynaud's disease is not known. It is a condition in which arterioles, usually in the fingers and toes, go into spasm, causing the skin to become discolored. It is often triggered by cold. Between 60 and 90 percent of Raynaud's disease cases occur in young women (*Merck Manual* 1997: 136).

20. According to Giddens (personal communication), if a patient, such as an adoptee, lacks a medical history, the doctor will often refuse to order various procedures because insurance companies claim a lack of back-up documentation to justify carrying out a series of tests.

21. It is especially common for women to be told that their pains are "in their head" if the symptoms cannot be assessed biomedically. See Finkler 1994a.

22. Risa noted that she could have petitioned the court to open her records on medical grounds. Under current state law, adoption records can be opened to

obtain the biological mother's family medical history, which suggests that the state recognizes the role of genetics in disease causation.

23. As will be seen in Chapter 9, a schizophrenia gene was presumably identified some years past, but subsequently this finding was retracted. This is a good example of how biomedical ideas enter the popular consciousness and are retained long after scientific retractions.

24. Hamer and Copeland 1998; Ridley 1997. Rice et al. (1999) have found that there was no evidence for a gene for homosexuality.

25. The two young women spoke Black English, whereas Liz's speech was distinctly standard midwestern dialect.

26. The notion that shared blood rather than reproduction defines kinship can be seen in the various surrogacy court decisions. See Dolgin's (1997) brilliant analysis.

27. Adoptees' amended birth certificates may lack certain specific information. According to Mira, unlike hers, her husband's birth certificate showed his mother's and father's names, their occupations, at what hospital he was born, the time of birth, who the attending physician was, and "all that stuff that my daughters', both my daughters' birth certificates, have on them. Mine has my adoptive parents' name, my adoptive name, and that's it. It has no weight, no time, no hospital, none of that stuff. It's totally different." Moreover, her certificate was printed on a different kind of paper.

28. Ronold did not know how the physician obtained his birth parents' medical histories.

Chapter 8. The Ideology of Genetic Inheritance in Contemporary Life: The Medicalization of Kinship

1. Hansen 1992; MacDonald 1992.

2. Broom and Woodward 1996: 358; Foucault 1975; Freidson 1970; see also Tomes 1990. Illich named a chapter in his book *Medical Nemesis* (1975) "The Medicalization of Life."

3. Halpern 1985; Mayall 1990; Estes 1988.

4. Diseases classified as mental disorders. Englehardt 1986: 191.

5. Rosenfield and Erchak 1988; Gabe and Lipshitz-Phillips 1984. On March 8, 1997 a prestigious research university in the South advertised the following: "Are you bothered by excessive shyness, timidity, fear of embarrassment, or speaking in front of people? Then you may be eligible for free treatment in a research study of a new medication and behavioral psychotherapy."

6. Bauman 1992: 149–50.

7. Tiefer 1994; *Merck Manual* 1997.

8. Ginsburg and Rapp 1991; Gurevich 1995; Johnson 1987; Kohler Riessman 1983; Martin 1987; Markens 1994, 1996; Ritenbaugh 1982. But see Bransen 1992, who argues that not all women have accepted the medicalization of their bodies. See also Martin 1987.

9. Bell 1987; Davis-Floyd 1992; Gonyea 1996; Jordan 1993; Lock 1993; Kaufert and Gilbert 1986; Klein and Dumble 1994; Worcester and Whatley 1992.

10. Sullivan 1993; Ritenbaugh 1982, Rodin et al. 1985.

11. Neustadter 1992.

12. Witzig 1996; Carey et al. 1991. But see also Wailoo 1996.

13. Englehardt 1986: 157.

14. Hansen 1992. The genetics of homosexuality is being currently debated and noted in Chapter 7 in Roberta's case.

15. Englehardt 1986: 190.

16. Finkler 1991, 1994b.

17. For a fuller discussion of anger as a moral emotion, see Finkler 1994b.

18. Griesemer 1994: 70; Lloyd 1994: 104.

19. This is not to say that Down's syndrome is uniformly regarded as normal in Mexico, since there is great variation along class lines concerning what is regarded normal and abnormal there. This is a special case of how medicalization molds reality.

20. An autosomal dominant disorder that usually affects a person's eye muscles around the age of 30 or later. The condition is marked by a drooping of the eyelids (ptosis), which affects the movement of the eyes and may result in double vision (*Merck Manual* 1997).

21. A condition characterized by multiple "cafe au lait spots," which are freckles within skin folds. In its benign form, other symptoms may include small bumps in the iris of the eye, which do not affect vision; and at its worst, it may cause skeletal deformities such as bowing of the lower legs or deformity of the bones around the eyes. In most cases it causes cosmetic problems; in its extreme form it produces disfigurement such as that of the "Elephant Man" (National Neurofibromatosis Foundation 1997).

22. But see Appleton 1995, who argues that alcoholism was medicalized not by biomedicine but by Alcoholics Anonymous. Which institution first medicalized alcoholism is less relevant to my present discussion than the fact that at present American culture is prone to regard any "deviant" condition in medical terms, and alcoholism as a disease. Arguably, in the fifteenth century alcoholism would not have been considered a medical problem by anyone, whether physicians or the population at large.

23. Broom and Woodward 1996, also Englehardt 1986. And see the case of Margarita in Finkler 1994a, an especially good example of how a medical diagnosis can bring coherence to a chaotic experience.

24. Bunkle 1993; Browner 1989; Doyal 1979, 1995; Finkler 1994a; Marieskind 1980; Yanoshik and Norsigian 1989.

25. Jordan 1993; see also Davis-Floyd 1996.

26. Foucault 1975; Szasz 1963.

27. Finkler 1991.

28. For example, in Mexico, while physicians may regard alcoholism as a disease, lay Mexicans usually refer to it as a vice (*un vicio*), signifying a moral transgression. Similarly, in the three cases I presented, the women did not accept their condition as diseases, even though they submitted to medical treatment. Significantly, in these cases the general practitioners who treated them for other conditions referred them to the genetics clinic, which encouraged them to be treated for these conditions.

29. Freidson 1970; Williams and Calnan 1996. Regarding alternative treatments, in the early 1990s approximately 33 percent of the U.S. population sought alternative therapy (Eisenberg et al. 1993). Significantly, and to the surprise of these same investigators, who reported in the *Journal of the American Medical Association* in 1998, the use of alternative therapies increased to 42.1 percent in 1997. See Eisenberg et al. 1998 as well as the entire November 11, 1998, issue of the *Journal of the American Medical Association*.

30. Kohler Riessman 1983; Shore 1992. On biomedicine and infertility, see Becker and Nachtigall 1992, 1994; Raymond 1993.

31. According to Raymond, there are 200 institutions in America that perform in vitro fertilization treatments (1993: 8). On a March 30, 1998, broadcast of the *McNeil-Lehrer NewsHour,* a discussion of disability suggested that women with AIDS and infertile women were equally disabled. Commentators on the program also made the point that toxic genes may eventually be counted as a disability.

32. Raymond 1993.

33. Scritchfield 1995.

34. Franklin 1997b: 138.

35. Raymond 1993: 38, 31; see also Davis-Floyd 1996.

36. Raymond 1993: 111.

37. Franklin 1997b: 210.

38. Bradish 1987; Duster 1990.

39. Hirsch 1993; Spallone and Steinberg 1987.

40. Hirsch 1993; Mead 1999; Shore 1992.

41. Raymond 1993.

42. Except, arguably, among elites in America. See Bellah et al. 1985; Domhoff 1983; Marcus and Hall 1992.

43. Finkler 1994a.

44. Giddens 1992: 104, 106–7.

45. *Science* (1993) describes how the BRCA-1 gene for breast cancer was discovered through blood samples and family histories taken from numerous extended families.

46. Bobinski 1996: 80. The reasoning is circular. If it is in the family it must be genetic; if it is genetic it must be in the family.

47. McAuliffe 1978, 1979.

48. The doctor-patient encounter is an especially powerful means by which professional ideologies are instilled in individuals' consciousness, cutting across class, race, and gender lines. Finkler 1991; Waitzkin 1991.

49. Jonsen 1996: 8–9. See also Hubbard and Wald 1997, who speak of the "healthy ill."

50. Nelkin 1992: 188.

51. But see Kaufert 1996.

52. Jonsen 1996: 10.

53. Serban 1989.

54. Green, Murton, and Strathern 1993.

55. Wexler 1979: 207. Huntington's disease is caused by a single dominant gene, and the odds are 50 percent that an individual will inherit the disease, which symptomatically becomes manifest at around age 35 or 40.

56. Lynch, Lynch, and Lynch 1979: 223.

57. This is not to say that people experiencing other genetically inherited diseases may not experience anger at the family because of their inheritance. The nature of the disease or the age of its onset may be a factor influencing people's response. In this sample of women with breast cancer, who have already had children, this was not the case.

58. Bellah et al. 1985; Taylor 1989; Tocqueville 1980.

59. Bellah et al. 1985; Giddens 1992.

60. For example, in Mexico, through the family, based on biogenetic ties, is the basic unit of existence, during doctor-patient encounters relatives were usually

not admitted, because the biomedical model of the doctor-patient encounter is based on the individual patient-doctor pair (Finkler 1991).

61. Jonsen 1996; Wexler 1992.

62. Wexler 1992: 228.

63. Important, the biomedical practice of organ transplantation also promotes kinship ties among persons who may have been alienated. In fact, the adoptees, including Ronold and Liz, noted their desire to find their blood kin if they will need a transplant in future. Organ transplant in the context of kinship requires study.

64. See Chapter 2. See also Witherspoon 1975; Finch and Mason 1993.

65. Minow and Shanley 1996: 7.

66. For a good example of this phenomenon see Chapter 9, n. 57.

Chapter 9. A Multidimensional Critique of Genetic Determinism

1. Collins 1999a.

2. Siebert 1995: 54. There are now computerized directories for use by doctors, which list 212 laboratories that can supposedly identify 275 genetic disorders. See, e.g., Flynn et al. 1996. The authors, however, observe that "Genomics has not led to a single blockbuster drug so far" (81).

3. Including fetuses. For example, on September 29, 1998, National Public Radio's *All Things Considered* reported on a new procedure called "pre-implantation genetic diagnosis," which permits doctors to detect genetic diseases before pregnancy even begins. Such tests have been used for Tay-Sachs, sickle cell anemia, and cystic fibrosis, and this test will become available for more common conditions like cancer and heart disease (National Public Radio 1998a).

4. Nelkin 1996a: 188.

5. In orthodox Jewish communities in the United States and Israel, where marriages are arranged, every potential marriage partner undergoes a test for Tay-Sachs and cystic fibrosis anonymously. If one of the potentially matched pair carries the gene for these diseases, the two people will never be introduced to each other. Yet, with the exception of Tay-Sachs, and possibly cystic fibrosis, most tests vary in accuracy, with false positives and false negatives.

6. For example, sexual selection is practiced in some countries, e.g., India.

7. Fox Keller 1992: 289, 1994; Duster 1990; Nelkin 1992: 180.

8. Allen 1996; Paul 1994; Weiner 1994.

9. Ponder 1997.

10. But see Berner 1996, who notes that using genetic information to exclude an individual in a group health plan from coverage is now prohibited. Nor may the person be charged more. See also Chap. 6, n. 6. Kolata 1997 reports that in one case a woman requested a prophylactic double mastectomy but failed to tell the insurer that she had been tested for a breast cancer gene. The insurer refused to pay on the grounds that they did not pay for preventive operations. When she reapplied and notified them that she had been tested, the company refused a second time on the grounds that having the gene was a preexisting condition.

11. Pinn and Jackson (1996: 553) strongly recommend that women be educated "about the specific scientific limitations of genetic testing for breast and ovarian cancer." For an incisive analysis of the perils of genetic testing see also Nelkin 1996b.

12. Lloyd 1994: 102.

13. Jonsen 1996: 18, 11–12.

14. Wexler 1992: 241, 242.

15. Lewontin 1992: 69. See also Hubbard 1990 and Chapter 4, n. 32.

16. Hamer and Copeland 1998: 301. They note that even if the project were officially stopped, most advanced research has been taken over by biotechnology start-up companies and by the giant pharmaceutical firms that usually end up owning them.

17. "We share virtually all our genes with apes. However, on average, a single related set of ape and human genes would differ in DNA sequence by about 10 percent. For a mouse, it is more like 20 to 30 percent." National Human Genome Research Institute 1998: 7.

18. Hubbard and Wald 1997; Billings, Beckwith, and Alper 1992.

19. Winkler and Anderson 1990.

20. Fox Keller 1994: 96.

21. Hubbard and Wald 1997.

22. Livingston 1958.

23. Ethnicity and race are highly problematic cultural categories; however, in the epidemiological literature they loom large as explanatory of disease etiologies. See Witzig 1996.

24. Perera 1997.

25. Jacob 1973; Perera 1997.

26. Fearon 1997.

27. Hubbard and Wald 1997.

28. Davis et al. 1997: 115.

29. Lloyd 1994: 109.

30. Hubbard and Wald 1997: 76; Lloyd 1994: 109; Spanier 1995.

31. Hubbard and Wald 1997.

32. Krieger and Fee 1994: 15.

33. Hubbard and Wald 1997: 27.

34. Lewontin 1992: 51.

35. Hubbard 1995b. Hubbard and Wald 1997.

36. Griesemer 1994; Hubbard and Wald 1997.

37. Hubbard 1995b: 45, 46. Not surprisingly, Hubbard and Wald (1997) believe that the HGP project is a waste of money.

38. Hubbard and Wald 1997: 101.

39. Griesemer 1994: 83. See also Alper 1998.

40. Lewontin, Rose, and Kamin 1984; Lewontin 1992.

41. McKeown 1985.

42. Lewontin 1992: 30, 47.

43. Spanier 1995; McKeown 1985.

44. In a recent etiological study of Parkinson's disease, Tanner et al. (1999) conducted an extensive twin study, the results of which led them to reject the genetic hypothesis. These researches showed that Parkinson's, contrary to the prevailing genetic theories, has an environmental etiology, particularly when its onset is after the age of 50. The authors conclude that the next challenge is to identify the nongenetic risk factors for Parkinson's disease.

45. Nelkin 1996a: 139.

46. Jacob 1973: 224; Lewontin, Rose, and Kamin 1984.

47. Jim Evans and Cecile Skrzynia, personal communication; Spanier 1995.

48. Fox Keller 1992; Lewontin 1992; Spanier 1995; Wingerson 1990.

49. Gould 1996: 361, 32.

50. The discovery of a gene for Huntington's disease "does not imply the existence of a gene for high intelligence, or low aggressivity, or high propensity for xenophobia, or special attraction to faces, bodies, or legs of a sexual partner — or for any other general feature that might be distributed as a bell curve in the full population. We commit a classic category mistake if we equate the causes of normal variation with the reasons for pathologies." Ibid., 33.

51. Gould 1996 writes this as a father of an autistic child.

52. Cullinan 1989: 79.

53. Forstenzer and Roye 1989: 170, 171.

54. Wexler 1992: 232.

55. Elsewhere (Finkler 1991, 1994a) I introduced and developed the concept of *life's lesions,* which suggests that human afflictions embody a person's biographical adversities, including experience of moral contradictions, that life's lesions become inscribed on the body and expressed symptomatologically. Life's lesions can be as virulent as any virus or pathogen. My reference point, however, is disorders that are not life threatening rather than such grave diseases as breast cancer.

56. Fox Keller 1986.

57. Cassell 1991; Kleinman 1998; Kleinman and Kleinman 1991. A persuasive example too is a 1991 article in *Health* by Carey et al., who report that, while it is accepted that economic hardship, racial discrimination, and salty and high fat diets are used to explain the fact that African Americans are twice as likely as whites to suffer from high blood pressure, a California doctor found evidence that the increased risk for some is in their genes.

58. Pinto-Correia 1997. The theory of preformation, accepted for over a hundred years from its inception, proposed that all living beings were preformed inside their progenitors, replicating themselves from generation to generation.

59. The idea that genetic determinism is parallel to the theological concept of being born with original sin obviously requires further development; and is outside the scope of this book. I note it here only for the reader's consideration. The Catholic notion that life begins at conception because of genetics lays down the blueprint for an individual. See Shore 1992.

Conclusion

1. See Thomson 1994 for how widespread the dilemma is.

2. Lewontin 1992: 31–32.

3. Lloyd 1994.

4. Hood 1992.

5. Glaring examples of the primacy of genetics over culture abound, including the founding of sperm banks that use semen from "geniuses" and college-educated men, preferably medical students. Moreover, as we saw in Chapter 7, there is a recent trend to open sealed adoption records. The issue of sealed adoptions is highly contested. Not surprisingly, it was only in the 1970s that a movement arose "rallying around the sealed records bandwagon" (Babb 1996; also Grimm 1999). In 1978, the American Adoption Congress was formed as a nonprofit umbrella organization "to bring together the multitude of search and support groups" (Grimm 1999) concerning open records and related issues, coinciding with the explosion in genetic research.

Significantly, in present day American society there is a trend away from adoption toward the new reproductive technologies because the parents are assured of a genetic link to the offspring (Belkin 1997). In fact, Stolberg 1997 reports that for in vitro fertilization one of the most common techniques is to use egg donors, but that means that the woman will not have a genetic connection to her offspring. By doing so, "couples in their baby-making fervor are not thinking through the moral implications of having children whose genetic roots are different from their own" (p. 24). According to this view genetics is equivalent to morality and a person's moral roots are lodged in the gene.

6. Hubbard and Wald 1997.

7. A guest reported on a *Science Friday* program (National Public Radio 1998b) that in the near future human beings will be implanted with a chip that will carry every aspect of their identity, including a description of their personalities and potential diseases.

8. The move toward cosmetic surgery may eventually lure the person into becoming a patient, nevertheless.

9. In the nineteenth century, certain diseases were considered prestigious—for example, tuberculosis, which served as a metaphor for an artistic personality (see Sontag 1978). Hemophilia may have been a mark of nobility, and obesity, before it became medicalized, was a mark of wealth. Sickle cell anemia is a mark traditionally associated with African American descent. See Wailoo 1996.

10. See also Yoxen 1986.

11. See especially Allen 1996, who cogently likens the current trends in genetics to those in Germany in the 1930s.

12. Bowler 1989: 169–70. And see Griesemer's (1994) analogy between the HGP and the discovery of the New World. Bowler (1989) observes that the genetic concepts of the nineteenth century flourished within a context of laissez faire economics. Fox Keller 1992, Lewontin 1992, and Allen 1996 all similarly attribute the emphasis on genetics in contemporary society to laissez faire economics and to current economic disparities.

13. Yoxen 1984.

14. Fox Keller 1994.

15. Lewontin 1992: 53, 72. See also Rifkin (1998) for a penetrating discussion of the numerous political and economic consequences of the biotechnology industry.

16. One could carry Lewontin's economic argument a step farther. For example, the ideology of genetic inheritance could be viewed as an onslaught on the institution of the family, which has been maligned for its toxicity, if we assume that in advanced capitalist society the family has outlived its usefulness as a socializing unit, remaining as a labor producing unit.

17. For example, when it is proclaimed that the propensity to smoke or drink is rooted in a genetic predisposition, the tobacco companies or distillers are absolved from any responsibility. Hubbard and Wald 1997; Nelkin and Lindee 1995.

18. Significantly, in my study of biomedical practice in Mexico (Finkler 1991), most of the physicians in the sample, if they lacked a justification for a diagnosis, would attribute the disease to stress. Stress, like heredity, has become a reductionist category to explain any kind of sickness for which physicians lack a clear etiology, ignoring, in the Mexican case, the miserable poverty in which the patients existed.

19. Rosenberg 1976.

20. Rothman 1994 (tuberculosis), Macale 1995 (hysteria), Hubbard and Wald 1997 (pellagra).

21. For a discussion of causality see Griesemer 1994 and Cranor 1994, who analyze the distinction between proximate and ultimate causalities in medicine.

22. Gorovitz and MacIntyre 1976; Pellegrino and Thomasma 1981.

23. For instance, a woman in my study of Mexican physicians asked the attending doctor why she, but not her neighbor, suffered from an ovarian disorder, when both of them had given birth to an equal number of children and lived under the same conditions of poverty and environmental degradation. The physician remained speechless. Finkler 1991.

24. Bauman 1992: 153.

25. Schneider 1984: 193.

26. For references on this topic see Chapter 1 n. 61, also Martin 1987, 1997.

27. Schneider 1980: 53. See Chapter 3 for exact quote.

28. Tocqueville 1980: 507.

29. There is no one overarching explanation for the decline of family and kin in modern society, although undoubtedly socioeconomic and political processes contributed most to the mobility of the family. See Chapter 2.

30. Bauman 1992: 42. See also Finkler 1994a.

31. Finch and Mason 1993; Witherspoon 1975; Freeman 1968.

32. McCarthy and Loren 1997, Chapter 10.

33. Bauman 1992: 198.

34. Witness the recent unearthing of the "Unknown Soldier." Nothing presumably remains unknown (Myers 1998).

35. Tocqueville 1980: 507.

36. Harvey 1989.

37. See also M. Strathern 1992b on this point.

38. Finkler 1991, 1994a.

39. The individual is usually held responsible for various diseases, for example, diabetes linked with obesity, obesity itself, and general ill health, is associated with bad habits: smoking, drinking, and overeating (McKeown 1985), even though these conditions are also regarded as genetic or having a genetic predisposition. See Hood 1992. The assumption is that when people are guided by knowledge of risk factors and live a morally proper lifestyle (meaning avoidance of risk factors), they will remain healthy, but in the final analysis the risk-averse lifestyle fails to protect the person from affliction.

40. Rothman (1986) discusses the "illusion of choice."

41. There is another difference between past eugenic conceptualizations and contemporary notions about genetic engineering: we can choose to be genetically engineered through genetic testing; in this manner we can exercise our freedom, unlike during the reign of eugenics, when it was illegal for certain groups to breed or to interbreed. But there is yet another important distinction between classical eugenics and current conceptualizations, as seen through the HGP. No matter how critical one may be of eugenics and its evils, Galton and the eugenicists of his time did regard human beings as social beings desirous of improving society, whereas contemporary genetics reduces the human being to a biochemical, atomistic creature, reflecting our extreme emphasis on biologism and individualism. See also Fox Keller 1992: 295.

42. See Chapter 3, n. 80, and the *Johnson v. Calvert* case in Dolgin 1997.

43. Conrad 1997; Nelkin and Lindee 1995.

44. Cranor 1994 (entire volume); Hubbard and Wald 1997; Fox Keller 1992; Lewontin, Rose, and Kamin 1984; Lewontin 1992; Nelkin and Lindee 1995.

45. See Cherlin and Furstenberg 1994, who discuss the recent prevalence of stepfamilies in the United States, among whom kinship bonds are highly fragile.

46. Finkler 1991, 1994a.

47. Finkler 1999.

48. In Mexico, for example, belief in heredity forms part of the folk attributions for some diseases, including some cancers (Finkler 1991). However, as I noted in the Preface, all the women I interviewed who had suffered from breast cancer believed it was caused by a blow.

49. Dumars and Chea 1989: 164–65.

50. Richter 1972.

51. Kuhn 1970.

References

Adato, Allison
1995   "Living in Legacy." *Life* 18(4): 60.
Allen, Garland
1996   "Science Misapplied: Eugenics Age Revisited." *Technological Review* (August/September): 23–31.
Alper, Joseph
1998.   "Genes, Free Will, and Criminal Responsibility." *Social Science and Medicine* 46: 1599–1611.
Alter, Jonathan
1998   "Clinton on the Couch." *Newsweek,* February 2: 31.
American Psychiatric Association
1994   *Diagnostic and Statistical Manual of Mental Disorders,* 4th ed. (DSMV IV) Washington, D.C.: American Psychiatric Association. 13: 24.
Andersen, Robert
1993   *Second Choice: Growing Up Adopted.* Chesterfield, Mo.: Badger Hill Press.
Angell, Marcia
1997   "Overdosing on Health Risks." *New York Times Magazine,* May 4: 44.
Appleton, Lynn M.
1995   "Rethinking Medicalization: Alcoholism and Anomalies." In *Images of Issues: Typifying Contemporary Social Problems,* ed. Joel Best. New York: Aldine de Gruyter. Pp. 59–80.
Associated Press
1996   "Genealogy Passion Results in Founding of a Vidalia Library." *Chattanooga Times,* December 12: F6.
Babb, Anne
1996   "Adoptees in Search in the United States." *The Decree* (publication of the American Adoption Congress; no page numbers).
Bartholet, Elizabeth
1993   *Family Bonds: Adoption and the Politics of Parenting.* Boston: Houghton Mifflin.
Bauman, Zygmunt
1992   *Mortality, Immortality, and Other Life Strategies.* Stanford, Calif.: Stanford University Press.

Becker, Gay and Robert Nachtigall
  1992   "Eager for Medicalization: The Social Production of Infertility as Disease." *Sociology of Health and Illness* 14: 456–71.
  1994   " 'Born to Be a Mother': The Cultural Construction of Risk in Infertility Treatment in the U.S." *Social Science and Medicine* 39: 507–18.
Begleiter, Henri, Theodore Reich, Victor Hesselbrock, Bernice Poriesz, Ting-Kai Li, Mark A. Schuckit, Howard J. Edenberg, and John P. Rice
  1995   "The Collaborative Study on the Genetics of Alcoholism: The Genetics of Alcoholism." *Alcohol Health and Research World* 19(3): 228.
Begley, Sharon
  1996   "Holes in Those Genes: Not Even DNA Can Live Up to All the Hyped Claims." *Newsweek,* January 15: 57.
  1997   "Infidelity and the Science of Cheating." *Newsweek,* December 30/January 6: 57–59.
  1998   "New Hope for Women at Risk." *Newsweek,* April 20: 68.
Belkin, Lisa
  1997   "Pregnant with Complications." *New York Times Magazine,* October 26: 34.
  1999   "What the Jumans Didn't Know About Michael." *New York Times Magazine,* March 14: 42–49.
Bell, Susan
  1987   "Changing Ideas: The Medicalization of Menopause." *Social Science and Medicine* 24: 535–42.
Bellah, Robert N., Richard Madsen, William M. Sullivan, Ann Swidler, and Steven M. Tipton
  1985   *Habits of the Heart: Individualism and Commitment in American Life.* Berkeley: University of California Press.
Berliner, Howard
  1975   "A Larger Perspective on the Flexner Report." *International Journal of Health Services* 5: 573–91.
Berner, Lynn Sargent
  1996   "As Genetics Soars, Congress Stalls." *Journal of Women's Health* 5: 291–93.
Bernstein, Peter L.
  1996   *Against the Gods: The Remarkable Story of Risk.* New York: John Wiley.
Billings, Paul R., Jonathan Beckwith, and Joseph S. Alper
  1992   "The Genetic Analysis of Human Behavior: A New Era." *Social Science and Medicine* 35: 227–38.
Black, Henry Campbell
  1990   *Black's Law Dictionary.* 6th ed. St. Paul, Minn.: West Publishing Co.
Blakeslee, Sandra
  1997   "Accounting for Taste." *New York Times,* February 23.
Bluman, Leslie
  1998   "Duke, UNC Study Increased Cancer Risk Among Ashkenazi Jewish Women." *Menorah* (January–February): 14.
Bobinski, Mary Anne
  1996   "Genetics and Reproductive Decision Making." In *The Human Genome Project and the Future of Health Care,* ed. Thomas H. Murray, Mark A. Rothstein, and Robert F. Murray, Jr. Bloomington: Indiana University Press, Pp. 79–112.

Bodmer, Walter F. and Robin McKie
 1994   *The Book of Man: The Human Genome Project and the Quest to Discover Our Genetic Heritage*. New York: Scribner.
Bounds, Wendy
 1996   "One Family's Search for a Faulty Gene." *Wall Street Journal*, August 15: B1.
Bourdieu, Pierre
 1977   *Outline of a Theory of Practice*. Trans. Richard Nice. Cambridge: Cambridge University Press.
Bourguignon, Erika
 1996   "Vienna and Memory: Anthropology and Experience." *Ethos* 24: 374–87.
Bowler, Peter J.
 1989   *The Mendelian Revolution: The Emergence of Hereditarian Concepts in Modern Science and Society*. Baltimore: Johns Hopkins University Press.
Boyarin, Jonathan
 1994   "Space, Time, and the Politics of Memory." In *Remapping Memory: The Politics of Timespace*, ed. Boyarin. Minneapolis: University of Minnesota Press.
Bradish, Paul
 1987   "From Genetic Counseling and Genetic Analysis to Genetic Ideal and Genetic Fate?" In *Made to Order: The Myth of Reproductive and Genetic Progress*, ed. Patricia Spallone and Deborah Lynn Steinberg. Oxford: Pergamon Press. Pp. 94–101.
Brandt, Allan M.
 1997   "Behavior, Disease, and Health in the Twentieth-Century United States: The Moral Valence of Individual Risk." In *Morality and Health: Interdisciplinary Perspectives*, ed. Allan M. Brandt and Paul Rozin. New York: Routledge. Pp. 53–79.
Bransen, Els
 1992   "Has Menstruation Been Medicalized? Or Will It Never Happen?" *Sociology of Health and Illness* 14: 98–110.
Brooke, Jill and John Metaxas
 1997   "How to Track Down Clues About Family Histories." *CNN Your Money*, transcript 97021505V33, February 15.
Broom, Dorothy H. and Roslyn V. Woodward
 1996   "Medicalization Reconsidered: Toward a Collaborative Approach to Care." *Journal of Health and Illness* 18: 357–78.
Browner, Carole H.
 1989   "Women, Household, and Health in Latin America." *Social Science and Medicine* 28: 461–73.
Brownlee, Shannon
 1994   "Hunting a Killer Gene." *U.S. News and World Report* 117 (8), September 26: 76.
Brownlee, Shannon, Gareth G. Cook, and Viva Hardigg
 1994   "Tinkering with Destiny." *U.S. News and World Report* 117 (8), September 26: 58.
Brownlee, Shannon and Joanne Silberner
 1991   "The Age of Genes." *U.S. News and World Report* 111 (19): 64.
Buchanan, Emily
 1997   "Playing God with People's Lives." *Guardian Weekly*, March 23: 30.

Bunkle, Phillida
  1993 "Calling the Shots? The International Politics of Depo-Provera." In *The "Racial" Economy of Science: Toward a Democratic Future,* ed. Sandra Harding. Bloomington: Indiana University Press. Pp. 287–302.
Cancian, Francesca M.
  1985 "Gender Politics: Love and Power in the Private and Public Spheres." In *Gender and the Life Course,* ed. Alice S. Rossi. New York: Aldine. Pp. 253–64.
Carey, Benedict, Mary Hossfeld, and Laura Fraser
  1991 "Inherited Pressure: Hypertension in African Americans." *Health* 5 (7): 13.
Carey, John, Naomi Freundlich, Julia Flynn, and Neil Gross
  1997 "The Biotech Century." *Business Week,* March 10: 78–90.
Carlton, John G.
  1997 "Genetic Testing for Diseases Sparks Debate over Insurance." *St. Louis Post-Dispatch,* March 17: 1A.
Carsten, Janet
  1995 "The Substance of Kinship and the Heat of the Hearth: Feeding, Personhood, and Relatedness Among Malays in Pulau Langkawi." *American Ethnologist* 22 (2): 223–41.
Cassell, Eric J.
  1991 *The Nature of Suffering and the Goals of Medicine.* New York: Oxford University Press.
Cherlin, Andrew J. and Frank F. Furstenberg, Jr.
  1994 "Stepfamilies in the United States: A Reconsideration." *Annual Review of Sociology* 20: 359–81.
Cloninger, C. Robert, Soren Sigvardsson, and Michael Bohman
  1996 "Type I and Type II Alcoholism: An Update." *Alcohol Health and Research World* 20 (1): 18.
Coleman, Brenda
  1998 "Gene Defect, Breast Cancer Link Rare, Researchers Report." *Durham Herald-Sun,* March 25.
Collier, Jane Fishburne and Sylvia Junko Yanagisako
  1987 "Introduction." In *Gender and Kinship: Essays Toward a Unified Analysis,* ed. Jane Fishburne Collier and Sylvia Junko Yanagisako. Stanford, Calif.: Stanford University Press.
Collins, Francis
  1999a "Designer Genes: The Ethical and Social Implications of Genetic Research." Keynote address, James M. Johnson Scholars Issues Forum, University of North Carolina at Chapel Hill, April 15.
  1999b "Genetics and Faith." Lecture, Christian Physicians Association of North Carolina, University of North Carolina at Chapel Hill, April 16.
Connerton, Paul
  1989 *How Societies Remember.* Cambridge: Cambridge University Press.
Conrad, Peter
  1997 "Public Eyes and Private Genes: Historical Frames, News Constructions, and Social Problems." *Social Problems* 44: 139–54.
Consumer Reports
  1996 "Family History: What You Don't Know Can Kill You." September 6, 97.
Cool, Lisa Collier
  1994 "Finding My Parents Saved My Life!" *Good Housekeeping* 219: 62.

Cranor, Carl F., ed.
  1994   *Are Genes Us? The Social Consequences of the New Genetics.* New Brunswick, N.J.: Rutgers University Press.
Cullinan, Alice L.
  1989   "Psychological Impact of Genetic Disease on Individual, Family, and Societal Systems." In *Genetic Disease: The Unwanted Inheritance,* ed. John D. Rainer, Sylvia P. Rubin, Michael K. Bartalos, Jack Emidman, Austin H. Kutscher, Kwame Anyane-Yeboa, Phyllis Tterka, and Joanne Malin. New York: Haworth Press. Pp. 77–86.
Dateline
  1998   "Shyness Treated as Genetic, Treated by Prozac." March 17.
Davis, Devra Lee, Debprah Axelrod, Michael P. Osborne, Nitin Telang, H. Leon Bradlow, and Elana Sittner
  1997   "Avoidable Causes of Breast Cancer: The Known, the Unknown, and the Suspected." In *Cancer: Genetics and the Environment,* ed. H. Leon Bradlow, Jack Fishman, and Michael P. Osborne. Annals of the New York Academy of Sciences 833. New York: New York Academy of Sciences. Pp. 112–28.
Davis-Floyd, Robbie E.
  1992   *Birth as an American Rite of Passage.* Berkeley: University of California Press.
  1996   "The Technocratic Body and the Organic Body: Hegemony and Heresy in Women's Birth Choices." In *Gender and Health: An International Perspective,* ed. Carolyn F. Sargent and Caroline B. Brettell. Upper Saddle River, N.J.: Prentice-Hall. Pp. 123–66.
Delaney, Carol
  1986   "The Meaning of Paternity and the Virgin Birth Debate." *Man* 21: 494–513.
  1991   *The Seed and the Soil: Gender and Cosmology in Turkish Village Society.* Berkeley: University of California Press.
Demos, John
  1977   "The American Family and Social Change." In *Family in Transition: Rethinking Marriage, Sexuality, Child Rearing, and Family Organization,* ed. Arlene Skolnick and S. Jerome Skolnick. Boston: Little, Brown. Pp. 59–77.
Dewey, John
  1929   *Experience and Nature.* New York: W. W. Norton.
Dolgin, Janet L.
  1997   *Defining the Family: Law, Technology, and Reproduction in an Uneasy Age.* New York: New York University Press.
Domhoff, G. William
  1983   *Who Rules America Now? A View for the '80s.* Englewood Cliffs, N.J.: Prentice-Hall.
Doria, John J.
  1995   "Gene Variability and Vulnerability to Alcoholism." *Alcohol Health and Research World* 19 (3): 245.
Douglas, Mary
  1970/1992   *Natural Symbols: Explorations in Cosmology.* New York: Vintage Books.
Doyal, Lesley
  1979   *The Political Economy of Health.* Boston: South End Press.

1995   *What Makes Women Sick: Gender and the Political Economy of Health.* New Brunswick, N.J.: Rutgers University Press.

Duby, Georges, Dominique Barthelemy, and Charles de la Roncière
1987   "Portraits." In *A History of Private Life.* Vol. 2, *Revelations of the Medieval World,* ed. Georges Duby. Cambridge, Mass.: Harvard University Press. Pp. 303–10.

Dumars, Kenneth W. and Chanthan S. Chea
1989   "The Cham: A Population Isolate." In *Genetic Disease: The Unwanted Inheritance,* ed. John D. Rainer, Sylvia P. Rubin, Michael K. Bartalos, Jack Emidman, Austin H. Kutscher, Kwame Anyane-Yeboa, Phyllis Tterka, and Joanne Malin. New York: Haworth Press. Pp. 153–68.

Durham Herald-Sun
1997   "Study Changes Course on Anxiety Gene Find." May 1.

Durkheim, Emile
1933/1964   *The Division of Labor in Society.* New York: Free Press.

Duster, Troy
1990   *Backdoor to Eugenics.* London: Routledge.

The Economist
1995   "Biotechnology and Genetics, Breaking Nature's Limits." Special insert, 334, February 25: 3–18.

Edwards, Jeanette
1993   "Explicit Connections: Ethnographic Enquiry in North-West England." In *Technologies of Procreation: Kinship in an Age of Assisted Conception,* ed. Jeanette Edwards, Sarah Franklin, Eric Hirsch, Frances Price, and Marilyn Strathern. Manchester: Manchester University Press. Pp. 42–66.

Eisenberg, David M.
1998   "Trends in Alternative Medicine Use in the United States 1990–1997: Results of a Follow-Up National Survey." *Journal of the American Medical Association* (November 11).

Eisenberg, David et al.
1993   "Unconventional Medicine in the United States." *New England Journal of Medicine* (January 28): 246–83.

Elmer-Dewitt, Philip
1994   "The Genetic Revolution." *Time* 143 (3): 46.

Engelhardt, H. Tristram, Jr.
1986   *The Foundation of Bioethics.* New York: Oxford University Press.

Estes, Carroll
1988   "The Biomedicalization of Aging: Dangers and Dilemmas." American Sociological Association: Association Paper 88S20430.

Evans-Pritchard, E. E.
1951/1990   *Kinship and Marriage Among the Nuer.* Oxford: Clarendon Press.
1962   "Heredity and Gestation as the Azande See Them." In Evans-Pritchard, *Social Anthropology and Other Essays.* New York: Free Press. Pp. 243–56.

Evens, Terrence M. S.
1989   "The Nuer Incest Prohibition and the Nature of Kinship: Alterlogical Reckoning." *Cultural Anthropology* 4: 323–46.

Fearon, Eric R.
1997   "Human Cancer Syndromes: Clues to the Origin and Nature of Cancer." *Science* 278, November 7: 1043–50.

Feldman, Miriam Karmel
1998   "Is DNA Destiny?" *Utne Reader,* March–April: 12.

Finch, Janet and Jennifer Mason
1993   *Negotiating Family Responsibilities.* London: Routledge.
Finch, Steven
1996   "To See Your Future Look into Your Past." *Health* 10(6): 92.
Finkler, Kaja
1974   *Estudio comparativo de la economía de dos comunidades de México.* Sepini 23.
        México: Instituto Nacional Indigenista.
1984   "The Nonsharing of Medical Knowledge Among Spiritualist Healers
        and Their Patients: A Contribution to the Study of Intra-Cultural Diver-
        sity and Practitioner-Patient Relationship." *Medical Anthropology* 3: 195–
        209.
1985/1994 *Spiritualist Healers in Mexico: Successes and Failures of Alternative
           Therapeutics.* South Hadley, Mass.: Praeger/Bergin and Garvey;
           reprint Salem, Mass.: Sheffield Publishing Co.
1991   *Physicians at Work, Patients in Pain: Biomedical Practice and Patient Response
        in Mexico.* Boulder, Colo.: Westview Press.
1994a   *Women in Pain: Gender and Morbidity in Mexico.* Philadelphia: University
        of Pennsylvania Press.
1994b   "Sacred and Biomedical Healing Compared." *Medical Anthropological
        Quarterly* 8: 179–97.
1996   "Factors Influencing Patient Perceived Recovery in Mexico." *Social Sci-
        ence and Medicine* 42: 199–207.
1999   "Diffusion Reconsidered: The Case of the Cross Cultural Transforma-
        tion of Biomedical Practice." *Medical Anthropology* 19 (1).
Fischer, Claude S.
1982   "The Dispersion of Kinship Ties in Modern Society: Contemporary
        Data and Historical Speculation." *Journal of Family History* (Winter):
        353–75.
Flynn, Julia et al.
1996   "Is Smithkline's Future in Its Genes?" *Business Week,* March 4: 80–81.
Forstenzer, Frances K. and David P. Roye
1989   "Psychological Implications of Genetic Factors in Scoliosis." In *Genetic
        Disease: The Unwanted Inheritance,* ed. John D. Rainer, Sylvia P. Rubin, Mi-
        chael K. Bartalos, Jack Emidman, Austin H. Kutscher, Kwame Anyane-
        Yeboa, Phyllis Tterka, and Joanne Malin. New York: Haworth Press.
Fortes, Meyer
1970   *Kinship and the Social Order: The Legacy of Lewis Henry Morgan.* London:
        Routledge and Kegan Paul.
Foster, George M. and Barbara Gallatin Anderson
1978   *Medical Anthropology.* New York: Wiley.
Foucault, Michel
1975   *The Birth of the Clinic: An Archaeology of Medical Perception.* Trans. A. M.
        Sheridan-Smith. New York: Vintage Books.
Fox, Robin
1992   "Comments." *Current Anthropology* 33: 303–4.
1993   *Reproduction and Succession: Studies in Anthropology, Law, and Society.* New
        Brunswick, N.J.: Transaction Publishers.
Fox Keller, Evelyn
1986   "Making Gender Visible in the Pursuit of Nature's Secrets." In *Feminist
        Studies/Critical Studies,* ed. Teresa de Lauretis. Bloomington: Indiana
        University Press. Pp. 67–77.

1992   "Nature, Nurture, and the Human Genome Project." In *The Code of Codes: Scientific and Social Issues in the Human Genome Project*, ed. Daniel J. Kevles and Leroy Hood. Cambridge, Mass.: Harvard University Press. Pp. 281–99.

1994   "Master Molecules." In *Are Genes Us? The Social Consequences of the New Genetics*, ed. Carl F. Cranor. New Brunswick, N.J.: Rutgers University Press. Pp. 89–98.

Franklin, Sarah

1993   "Making Representations: The Parliamentary Debate on the Human Fertilization and Embryology Act." In *Technologies of Procreation: Kinship in an Age of Assisted Conception*, ed. Jeanette Edwards, Sarah Franklin, Eric Hirsch, Frances Price, and Marilyn Strathern. Manchester: Manchester University Press. Pp. 96–131.

1995   "Romancing the Helix: Nature and Scientific Discovery." In *Romance Revisited*, ed. Lynne Pearce and Jackie Stacey. London: Lawrence and Wishart. Pp. 63–77.

1997a "Making Sense of Missed Conceptions." In *Situated Lives: Gender and Culture in Everyday Life*, ed. Louise Lamphere, Helena Ragoné, and Patricia Zavella. New York: Routledge. Pp. 99–109.

1997b *Embodied Progress: A Cultural Account of Assisted Conception*. New York: Routledge.

Freeman, J. D.

1968   "On the Concept of the Kindred." In *Kinship and Social Organization*, ed. Paul Bohannan and John Middleton. American Museum Sourcebooks in Anthropology. Garden City, N.Y.: Natural History Press. Pp. 255–72.

Freidson, Eliot

1970   *Profession of Medicine: A Study of the Sociology of Applied Knowledge*. New York: Harper and Row.

Freundlich, Naomi

1997   "Finding a Cure in DNA?" *Business Week*, March 10: 90–92.

Fujimura, Joan H.

1996   *Crafting Science: A Sociohistory of the Quest for the Genetics of Cancer*. Cambridge, Mass.: Harvard University Press.

Gabe, Jonathan and Susan Lipshitz-Phillips

1984   "Tranquillisers as Social Control." *Sociological Review* 32: 524–47.

Geertz, Clifford

1973   *The Interpretation of Cultures: Selected Essays*. New York: Basic Books.

Giddens, Anthony

1984   *The Constitution of Society: Outline of the Theory of Structuration*. Berkeley: University of California Press.

1990   *The Consequences of Modernity*. Stanford, Calif.: Stanford University Press.

1991   *Modernity and Self-Identity: Self and Society in the Late Modern Age*. Stanford, Calif.: Stanford University Press.

1992   *The Transformation of Intimacy: Sexuality, Love, and Eroticism in Modern Societies*. Stanford, Calif.: Stanford University Press.

Ginsburg, Faye and Rayna Rapp

1991   "The Politics of Reproduction." *Annual Review of Anthropology* 20: 311–43.

Glausiusz, Josie

1995a "A Gene for Breast Cancer." *Discover*, January: 99.

1995b   "Anastasia, Nyet." *Discover,* January: 99.
1996   "The Genes of 1995." *Discover,* January: 32–33.
Gold, Michael
1994   "Adoption as a Jewish Option." In *The Jewish Family and Jewish Continuity,* ed. Steven Bayme and Gladys Rosen. Hoboken, N.J.: KTAV. Pp. 173–80.
Gonyea, Judith
1996   "Finished at Fifty: The Politics of the Menopause and Hormone Replacement Therapy." *American Journal of Preventive Medicine* 12 (September–October): 415–19.
Goode, William Josiah
1970   *World Revolution and Family Patterns.* New York: Free Press.
1977   "World Revolution and Family Patterns." In *Family in Transition: Rethinking Marriage, Sexuality, Child Rearing, and Family Organization,* ed. Arlene S. Skolnick and Jerome H. Skolnick. Boston: Little, Brown. Pp. 47–58.
Gorovitz, Samuel and Alasdair MacIntyre
1976   "Toward a Theory of Medical Fallibility." *Journal of Medicine and Philosophy* 1: 51–71.
Gottlieb, Beatrice
1993   *The Family in the Western World from the Black Death to the Industrial Age.* New York: Oxford University Press.
Gough, E. Kathleen
1968   "The Nayars and the Definition of Marriage." In *Marriage, Family, and Residence,* ed. Paul Bohannan and John Middleton. American Museum Sourcebooks in Anthropology. Garden City, N.Y.: Natural History Press. Pp. 49–72.
Gould, Stephen Jay
1996   *The Mismeasure of Man.* New York: W. W. Norton.
1998   "The Internal Brand of the Scarlet." *Natural History* 3: 24–78.
Graburn, Nelson H. H., ed.
1970   *Readings in Kinship and Social Structure.* New York: Harper and Row.
Grady, Denise
1994   "The New Way to Predict Your Future Health." *Redbook* 183: 32.
Gramsci, Antonio
1971   *Selections from the Prison Notebooks.* Ed and trans. Quentin Hoare and Geoffrey Nowell Smith. London: Lawrence and Wishart.
Granner, Daryl K.
1988   "Nucleic Acid Structure and Function." In *Harper's Biochemistry,* 22nd ed., ed. Robert K. Murray et al. Norwalk, Conn.: Appleton and Lange. Pp. 366–82.
Green, Josephine, Frances Murton, and Helen Statham
1993   "Psychosocial Issues Raised by a Familial Ovarian Cancer Register." *Journal of Medical Genetics* 30 (March): 575–79.
Griesemer, James R.
1994   "Tools for Talking: Human Nature, Weismannism, and the Interpretation of Genetic Information." In *Are Genes Us? The Social Consequences of the New Genetics,* ed. Carl F. Cranor. New Brunswick, N.J.: Rutgers University Press.
Grimm, Shea
1999   "Sealed Records and Adoption Reform: An Historical Perspective."

Web site: ⟨www.bastards.org/activism/reform.htm⟩. Also ⟨www.ibar.com/voices/activism/history.htm⟩.

Groopman, Jerome
1998   "Decoding Destiny." *New Yorker,* February 9.

Gros, François
1989   *The Gene Civilization.* Trans. Lee F. Scanlon. New York: McGraw-Hill.

Gross, Daniel R.
1992   *Discovering Anthropology.* Mountain View, Calif.: Mayfield.

Gurevich, Maria
1995   "Rethinking the Label: Who Benefits from the PMS Construct?" *Women and Health* 23: 67–98.

Hacker, Andrew
1997   "The War over the Family." *New York Review of Books,* December 4: 34–38.

Hacking, Ian
1975   *The Emergence of Probability.* Bristol: Cambridge University Press.

Hahn, Robert and Arthur Kleinman
1983   "Biomedical Practice and Anthropological Theory: Frameworks and Directions." *Annual Review of Anthropology* 12: 305–33.

Haller, Mark H.
1984   *Eugenics: Hereditarian Attitudes in American Thought.* New Brunswick, N.J.: Rutgers University Press.

Halpern, Sydney Ann
1985   "Medicalization Through Specialization." Society for the Study of Social Problems Association Paper 85S16990.

Hamer, Dean and Peter Copeland
1998   *Living with Our Genes: Why They Matter More Than You Think.* New York: Doubleday.

Hamilton, Joan O'C. and Julie Flynn
1997   "When Science Fiction Becomes Social Reality." *Business Week,* March 10: 84–85.

Hansen, Bert
1992   "American Physicians' 'Discovery' of Homosexuals, 1880–1900: A New Diagnosis in a Changing Society." In *Framing Disease: Studies in Cultural History,* ed. Charles E. Rosenberg and Janet Golden. New Brunswick, N.J.: Rutgers University Press. Pp. 104–33.

Haraway, Donna J.
1991   *Simians, Cyborgs, and Women: The Reinvention of Nature.* New York: Routledge.

Harris, C. C.
1990   *Kinship.* Minneapolis: University of Minnesota Press.

Hartman, Lynn C. et al.
1999   "Efficacy of Bilateral Prophylactic Mastectomy in Women with a Family History of Breast Cancer." *New England Journal of Medicine* 340: 77–84.

Hartouni, Valerie
1997   *Cultural Conceptions: On Reproductive Technologies and the Remaking of Life.* Minneapolis: University of Minnesota Press.

Harvey, David
1989   *The Condition of Postmodernity: An Enquiry into the Origins of Cultural Change.* Cambridge: Blackwell.

Hawley, Janet
1997   "Dread Locked." *Good Weekend,* May 31: 12.

Herbert, Bob
    1999   "How Many Innocent Prisoners?" *New York Times,* July 18: 47.
Herbert, Wray
    1997   "Politics of Biology: How the Nature vs. Nurture Debate Shapes Public Policy—and Our View of Ourselves." *U.S. News and World Report,* April 21: 72–80.
Herlihy, David
    1985   *Medieval Households.* Cambridge, Mass.: Harvard University Press.
Higgins, Ean
    1997   "Study Links Men's Bad Behaviour to What's in Their Genes," *The Australian,* June 14: 12.
Hirsch, Eric
    1993   "Negotiated Limits: Interviews in South-East England." In *Technologies of Procreation: Kinship in an Age of Assisted Conception,* ed. Jeanette Edwards, Sarah Franklin, Eric Hirsch, Frances Price, and Marilyn Strathern. Manchester: Manchester University Press. Pp. 67–95.
Holden, Constance
    1991   "Probing the Complex Genetics of Alcoholism." *Science* 251: 163–64.
Holy, Ladislav
    1996   *Anthropological Perspectives on Kinship.* Chicago: Pluto Press.
Hood, Leroy
    1992   "Biology and Medicine in the Twenty-First Century." In *The Code of Codes: Scientific and Social Issues in the Human Genome Project,* ed. Daniel J. Kevles and Leroy Hood. Cambridge, Mass.: Harvard University Press. Pp. 136–63.
Hornblower, Margot
    1999   "Roots Mania." *Time,* April 19: 55–69.
Hubbard, Ruth
    1990   *The Politics of Women's Biology.* New Brunswick, N.J.: Rutgers University Press.
    1995a "Human Nature." In *Biopolitics: A Feminist and Ecological Reader on Biotechnology,* ed. Vandana Shiva and Ingunn Moser. London: Zed Books, Pp. 27–37.
    1995b "Genes as Causes." In *Biopolitics: A Feminist and Ecological Reader on Biotechnology,* ed. Vandana Shiva and Ingunn Moser. London: Zed Books. Pp. 38–51.
    1998   "Outwitting Destiny." *New Yorker* (*The Mail*), March 16.
Hubbard, Ruth and Elijah Wald
    1997   *Exploding the Gene Myth: How Genetic Information Is Produced and Manipulated by Scientists, Physicians, Lawyers, Insurance Companies, Educators, and Law Enforcers.* Boston: Beacon Press.
Illich, Ivan
    1975   *Medical Nemesis.* London: Marion Boyars.
Ingleby, David
    1982   "The Social Construction of Mental Illness." In *The Problem of Medical Knowledge: Examining the Social Construction of Medicine,* ed. Peter Wright and Andrew Treacher. Edinburgh: Edinburgh University Press. Pp. 123–43.
Inhorn, Marcia
    1994   *Quest for Conception: Gender, Infertility, and Egyptian Medical Traditions.* Philadelphia: University of Pennsylvania Press.

Jacob, François
  1973   *The Logic of Life: A History of Heredity.* Trans. Betty Spillman. New York: Pantheon.
Jaroff, Leon
  1989   "The Gene Hunt; Scientists Launch a $3 Billion Project to Map the Chromosomes and Decipher the Complete Instructions for Making a Human Being." *Science* March 20: 62.
  1994   "Battle for Gene Therapy." *Time* 143 (3): 56.
  1996   "Keys to the Kingdom." *Time* Special Issue 148 (14): 24–29.
Johns Hopkins Medical Letter
  1999   "Surgery to Prevent Breast Cancer?" *Health After 50* 9 (3): 1.
Johnson, Thomas M.
  1987   "Premenstrual Syndrome as a Western Culture-Specific Disorder." *Culture, Medicine, and Psychiatry* 11: 337–56.
Jonsen, Albert R.
  1996   "The Impact of Mapping the Human Genome on the Patient-Physician Relationship." In *The Human Genome Project and the Future of Health Care,* ed. Thomas H. Murray, Mark A. Rothstein, and Robert F. Murray, Jr. Bloomington: Indiana University Press. Pp. 1–20.
Jordan, Brigitte
  1993   *Birth in Four Cultures: A Cross-Cultural Investigation of Childbirth in Yucatan, Holland, Sweden, and the United States.* 4th ed., rev. Robbie Davis-Floyd. Prospect Heights, Ill: Waveland Press.
Jordanova, L. J.
  1980   "Natural Facts: A Historical Perspective on Science and Sexuality." In *Nature, Culture, and Gender,* ed. Carol P. MacCormack and Marilyn Strathern. Cambridge: Cambridge University Press. Pp. 42–69.
Judson, Horace Freeland
  1992   "A History of the Science and Technology Behind Gene Mapping and Sequencing." In *The Code of Codes: Scientific and Social Issues in the Human Genome Project,* ed. Daniel J. Kevles and Leroy Hood. Cambridge, Mass.: Harvard University Press. Pp. 37–82.
Kass, Leon R.
  1998   Review of Bryan Appleyard, *Brave New Worlds: Staying Human in the Genetic Future. New York Times Book Review,* August 23: 7.
Kaufert, Patricia A.
  1996   "Women and the Debate over Mammography: An Economic, Political, and Moral History." In *Gender and Health: An International Perspective,* ed. Carolyn F. Sargent and Caroline B. Brettell. Upper Saddle River, N.J.: Prentice-Hall. Pp. 167–86.
Kaufert, Patricia and Penny Gilbert
  1986   "Women, Menopause, and Medicalization." *Culture, Medicine, and Psychiatry* 10: 7–21.
Keesing, Roger M.
  1975   *Kin Groups and Social Structure.* New York: Holt, Rinehart and Winston.
Kevles, Daniel J.
  1985   *In the Name of Eugenics: Genetics and the Uses of Human Heredity.* New York: Knopf.
Kevles, Daniel J. and Leroy Hood
  1992a "Out of Eugenics: The Historical Politics of the Human Genome." In *The Code of Codes: Scientific and Social Issues in the Human Genome Project,*

ed. Daniel J. Kevles and Leroy Hood. Cambridge, Mass.: Harvard University Press. Pp. 3–36.

Kevles, Daniel J. and Leroy Hood, eds.
1992b   *The Code of Codes: Scientific and Social Issues in the Human Genome Project.* Cambridge, Mass.: Harvard University Press.

Kiernan, Vincent
1997   "Gene Active in Women Fosters Social Behavior." *Chronicle of Higher Education,* June 20: A14.

Klapisch-Zuber, Christiane
1996   "Family Trees and the Construction of Kinship in Renaissance Italy." In *Gender, Kinship, Power: A Comparative and Interdisciplinary History,* ed. Mary Jo Maynes, Ann Waltner, Birgitte Soland, and Ulrike Strasser. New York: Routledge.

Klein, Renate and Lynette Dumble
1994   "Disempowering Midlife Women: The Science and Politics of Hormone Replacement Therapy." *Women's Studies International Forum* 17: 327–43.

Kleinman, Arthur
1980   *Patients and Healers in the Context of Culture.* Berkeley: University of California Press.
1988   *The Illness Narratives: Suffering, Healing, and the Human Condition.* New York: Basic Books.

Kleinman, Arthur and Joan Kleinman
1991   "Suffering and Its Professional Transformation: Toward an Ethnography of Interpersonal Experience." *Culture, Medicine, and Psychiatry* 15: 275–301.

Kohler Riessman, Catherine
1983   "Women and Medicalization: A New Perspective." *Social Policy* (Summer): 3–18.

Kolata, Gina
1997   "Advent of Testing for Breast Cancer Genes Leads to Fears of Discrimination." *New York Times,* February 4.
1998   "Infertile Foreigners See Opportunity in U.S." *New York Times,* January 4.

Krieger, Nancy and Elizabeth Fee
1994   "Man-Made Medicine and Women's Health: The Biopolitics of Sex/Gender and Race/Ethnicity." *International Journal of Health Services* 24: 265–83.

Kuhn, Thomas
1970   *The Structure of Scientific Revolutions.* Chicago: University of Chicago Press.

Latour, Bruno and S. Woolgar
1979   *Laboratory Life: The Social Construction of Scientific Fact.* Beverly Hills, Calif.: Sage.

Leach, E. R.
1961   *Rethinking Anthropology.* London: Athlone Press.

Leonardo, Micaela
1992   "The Female World of Cards and Holidays: Women, Families, and the Work of Kinship." In *Rethinking the Family: Some Feminist Questions,* ed. Barrie Thorne with Marilyn Yalom. Boston: Northeastern University Press. Pp. 246–61.

Lévi-Strauss, Claude
  1969   *The Elementary Structure of Kinship*. Ed. Rodney Needham. Boston: Beacon Press.
Lewontin, R. C.
  1992   *Biology as Ideology*. New York: HarperPerennial.
Lewontin, R. C., Steven Rose, and Leon J. Kamin
  1984   *Not in Our Genes: Biology, Ideology, and Human Nature*. New York: Pantheon.
Lieberman, Leonard, Larry T. Reynolds, and Douglas Friedrich
  1992   "The Fitness of Human Sociobiology: The Future Utility of Four Concepts in Four Subdisciplines." *Social Biology* 39: 158–69.
Livingstone, Frank B.
  1958   "Anthropological Implications of Sickle Cell Gene Distribution in West Africa." *American Anthropologist* 60: 533–62.
Lloyd, Elisabeth A.
  1994   "Normality and Variation. The Human Genome Project and the Ideal Human Type." In *Are Genes Us? The Social Consequences of the New Genetics*, ed. Carl F. Cranor. New Brunswick, N.J.: Rutgers University Press. Pp. 99–112.
Lock, Margaret M.
  1980   *East Asian Medicine in Urban Japan: Varieties of Medical Experience*. Berkeley: University of California Press.
  1986   "Plea for Acceptance: School Refusal Syndrome in Japan." *Social Science and Medicine* 23: 99–112.
  1993   *Encounters with Aging: Mythologies of Menopause in Japan and North America*. Berkeley: University of California Press.
Lock, Margaret and Deborah Gordon
  1988   *Biomedicine Examined*. Dordrecht: Kluwer Academic.
López-Beltrán, Carlos
  1994   "Forging Heredity: From Metaphor to Cause, a Reification Story." *Studies in History and Philosophy of Science* 25: 211–35.
Lowie, Robert H.
  1948   *Social Organization*. New York: Rinehart.
Lubinsky, Mark S.
  1993   "Degenerate Heredity: The History of a Doctrine in Medicine and Biology." *Perspectives in Biology and Medicine* 37: 74–90.
Ludmerer, Kenneth M.
  1972   *Genetics and American Society: An Historical Appraisal*. Baltimore: Johns Hopkins University Press.
Lynch, H. T., Patrick Lynch, and Jane Lynch
  1979   "Genetic Counseling and Cancer." In *Genetic Counseling: Psychological Dimensions*, ed. Seymour Kessler. New York: Academic Press. Pp. 221–42.
MacDonald, Michael
  1992   "The Medicalization of Suicide in England: Laymen, Physicians, and Cultural Change, 1500–1870." In *Framing Disease: Studies in Cultural History*, ed. Charles E. Rosenberg and Janet Golden. New Brunswick, N.J.: Rutgers University Press. Pp. 85–103.
Maine, Henry
  1861/1970   "The Primitive Family and the Corporation." Reprinted in *Read-

ings in Kinship and Social Structure, ed. Nelson H. H. Graburn. New York: Harper and Row. Pp. 11–12.

1861/1931   *Ancient Law*. London: Oxford University Press.

Mair, Lucy
  1971   *Marriage*. London: Penguin.

Malinowski, Bronislaw
  1922   *Argonauts of the Western Pacific*. New York: E. P. Dutton.
  1929/1962   *The Sexual Life of Savages*. New York: Harcourt, Brace and World.
  1930/1970   "Kinship." Reprinted in *Readings in Kinship and Social Structure*, ed. Nelson H. H. Graburn. New York: Harper and Row.

Marcus, George E. with Peter Dobkin Hall
  1992   *Lives in Trust: The Fortunes of Dynastic Families in Late Twentieth-Century America*. Boulder, Colo.: Westview Press.

Marieskind, Helen I.
  1980   "The Impact of Technology on Women's Health Care." Chapter 7 in Marieskind, *Women in the Health System: Patients, Providers, and Programs*. St. Louis: C. V. Mosby. Pp. 235–82.

Markens, Susan
  1994   "Dr. Jekyll and Ms Hyde: A Political and Cultural Critique of PMS." American Sociological Association Paper 94S30544.
  1996   "The Problematic of 'Experience': A Political and Cultural Critique of PMS." *Gender and Society* 10: 42–58.

Marks, Jonathan
  1995   *Human Biodiversity: Genes, Race, and History*. Chicago: Aldine.

Martin, Emily
  1987   *The Woman in the Body: A Cultural Analysis of Reproduction*. Boston: Beacon Press.
  1997   "The Egg and the Sperm." In *Situated Lives: Gender and Culture in Everyday Life*, ed. Louise Lamphere, Helena Ragoné, and Patricia Zavella. New York: Routledge. Pp. 85–98.

Marty, Martin E.
  1996   "Slightly Extraordinary Genes." *Christian Century* 113, February 7: 183.

Matthews, Kathy
  1999   "Diary of a C-Scope." *Persona* (New York: Condé Nast), June: 27–28.

Mayall, Berry
  1990   "Childcare and Childhood." *Children and Society* 4 (Winter): 374–85.

McAuliffe, William E.
  1978   "Studies of Process-Outcome Correlations in Medical Care Evaluations: A Critique." *Medical Care* 26: 907–30.
  1979   "Measuring the Quality of Medical Care: Process Versus Outcome." *Milbank Memorial Fund Quarterly/Health and Society* 57: 118–52.

McCarthy, Peggy and Jo An Loren, eds.
  1997   *Breast Cancer? Let Me Check My Schedule: Ten Remarkable Women Meet the Challenge of Fitting Breast Cancer into Their Very Busy Lives*. Boulder, Colo.: Westview Press.

McKeown, Thomas
  1985   *The Role of Medicine: Dream, Mirage, or Nemesis*. Princeton, N.J.: Princeton University Press.

McKusick, Victor A.
  1998   *Mendelian Inheritance of Man: A Catalog of Human Genes and Genetic Disorders*. 12th ed. Baltimore: Johns Hopkins University Press.

Mead, Rebecca
  1999.   "Eggs for Sale." *New Yorker,* August 9: 56–65.
Merck Manual of Diagnosis and Therapy
  1977. 13th ed. Merck Sharp and Dohme Research Laboratories, Division of Merck and Co.
Merck Manual of Medical Information (ed Horne)
  1997   Merck Research Laboratories. Division of Merck and Co.
Metzler, Kristan
  1994   "The Apple Doesn't Fall Far in Families Linked to Crime." *Insight on the News* 10 (35): 17.
Meyer, Michele
  1997   "Inheriting Your Health: Genetic Testing for Diseases." *Better Homes and Gardens* 75 (2): 58.
Micale, Mark S.
  1995   *Approaching Hysteria: Disease and Its Interpretations.* Princeton, N.J.: Princeton University Press.
Milunsky, Aubrey
  1992   *Heredity and Your Family's Health.* Baltimore: Johns Hopkins University Press.
Minow, Martha and Mary Lyndon Shanley
  1996   "Relational Rights and Responsibilities: Revisioning the Family in Liberal Political Theory and Law." In *The Family and Feminist Theory,* ed. Ellen K. Feder and Eva Feder Kittay. Special Issue, *Hypatia: A Journal of Feminist Philosophy* 11 (1) (Winter): 4–29.
Mintz, Steven and Susan Kellogg
  1988   *Domestic Revolutions: A Social History of American Family Life.* New York: Free Press.
Modell, Judith
  1994   *Kinship with Strangers: Adoption and Interpretations of Kinship in American Culture.* Berkeley: University of California Press.
Monmaney, Terence
  1995   "Genetic Testing: Kids' Latest Rite of Passage." *Health* 9 (1): 46.
Morgan, Lewis Henry
  1870/1971   "The Comparative Study of Family Systems." Reprinted in *Readings in Kinship and Social Structure,* ed. Nelson H. H. Graburn. New York: Harper and Row. Pp. 12–18.
Morrow, David J.
  1997   "No Mere Distraction, But a Disorder." *New York Times,* September 2: 2.
MSNBC
  1998   "Motherhood in Question: Surrogates and Carriers." *The Fertility Race.* Part 4. April 21: 1–8. (www.msnbc.com/news/149876.asp).
Myers, Steven L.
  1998   "Laying to Rest the Last of the Unknown Soldiers." *New York Times,* May 3: 5.
Nash, Madeleine
  1994   "Riding the DNA Trail." *Time* 143(3): 54.
  1997   "Addicted: Why Do People Get Hooked? Mounting Evidence Points to Powerful Brain Chemical Called Dopamine." *Time,* May 5.
National Human Genome Research Institute
  1998   (www.ornl.gov/hgmis/faq/faqs1.html 4/20).

National Neurofibromatosis Association
1997   *Questions and Answers.* New York: National Neurofibromatosis Foundation.
National Public Radio
1997a   "Colon Cancer." *Morning Edition,* transcript 97032003-210, March 20.
1997b   "Genetics of Complex Traits." *Talk of the Nation Science Friday,* transcript 97021402-211, February 14.
1997c   "Prophylactic Mastectomies." *All Things Considered,* transcript 97041401-212, April 14.
1998a   "Report on Preimplantation Genetic Diagnosis." *All Things Considered,* September 29.
1998b   *Talk of the Nation Science Friday,* November 13.
Nelkin, Dorothy
1992   "The Social Power of Genetic Information." In *The Code of Codes: Scientific and Social Issues in the Human Genome Project,* ed. Daniel J. Kevles and Leroy Hood. Cambridge, Mass.: Harvard University Press. Pp. 177–90.
1996a   "The Politics of Predisposition: The Social Meaning of Predictive Biology." In *Biopolitics: The Politics of the Body, Race, and Nature,* ed. Agnes Heller and Sonja Puntscher Reikmann. Brookfield, Vt.: Avebury.
1996b   "The Social Dynamics of Genetic Testing: The Case of Fragile-X." *Medical Anthropology Quarterly* 10: 537–50.
Nelkin, Dorothy and M. Susan Lindee
1995   *The DNA Mystique: The Gene as a Cultural Icon.* New York: W. H. Freeman.
Nelkin, Dorothy and Laurence Tancredi
1989   *Dangerous Diagnostics: The Social Power of Biological Information.* New York: Basic Books.
Neustadter, Roger
1992   "Squatter's Rights in the Ovum: The Unborn as Patient." *Free Inquiry in Creative Sociology* 20: 199–204.
Ortner, Sherry
1974   "Is Female to Male as Nature Is to Culture?" In *Woman, Culture, and Society,* ed. Michelle Zimbalist Rosaldo and Louise Lamphere. Stanford, Calif.: Stanford University Press. Pp. 67–88.
Osherson, Samuel and Lorna Amara Singham
1981   "The Machine Metaphor in Medicine." In *Social Contexts of Health, Illness and Patient Care,* ed. Elliott G. Mishler, Lorna R. Amara Singham, et al. Cambridge: Cambridge University Press.
Ostrom, Carol
1997   "DNA Labs Offer New Test of Family Ties—More People Use Genetics to Learn Who's Related—and Who's Not." *Seattle Times,* March 14: A1.
Ottenheimer, Martin
1996   *Forbidden Relatives: The American Myth of Cousin Marriage.* Urbana: University of Illinois Press.
Paige, Karen Ericksen and Jeffery M. Paige
1981   *The Politics of Reproductive Ritual.* Berkeley: University of California Press.
Park, Andrew
1997   "Adoptees Seek Access to Genetic History." *News and Observer,* June 20.
Parkin, Robert
1997   *Kinship: An Introduction to Basic Concepts.* Oxford: Blackwell.

Paul, Diane B.
  1994 "Eugenic Anxieties, Social Realities, and Political Choices." In *Are Genes Us? The Social Consequences of the New Genetics,* ed. Carl F. Cranor. New Brunswick, N.J.: Rutgers University Press. Pp. 142–54.

Pellegrino, Edmund D. and David C. Thomasma
  1981 *A Philosophical Basis of Medical Practice: Toward a Philosophy and Ethic of the Healing Professions.* New York: Oxford University Press.

Peletz, Michael
  1995 "Kinship Studies in Late Twentieth-Century Anthropology." *Annual Review of Anthropology* 24: 343–72.

Pembrey, Marcus
  1996 "The New Genetics: A User's Guide." In *The Troubled Helix: Social and Psychological Implications of the New Human Genetics,* ed. Theresa Marteau and Martin Richards. Cambridge: Cambridge University Press. Pp. 63–81.

Perera, Frederica P.
  1997 "Environment and Cancer: Who Are Susceptible." *Science* 278, November 7: 1068–73.

Petchesky, Rosalind P.
  1987 "Fetal Images: The Power of Visual Culture in the Politics of Reproduction." In *Reproductive Technologies: Gender, Motherhood, and Medicine,* ed. Michelle Stanworth. Minneapolis: University of Minnesota Press.

Petersen, Alan
  1998 "The New Genetics and the Politics of Public Health." *Critical Public Health* 8: 59–72.

Petersen, Alan and Deborah Lupton
  1996 *The New Public Health: Health and Self in the Age of Risk.* London: Sage.

Pinn, Vivian W. and Debbie M. Jackson
  1996 "Advisory Committee to NIH Office Passes Resolutions." *Journal of Women's Health* 5: 549–53.

Pinto-Correia, Clara
  1997 *The Ovary of Eve: Egg and Sperm and Preformation.* Chicago: University of Chicago Press.

Pomata, Gianna
  1996 "Blood Ties and Semen Ties: Consanguinity and Agnation in Roman Law." In *Gender, Kinship, Power: A Comparative and Interdisciplinary History,* ed. Mary Jo Maynes, Ann Waltner, Birgitte Soland, and Ulrike Strasser. New York: Routledge. Pp. 43–66.

Ponder, Bruce
  1997 "Genetic Testing for Cancer Risk." *Science* 278, November 7: 1050–54.

Popenoe, David
  1993 "American Family Decline, 1960–1990: A Review and Appraisal." *Journal of Marriage and the Family* 55: 527–55.

Radcliffe-Brown, A. R.
  1952 *Structure and Function in Primitive Society.* London: Cohen and West.

Ragoné, Helena
  1994 *Surrogate Motherhood: Conception in the Heart.* Boulder, Colo.: Westview Press.
  1997 "Chasing the Blood Tie." In *Situated Lives: Gender and Culture in Everyday Life,* ed. Louise Lamphere, Helena Ragoné, and Patricia Zavella. New York: Routledge. Pp. 110–27.

Rapp, Rayna
1992   "Family and Class in Contemporary America: Notes Toward an Under-
        standing of Ideology." In *Rethinking the Family: Some Feminist Questions*,
        ed. Barrie Thorne with Marilyn Yalom. Boston: Northeastern University
        Press. Pp. 49–70.

Rather, L. J.
1978   *The Genesis of Cancer: A Study in th History of Ideas*. Baltimore: Johns
        Hopkins University Press.

Raymond, Janice G.
1993   *Women as Wombs: Reproduction Technologies and the Battle over Women's
        Freedom*. San Francisco: HarperSanFrancisco.

Redfield, Robert
1941   *The Folk Culture of Yucatan*. Chicago: Chicago University Press.

Reiser, David and David H. Rosen
1984   *Medicine as a Human Experience*. Baltimore: University Park Press.

Reiser, Stanley Joel
1978   *Medicine and the Reign of Technology*. Cambridge: Cambridge University
        Press.

Richards, Martin
1993   "The New Genetics: Some Issues for Social Scientists." *Sociology of Health
        and Illness* 15: 567–86.
1996   "Families, Kinship and Genetics." In *The Troubled Helix: Social and Psy-
        chological Implications of the New Human Genetics*, ed. Theresa Marteau
        and Martin Richards. Cambridge University Press. Pp. 249–73.

Richter, Maurice N., Jr.
1972   *Science as a Cultural Process*. Cambridge: Schenkman.

Rice, George, Carol Anderson, Neil Reisch, and George Ebers
1999   "Male Homosexuality: Absence of Linkage to Microsatellite Markers at
        Xq28." *Science* 284: 665–67.

Ridley, Matt
1997   *The Origins of Virtue: Human Instinct and the Evolution of Cooperation*. New
        York: Viking.

Rifkin, Jeremy
1998   "The Biotech Century: Human Life as Intellectual Property." *The Na-
        tion*, April 13: 11–19.

Ritenbaugh, Cheryl
1982   "Obesity as a Culture-Bound Syndrome." *Culture, Medicine, and Psychia-
        try* 6: 347–61.

Rivers, W. H. R.
1900   "A Genealogical Method of Collecting Social and Vital Statistics." *Jour-
        nal of the Royal Anthropological Institute* 30: 74–82.

Rodin, Judith et al.
1985   "Women and Weight: Normative Discontent." *Nebraska Symposium on
        Motivation* 32: 267–307.

Rodin, Mari
1992   "The Social Construction of Premenstrual Syndrome." *Social Science
        and Medicine* 35: 49–56.

Rosaldo, Renato
1994   "Subjectivity in Social Analysis." In *The Postmodern Turn*, ed. Steven
        Seidman. Cambridge: Cambridge University Press. Pp. 171–86.

Rosenberg, Charles E.
1976   *No Other Gods: On Science and American Social Thought.* Baltimore: Johns Hopkins University Press.

Rosenfied, Richard and Gerald Erchak
1988   "Learning Disabilities, Dyslexia, and the Medicalization of the Classroom." Society for the Study of Social Problems Association Paper 88S20306.

Rosser, Sue V.
1994   *Women's Health — Missing from U.S. Medicine.* Bloomington: Indiana University Press.

Rothman, Barbara Katz
1986   *The Tentative Pregnancy: Prenatal Diagnosis and the Future of Motherhood.* New York: Viking Press.

Rothman, Sheila M.
1994   *Living in the Shadow of Death: Tuberculosis and the Experience of Illness in America.* New York: Basic Books.

Rothstein, Edward
1998   "DNA Teaches History a Few Lessons of Its Own." *New York Times,* May 24: 5.

Rubin, Rita
1996   "Do You Have a Cancer Gene?" *U.S. News and World Report* 128, May 13: 66–68.

Sack, Catherine
1997 "Washington Diarist: Tropic of Cancer." *New Republic,* June 2.

Sahlins, Marshall D.
1968   *Tribesmen.* Englewood Cliffs, N.J.: Prentice Hall.
1976a   *Culture and Practical Reason.* Chicago: University of Chicago Press.
1976b   *The Use and Abuse of Biology: An Anthropological Critique of Sociobiology.* Ann Arbor: University of Michigan Press.

Scheffler, Harold W.
1991   "Sexism and Naturalism in the Study of Kinship." In *Gender at the Crossroads of Knowledge: Feminist Anthropology in the Postmodern Era,* ed. Micaela di Leonardo. Berkeley: University of California Press.

Schmidt, Mathew and Lisa Jean Moore
1998   "Constructing a 'Good Catch': Picking a Winner." In *Cyborg Babies: From Techno-Sex to Techno-Tots,* ed. Robbie Davis-Floyd and Joseph Dumit. New York: Routledge. Pp. 21–39.

Schneider, David Murray
1965   "Kinship and Biology." In *Aspects of the Analysis of Family Structure,* ed. Ansley J. Coale, Lloyd A. Fallers, Marion J. Levy, David M. Schneider, and Silvan S. Tomkins. Princeton, N.J.: Princeton University Press. Pp. 83–101.
1972   "What Is Kinship All About?" In *Kinship Studies in the Morgan Centennial Year,* ed. Priscilla Reining. Washington, D.C.: Anthropological Society of Washington. Pp. 32–63.
1980   *American Kinship: A Cultural Account.* 2nd ed. Chicago: University of Chicago Press.
1984   *A Critique of the Study of Kinship.* Ann Arbor: University of Michigan Press.
1992   "Comments." *Current Anthropology* 33: 307–10.

Science
1993   "Zeroing in on a Breast Cancer Susceptibility Gene." 259 (January 29): 622–23.

Schwartz, Howard Eilberg
    1996   "The Father, the Phallus, and the Seminal Word: Dilemmas of Patrilin-
            eality in Ancient Judaism." In *Gender, Kinship, Power: A Comparative and
            Interdisciplinary History,* ed. Mary Jo Maynes, Ann Waltner, Birgitte So-
            land, and Ulrike Strasser. New York: Routledge. Pp. 27–42.
Scritchfield, Shirley A.
    1995   "The Social Construction of Infertility: From Private Matter to Social
            Concern." In *Images of Issues: Typifying Contemporary Social Problems,* ed.
            Joel Best. New York: Aldine de Gruyter. Pp. 131–46.
Segalen, Martine
    1986   *Historical Anthropology of the Family.* Trans. J. C. Whitehouse and Sarah
            Matthews. Cambridge: Cambridge University Press.
Seligman, Daniel
    1994   "A Substantial Inheritance." *National Review* 46 (19): 56–60.
Serban, George E.
    1989   "Unwanted Inheritance: The Psychosocial Care of Progressive Genetic
            Illnesses." In *Genetic Disease: The Unwanted Inheritance,* ed. John D.
            Rainer, Sylvia P. Rubin, Michael K. Bartalos, Jack Emidman, Austin H.
            Kutscher, Kwame Anyane-Yeboa, Phyllis Tterka, and Joanne Malin. New
            York: Haworth Press. Pp. 199–202.
SerVaas, Cory
    1995   "Genetic Roots of Family Health." *Saturday Evening Post* 267: 42–45.
Shiloh, Shoshana
    1996   "Decision-Making in the Context of Genetic Risk." In *The Troubled He-
            lix: Social and Psychological Implications of the New Human Genetics,* ed.
            Theresa Marteau and Martin Richards. Cambridge: Cambridge Univer-
            sity Press. Pp. 82–103.
Shore, Chris
    1992   "Virgin Births and Sterile Debates." *Current Anthropology* 33: 295–314.
Shorter, Edward
    1977   *The Making of the Modern Family.* New York: Basic Books.
Shryock, Richard H.
    1936/1979   *The Development of Modern Medicine: An Interpretation of the Social and
            Scientific Factors Involved.* Madison: University of Wisconsin Press.
Siebert, Charles
    1995   "The DNA We've Been Dealt." *New York Times Magazine,* September 17:
            50–104.
Sixty Minutes
    1999   "Who Am I?" July 1.
Skuse, D. H., James Bishop, B. Coppin, P. Dalton, G. Aamondt-Leeper,
M. Bacarese-Hamilton, C. Creswell, R. McGurk, and P. Jacobs
    1997   "Evidence from Turner's Syndrome of an Imprinted X-Linked Locus
            Affecting Cognitive Function." *Nature* 387: 705–8.
Sontag, Susan
    1978   *Illness as Metaphor.* New York: Farrar, Straus and Giroux
Spallone, Patricia and Deborah Lynn Steinberg, eds.
    1987   *Made to Order: The Myth of Reproductive and Genetic Progress.* Oxford: Per-
            gamon Press.
Spanier, Bonnie B.
    1995   *Im/Partial Science: Gender Ideology in Molecular Biology.* Bloomington: In-
            diana University Press.

Stacey, Judith
　1990　*Brave New Families: Stories of Domestic Upheaval in Late Twentieth Century America.* New York: Basic Books.
Stepan, Nancy Leys
　1991　*The Hour of Eugenics: Race, Gender, and Nation in Latin America.* Ithaca, N.Y.: Cornell University Press.
Stolberg, Sheryl Gay
　1997　"For the Infertile, a High-Tech Treadmill." *New York Times,* December 14.
Stone, Lawrence
　1975　"The Rise of the Nuclear Family in Early Modern England." In *The Family in History,* ed. Charles E. Rosenberg. Philadelphia: University of Pennsylvania Press. Pp. 13–58.
Stone, Linda
　1997　*Kinship and Gender: An Introduction.* Boulder, Colo.: Westview Press.
Strathern, Andrew
　1972　*One Father, One Blood: Descent and Group Structure Among the Melpa People.* Canberra: Australian National University Press.
Strathern, Marilyn
　1992a　*After Nature: English Kinship in the Late Twentieth Century.* Cambridge: Cambridge University Press.
　1992b　*Reproducing the Future: Essays on Anthropology, Kinship, and the New Reproductive Technologies.* New York: Routledge.
　1995　"Displacing Knowledge: Technology and the Consequences for Kinship." In *Conceiving the New World Order: The Global Politics of Reproduction,* ed. Faye D. Ginsburg and Rayna Rapp. Berkeley: University of California Press. Pp. 346–64.
Sullivan, Deborah
　1993　"Cosmetic Surgery: Market Dynamics and Medicalization Research." *Sociology of Health Care* 10: 97–115.
Szasz, Thomas
　1963　*Law, Liberty, and Psychiatry: An Inquiry into the Social Uses of Mental Health Practices.* New York: Macmillan.
Tanner, Caroline M. et al.
　1999　"Parkinson Disease in Twins. An Etiologic Study." *Journal of the American Medical Association* 281: 341–46.
Taylor, Charles
　1989　*Sources of the Self: The Making of the Modern Identity.* Cambridge, Mass.: Harvard University Press.
Thom, Deborah and Mary Jennings
　1996　"Human Pedigree and the 'Best Stock': From Eugenics to Genetics?" In *The Troubled Helix: Social and Psychological Implications of the New Human Genetics,* ed. Theresa Marteau and Martin Richards. Cambridge: Cambridge University Press. Pp. 211–34.
Thompson, Larry
　1994　"The Breast Cancer Gene: A Woman's Dilemma." *Time* 143 (3): 52.
Thorne, Barrie
　1992　"Feminism and the Family: Two Decades of Thought." In *Rethinking the Family: Some Feminist Questions,* ed. Barrie Thorne with Marilyn Yalom. Boston: Northeastern University Press. Pp. 3–30.

Tiefer, Leonore
  1994   "The Medicalization of Impotence: Normalizing Phallocentrism." *Gender and Society* 8: 363–77.

Time
  1962   "Inheriting Bad Health." February 2: 37.

Tocqueville, Alexis de
  1840/1980   *Democracy in America.* Ed. Phillips Bradley. New York: Knopf.

Tomes, Nancy
  1990   "Historical Perspectives on Women and Mental Illness." In *Women, Health, and Medicine in America: A Historical Handbook,* ed. Rima D. Apple. New York: Garland.

Trawick, Margaret
  1992   *Notes on Love in a Tamil Family.* Berkeley: University of California Press.

Turning Point (ABC)
  1996   "Race for a Miracle: The Brad and Vicki Margus Story." Transcript 152, February 12.

Turner, Bryan S.
  1987   *Medical Power and Social Knowledge.* London: Sage.
  1992   *Regulating Bodies: Essays in Medical Sociology.* London: Routledge.

Turner, Leigh
  1997   "The Media and the Ethics of Cloning." *Chronicle of Higher Education,* September 26: B4.

Turner, Mark
  1987   *Death Is the Mother of Beauty: Mind, Metaphor, Criticism.* Chicago: University of Chicago Press.

Veciana-Suárez, Ana
  1996   "The Quest That May Save My Children's Lives." *Woman's Day* 59 (10): 36.

Veyne, Paul
  1987   "The Roman Empire." In *A History of Private Life.* Vol. 1, *From Pagan Rome to Byzantium,* ed. Paul Veyne. Cambridge, Mass.: Harvard University Press. Pp. 9–233, 551–644.

Wade, Nicholas
  1997   "Testing Genes to Save a Life Without Costing You a Job." *New York Times,* September 14.
  1998   "Scientist's Plan: Map All DNA Within 3 Years." *New York Times,* May 10.

Wailoo, Keith
  1996   "Genetic Marker of Segregation: Sickle Cell Anemia, Thalassemia, and Racial Ideology in American Medical Writing, 1920–1950." *History and Philosophy of the Life Sciences* 18: 305–20.

Waitzkin, Howard
  1991   *The Politics of Medical Encounters: How Patients and Doctors Deal with Social Problems.* New Haven, Conn.: Yale University Press.

Wall Street Journal
  1996   "Doctors Recommend Every Family Make Its Own Medical Tree." August 15: B5.

Wallace, Anthony F. C.
  1980   *Rockdale: The Growth of an American Village in the Early Industrial Revolution.* New York: Alfred A. Knopf.

Wardlow, Holly and Robert H. Curry
  1996   " 'Sympathy for My Body': Breast Cancer and Mammography at Two
          Atlanta Clinics." *Medical Anthropology* 16: 319–40.
Weinberg, Robert
  1996   "How Cancer Arises." *Scientific American* special issue, September: 62–
          70.
Weiner, Charles
  1994   "Anticipating the Consequences of Genetic Engineering: Past, Present,
          and Future." In *Are Genes Us? The Social Consequences of the New Genetics,*
          ed. Carl F. Cranor. New Brunswick, N.J.: Rutgers University Press. Pp.
          31–51.
Weismantel, Mary
  1995   "Making Kin: Kinship Theory and Zumbagua Adoptions." *American
          Ethnologist* 22 (4): 685–709.
Wertz, Dorothy
  1992   "Ethical and Legal Implications of the New Genetics: Issues for Discus-
          sion." *Social Science and Medicine* 35: 495–505.
Wexler, Nancy
  1979   "Genetic 'Russian Roulette': The Experience of Being 'At Risk' for
          Huntington's Disease." In *Genetic Counseling: Psychological Dimensions,*
          ed. Seymour Kessler. New York: Academic Press. Pp. 199–220.
  1992   "Clairvoyance and Caution: Repercussions from the Human Genome
          Project." In *The Code of Codes: Scientific and Social Issues in the Human
          Genome Project,* ed. Daniel J. Kevles and Leroy Hood. Cambridge, Mass.:
          Harvard University Press. Pp. 211–43.
Williams, Simon J. and Michael Calnan
  1996   "The 'Limits' of Medicalization? Modern Medicine and the Lay Popu-
          lace in 'Late' Modernity." *Social Science and Medicine* 42: 1609–20.
Willing, Richard
  1999   "Explosion of Technology Is Straining Family Ties." *USA Today,* July 29:
          A1–2.
Wingerson, Lois
  1990   *Mapping Our Genes: The Genome Project and the History of Medicine.* New
          York: Dutton.
Winkler, Mary G. and Karl E. Anderson
  1990   "Vampires, Porphyria, and the Media: Medicalization of a Myth." *Per-
          spectives on Biology and Medicine* 33: 598–611.
Witherspoon, Gary
  1975   *Navajo Kinship and Marriage.* Chicago: University of Chicago Press.
Witzig, Ritchie
  1996   "The Medicalization of Race: Scientific Legitimization of a Flawed So-
          cial Construct." *Annals of Internal Medicine* 125: 675–79.
Wolf, Eric R.
  1999   *Envisioning Power: Ideologies of Dominance and Crisis.* Berkeley: University
          of California Press.
Worcester, Nancy and Marianne Whatley
  1992   "The Selling of HRT: Playing on the Fear Factor." *Feminist Review* 41
          (Summer): 1–26.
Wright, Peter and Andrew Treacher
  1982   *The Problem of Medical Knowledge: Examining the Social Construction of Medi-
          cine.* Edinburgh: Edinburgh University Press.

Yanoshik, Kim and Judy Norsigian
    1989   "Contraception, Control, and Choice: International Perspectives." In *Healing Technology: Feminist Perspectives,* ed. Kathryn Strother Ratcliff. Ann Arbor: University of Michigan Press. Pp. 61–92.

Yanagisako, Sylvia J. and Jane F. Collier
    1990   "The Mode of Reproduction in Anthropology." In *Theoretical Perspectives on Sexual Difference,* ed. Deborah L. Rhode. New Haven, Conn.: Yale University Press. Pp. 131–44.

Young, Alan
    1981   "The Creation of Medical Knowledge: Some Problems in Interpretation." *Social Science and Medicine* 15B: 379–86.

Yoxen, Edward
    1986   *Unnatural Selection? Coming to Terms with the New Genetics.* London: Heinemann.

Zihlman, Adrienne L.
    1995   "Misreading Darwin on Reproduction: Reductionism in Evolutionary Theory." In *Conceiving the New World Order: The Global Politics of Reproduction,* ed. Faye D. Ginsburg and Rayna Rapp. Berkeley: University of California Press. Pp. 425–44.

Ziv, Laura
    1997   "I Gave Up My Breasts to Save My Life." *Cosmopolitan,* August: 187.

Index

Acknowledgments

I wish to acknowledge numerous people—first and foremost, all the participants in this study, who freely gave me their time and received me with patience and forbearance. I am most grateful for their willingness to share with me their experience, which contributed so much to my understanding of many of the issues discussed here. I owe a special debt to Cecile Skrzynia, of the Division of Hematology and Oncology of the School of Medicine at the University of North Carolina, Chapel Hill, for introducing me to the women who are presented in Chapters 5 and 6. Also my thanks to Jim Evans from the same division. I thank Robin Miller for introducing me to the group of adoptees. I especially wish to thank Lynn Giddens, who assisted me in meeting the adoptees presented in Chapter 8 and shared with me the wealth of her experience as an advocate for adoptees.

The project was supported by a fellowship from the Institute of Arts and Humanities, University of North Carolina, Chapel Hill; by a grant from the University of North Carolina Research Council and from University of North Carolina, Graduate School. My thanks to these institutions. Various people gave a close reading of the entire manuscript or individual chapters. I thank Terry Evens for his helpful observations on the entire manuscript. I am most grateful to Ruth Hubbard for her very close reading of Chapters 1, 4, 8, 9, and 10 and her invaluable comments and insights. My very special thanks to Fred Behrends and Joseph Schatzmuller for their careful reading of Chapters 2 and 3 and their insights on the historical aspects of these chapters and to Paul Leslie for his careful reading and comments on Chapter 4. Thanks too to Jennifer Drolet for her editorial assistance.

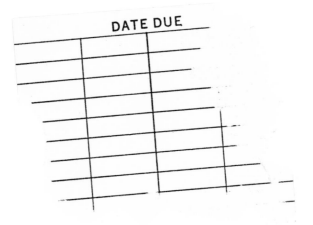

DATE DUE